INTRODUCTION TO HEALTH PROMOTION

INTRODUCTION TO HEALTH PROMOTION

Edited by

Anastasia Snelling

American University, Washington, DC, USA

Second Edition

JB JOSSEY-BASS™

A Wiley Brand

Published by John Wiley & Sons, Inc., Hoboken, New Jersey.
Published simultaneously in Canada.

For general information on our other products and services or for technical support, please contact our Customer Care Department within the United States at (800) 762-2974, outside the United States at (317) 572-3993 or fax (317) 572-4002.

Wiley also publishes its books in a variety of electronic formats. Some content that appears in print may not be available in electronic formats. For more information about Wiley products, visit our web site at www.wiley.com.

Library of Congress Cataloging-in-Publication Data:

Names: Snelling, Anastasia, 1957- editor.
Title: Introduction to health promotion / edited by Anastasia Snelling.
Description: Second edition. | Hoboken, New Jersey : Jossey-Bass, [2024] |
   Includes bibliographical references and index.
Identifiers: LCCN 2023012885 (print) | LCCN 2023012886 (ebook) | ISBN
   9781394155965 (paperback) | ISBN 9781394155989 (adobe pdf) | ISBN
   9781394155972 (epub)
Subjects: MESH: Health Promotion—methods | Health Promotion--trends |
   Health Behavior | Health Planning—methods | Preventive Health
   Services—methods | United States
Classification: LCC RA427.8 (print) | LCC RA427.8 (ebook) | NLM WA 590 |
   DDC 362.1—dc23/eng/20230508
LC record available at https://lccn.loc.gov/2023012885
LC ebook record available at https://lccn.loc.gov/2023012886

Cover Design: Wiley
Cover Images: © Tom Werner/Getty Images; Claudia Totir/Getty Images; MilanMarkovic78/Shutterstock

SKY10058215_102523

CONTENTS

Part Three HEALTH PROMOTION IN ACTION   221

TABLES AND FIGURES

Tables

Figures

A decade ago, Dr. Snelling brought the foundational text, *Introduction to Health Promotion*, to our community. A lot can change in 10 years. While the prevalence of smoking has reached a 50-year low, we sit more than move and "socialize" through computer and phone screens more than in person. We now face a loneliness and isolation epidemic, as memorialized by Dr. Vivek Murthy's (the surgeon general) advisory committee report.

The additional published research and societal changes (including those brought by the COVID-19 pandemic) warranted a second edition of Dr. Snelling's text. Furthermore, as our health care system continues down an unsustainable path and professionals across the spectrum are showing a greater interest in harnessing behavior change science, the field of health promotion continues to grow in importance.

While this text is fundamental for students in the field of health promotion, it is also an important resource for the plethora of professionals who've come to recognize over the course of their career that health promotion is a fundamental and essential part of their own work as well as the sustainability of our health care delivery system. Doctors, nurses, pharmacists, health coaches—health professionals across the spectrum are appreciating that their formal education painted a limited view of the possibilities individuals face that impact their health and well-being.

The boundary between our ability to make healthy choices and experience positive emotions and the influence of our family members, neighbors, coworkers, and communities is murky. Though there is a connection—a strong one. We are all influenced by the cultures within which we live, work, and play. Cultures are the shared behaviors, beliefs, and attitudes of a given group of people. A strong understanding of the content in this text will assuredly help the reader navigate supporting individuals as well as cultures.

Richard Safeer, M.D.
Chief Medical Director, Employee Health and
Well-Being, Johns Hopkins Medicine

Assistant Professor of General Internal Medicine and Pediatrics,
Johns Hopkins University School of Medicine

Assistant Professor of Health, Behavior and Society,
Johns Hopkins Bloomberg School of Public Health

Author of *A Cure for the Common Company,
A Well-Being Prescription for a Happier,
Healthier and More Resilient Workforce*

The health promotion field emerged during the second half of the twentieth century as medicine and science became successful in treating infectious diseases with antibiotics, advancing maternal and child health, and improving sanitation practices. These gains significantly improved the quality and quantity of life for all. Yet, now we face the next medical crisis: chronic disease. Medicine and science research have continued to manage disease conditions through a number of procedures, surgeries, and pharmaceuticals. All of these approaches come with a very high cost to the individual through reduced quality of life and economic cost to organizations and the federal government responsible for providing health insurance. At this time, health care costs account for 18.3% of the gross domestic product. This means that the United States spends almost eighteen cents of every dollar on providing health care to Americans. Controlling these health care costs is a continuing priority for the nation. Consider that over 70% of all health care costs are related to chronic disease and that many risk factors for chronic disease are considered modifiable, such as tobacco use, physical inactivity, food choices, and managing stress. These modifiable risk factors are the core behaviors that the field of health promotion focuses on to improve the quality of people's lives and manage rising health care costs.

Changing individual and societal health behavior is a very complex process. Since the 1980s, more research has shown that for individuals to successfully adopt healthy behaviors, social, behavioral, and environmental factors also must be part of the process of change. The healthy choice must be the easy choice in our homes, schools, worksites, and communities. The vision is to live in a country where a culture of health is seen, practiced, and supported throughout the life span.

The unique contribution of this book is to introduce students to the individual and societal forces that have transformed the factors that influence one's health, including social and physical environments, medical advances, personal lifestyle choices, and legislation. The book identifies and discusses the innovative health campaigns, strategies, and policies that are being implemented and enacted to improve health behaviors and practices that ultimately improve the quality of life.

It is my desire that the writings in this book inspire you to either embark on a career in health promotion or, at the very least, provide you with an understanding of the ways in which many disciplines intersect with health promotion, so that whatever discipline you study, you will better understand how your work interacts with the promotion of health. Almost every discipline intersects with the field of health promotion. Further, health promotion professionals do not work in isolation. The nature of health promotion is to work across multiple disciplines to design and develop strategies that use the best knowledge we know and apply it to health behaviors. Table P.1 lists diverse areas of study and identifies the

Table P.1   Disciplines and the Relationship with Health Fields

Discipline	Contribution	Example
Communication and marketing	Social marketing campaigns	Campaigns to reduce smoking or promote physical activity
Public policy	Local, state, and national policy promoting health	Affordable Care Act
Human resources	Health benefits offered through employers	Worksite health
Biology	Understanding the changes in the body from food and exercise	Healthy behavior identification
Psychology	Understanding why people make the choices they do and how to facilitate behavior change	Health promotion models
Sociology	Understanding how human society functions and influences behavior	Health promotion models
Medicine and allied health	Monitoring health, identifying risk factors, and restoring health	Annual physicals; clinical preventive services
Economics	Behavioral economics	Encouraging healthy food choices

related work of health promotion, whether you study exercise or nutrition science to understand how to advise consumers on health behaviors to improve their health status or if you study communication or marketing to design health campaigns that inform the general public about health risks associated with smoking or drinking and driving or public policy to understand or evaluate how public health policy decreases health disparities by providing consumers with healthful foods or access to affordable health care.

This introductory textbook for health promotion students is designed and written to be distinctly different from other textbooks. It provides readers with an in-depth examination of the forces that have changed our lifestyles and environments over the past century, which in turn have resulted in changes in individual health behaviors that affect the onset of chronic conditions. During this same time frame, there were also considerable medical advances, improving early detection of disease and developing progressive treatments for chronic conditions. These changes are ones that health promoters must understand and address. Ultimately, the framework for the development of social and physical environments that support healthy lifestyle choices will guide the transformation of communities where people are empowered to make healthy choices, so they can live longer lives free of preventable disease, disability, and premature death.

The book is divided into three parts. Part 1, "The Foundation of Health Promotion," introduces the framework of health promotion and provides the student with a number of key terms, models, and trends related to the field. Chapter 2 introduces health behavior change theories that offer constructs on how individuals approach personal behavior change, that is, the essence of health promotion—engaging individuals to actively promote their own health through daily actions such as being physically active or selecting healthy foods to eat. Program planning models (chapter 3) are essential tools to successfully reach large groups of people through social marketing campaigns to interventions to enacting policies to create environments in which people can practice healthy behaviors.

Part 2, "Health Behaviors," describes those actions that promote health and prevent disease. These chapters introduce the short history of how tobacco use, eating, physical activity, and emotional health has evolved as a result of the changes in our social and physical environments. These chapters provide a comprehensive discussion of the health behaviors that influence the onset of chronic disease in our country and how and why these behaviors have changed over time. Chapter 8 highlights the important role clinical preventive services also have in promoting health by monitoring chronic disease development and overall health status. Health promotion professionals are promoting healthful living; hence, the inclusion of preventive services (immunizations and age-appropriate screenings) available through the medical community needs to be understood and promoted.

These health behavior chapters examine how changes in our environment and society over the past several decades have affected behaviors and how those changed behaviors affect health and disease. By understanding the historical perspective of each of these behaviors, health promotion professionals will possess a richer context for their work, understanding that multiple forces have shaped, and continue to affect, the health of individuals and our society. Health behavior change is complex; in order to advance innovative solutions, it is critical that health promoters fully understand the history of these behaviors. Within each chapter, examples of policies and programs that exemplify health promotion in action are provided.

Part 3, "Health Promotion in Action," presents how state and federal governments engage in promoting healthful living for their consumers, what associations and certifications support the health promotion profession, where health promotion is taking place and the job opportunities available for this profession, and closing out with future trends in health promotion as we move through the twenty-first century. There are a plethora of national activities that promote health and prevent disease. The federal agencies monitor health status, provide broad guidelines, conduct research, and fund programs to promote health. Collectively, there are thousands of federal employees who work across disciplines to study or implement new approaches to improve the health of our society.

Chapter 10 discusses the setting where health promotion takes place, which further exemplifies that health promotion is beginning to be seen everywhere, such as in day care centers, schools, colleges, worksites, food stores, retirement homes, and communities. Again, thousands of professionals believe in the vision of a country in which people practice healthy behaviors every day because the healthy choice is the easy choice. Staying current within the discipline will be important after you graduate. Chapter 11 discusses associations, journals, and certifications that provide important information for your life beyond the borders of an academic institution. In time, reading a textbook or listening to a professor's lecture will be in the past. But as a professional, you will need to stay current, and this chapter is full of associations and journals that will facilitate your continued professional development. The final chapter is a look into the future, predicting some trends that will help to create a culture of health to ensure that the Healthy People 2030 goals to "attain high-quality, longer lives free of preventable disease, to improve the health of all groups, to create social and physical environments that promote good health for all, and to promote healthy behaviors across all life stages" will be achieved.

At the end of each chapter, the student will find a brief summary and list of key terms of the information presented in the chapter. After the summary and key terms are a list of student questions and activities. Both the questions and activities are written to extend the learning and understanding of the material presented in the chapter. By completing the questions and activities, students will gain a deeper understanding of the breadth and depth of the health promotion field. All references used in each chapter are at the end, and students are encouraged to seek out these articles, book chapters, and books for additional information.

My goal for this textbook is to enhance the academic preparation of students who are pursuing degrees in health promotion, public health, health education, and other degrees that address or affect the health status of individuals, communities, and societies nationally as well as around the world. Although this textbook focuses on behaviors, trends, and resources in the United States to promote health, many of them are applicable to cultures and settings around the world. There is a universal desire to live a healthful life, and this desire can be found in people of every age, gender, race, and ethnicity.

The book provides a foundation of knowledge for the health promotion professional. Many students are excited to learn such a field exists and ask where they can begin. My response is always with themselves! Being a role model and learning to practice what health promotion professionals teach is a great starting point. I do not expect that you will set a perfect example of health every day, but by practicing health-promoting behaviors, you will personally experience the process and the benefits and become healthy as a result.

An instructor's supplement is available at www.josseybass.com/go/snelling. Additional materials such as videos, podcasts, and readings can be found at www.josseybasspublichealth .com. Comments about this book are invited and can be sent to publichealth@wiley.com.

Acknowledgments

I would like to first thank all of the contributing authors of this book whose expertise in their respective areas has enhanced the content in this book. Many of the contributing authors have spent time at American University, and the health promotion programs have been enriched as a result of their work. Also, I would like to thank all the faculty, staff, and students in the Department of Health Studies at American University for their encouragement and support along this journey.

I would also like to thank Wiley for producing this book with me. The entire team has been valuable in making this a reality.

Finally, this book is dedicated to my family, who inspire me to make a difference in people's lives through my work. My husband, Roger; my children, Trevor, Anastasia, and Amelia;

my parents, John and Amelia Mustone; my siblings, John, Lisa, Paul, Mary Ellen, and Jessica; and my extended Mustone and Snelling family members. May we all live a life full of love, happiness, and good health!

> *To laugh often and much; to win the respect of intelligent people and the affection of children; to earn the appreciation of honest critics and endure the betrayal of false friends; to appreciate beauty; to find the best in others; to leave the world a bit better, whether by a healthy child, a garden patch or a redeemed social condition; to know even one life has breathed easier because you have lived. This is to have succeeded.*
>
> Ralph Waldo Emerson

PREFACE TO SECOND EDITION

Much has changed since the first edition of this book was published and more than ever, individuals, communities, and society, we need health promotion activities, programs, and policies to improve the quality of health for all. The COVID-19 pandemic, a once-in-a-century event, landed in the United States in 2020 and forced universal lockdown for most Americans. The term lockdown has brought on a whole new meaning to us and one that people do not wish to live through again. There are many key takeaways that will be studied for years to come. One outcome is that over a million people in the US alone died from COVID, and those who had pre-existing conditions suffered the most.

Related to health promotion, it is clear that promoting health holistically is evolving and many of the contributors have updated the chapters to reflect these experiences. The pandemic also shone a light on the health disparities that have been always existed but were only exacerbated as a result of the pandemic. The chapters in the book begin the discussion of issues around health disparities and innovative programs being implemented in communities to provide tailored programming to meet people in their own communities. Community engagement that leads to community-driven programs will be the transformation necessary to successfully address health disparities. Creating a society where health is attainable in every home, school, worksite, and community will take creative policy and program leaders who are ready to make a difference in this changing world.

Anastasia Snelling
September 2023

Dr. Anastasia Snelling is a professor and Chair of the Department of Health Studies at American University. She has been a member of the Academy of Nutrition and Dietetics as a registered dietitian for over thirty years and a fellow of the American College of Nutrition. Dr. Snelling's book, *Introduction to Health Promotion*, was released through Jossey Bass Publisher in 2014 and a second edition released in 2023.

She directs the Healthy Schools, Healthy Communities Lab that is rooted in a community engagement and equity model to increase the impact of policies and programs through a community-driven approach. This work is done in under-resourced neighborhoods in Washington, DC, in collaboration with community leaders. Grounded in the Social Ecological Model, her work in schools and communities impacts different levels of influence that can improve the health and food environment, leading to improved health and weight status. By addressing the needs of children and adults within their social, economic, and cultural contexts, she works with them to advance health of individuals and communities.

Dr. Snelling has received over forty grants from federal and local government, nonprofit food and health organizations, and foundations. The outcomes of her research activities are presented at national and international conferences. She has over hundred publications, and her work appears in many highly regarded journals focusing on nutrition, public health, and school and community health. She has appeared on *C-Span* to discuss food labeling regulation, and her opinions and expertise have appeared in such media outlets as *Education Week*, the *Washington Post, US World and News Report*, and *Fox Business News*.

Jennifer Childress is the owner of Patina Esprit Wellness, LLC, where she provides health coaching, personal training, and consulting services to her clients. In addition to her training and coaching practice, Jen also serves as an independent consultant to the Alliance to Make US Healthiest, where she works on implementing and advancing the HealthLead Workplace Accreditation Program. Jen has a master's degree in health promotion management (American University, Washington, DC) and holds certificates in personal fitness training (Aerobics and Fitness Association of America [AFAA]), coaching (Coach Training Alliance), and health education (National Commission for Health Education Credentialing [NCHEC]).

She has been an author on articles published in the *American Journal of Public Health*, the *North Carolina Medical Journal*, and the Wellness Councils of America (WELCOA) *Absolute Advantage*. Jen has taught as an adjunct professor in the Department of Health and Physical Education at Grand View University in Des Moines, Iowa. She is involved within the business community and has served on the National Board of the American Business Women's Association (ABWA). **Laurie DiRosa** is an Associate Professor in the Department of Health, Nutrition, and Exercise Sciences at Immaculata University, teaching undergraduate and graduate health and exercise science courses. She also is the Director of a pro-bono program titled GetFIT@IU, which is a fitness program that serves individuals with intellectual and developmental disabilities utilizing undergraduate exercise science students to provide one-to-one training in strength, flexibility, and balance. She is the author of a unique health coaching program founded on motivational interviewing that is tailored specifically for health professionals and continually trains undergraduate and graduate health profession students and community laypersons in public health in these skills. Dr. DiRosa holds an EdD from Wilmington University, an MS in health promotion management from American University, and a BS in exercise and sport science from Ursinus College.

Jill Dombrowski has been a Clinical Assistant Professor at The Catholic University of America (CUA) in the School of Nursing since 2006. Dr. Dombrowski holds a BSN from Georgetown University and an MSN and PhD from The Catholic University of America, as well as an MS from American University in Health/Fitness Management. Her clinical background includes critical care and occupational health nursing. She teaches undergraduate, graduate, and doctoral-level health promotion courses and coordinates wellness committees for faculty and staff, as well as students. Dr. Dombrowski's research interests include worksite health promotion interventions, physical activity in working mothers, motivational interviewing, and mindfulness.

Dr. David Hunnicutt, former CEO of WELCOA, is now the Principal of DHI—a leadership training and consulting company whose mission is to help leaders get the right results the right way.

With a reputation for being a simplifier and a sense-maker, Dr. Hunnicutt has the proven ability to take difficult and complicated business concepts and make them understandable, useful, and impactful.

He is the chief architect of a number of nationally recognized leadership, culture-building, and well-being frameworks—including his newest initiative, Great at Work®.

Embraced and adopted by hundreds of CEOs, senior executives, managers, consultants, and boards of directors from Fortune 500's to smaller, privately held firms, David's business approaches have helped leaders of all kinds to transform their organizations and change their employees' lives for the better.

An exceptional communicator, David has been invited to share his perspectives and approaches with some of the best organizations in the US. Over the last two decades, he has delivered more than 500 keynote addresses.

Michelle Kalicki received her BS in sport management from the University of Florida and her MS in health promotion management from American University. Her work has included projects to research children's eating behaviors in elementary schools, to improve staff well-being in early childhood settings, and to facilitate the development of health ministries in churches. She is passionate about creating a culture where health is prioritized at the individual to policy levels.

Casey Korba is director of policy at Aledade, Inc. Her areas of focus include advocating at the federal and state levels for policies that help independent primary care practices and Community Health Centers thrive in value-based care so that they can succeed in population health and improving the health of their communities. Before Aledade, Casey led research on health equity, telehealth, and value-based care for the Deloitte Center for Health Solutions. Casey received a BA in English literature from Dickinson College and an MS in health promotion management at American University.

Marty Loy has served as professor of Health Promotion, dean of the College of Professional Studies, and most recently as provost at the University of Wisconsin–Stevens Point. His teaching and research are in the areas of stress management, including mindfulness meditation, and childhood grief and loss. Marty won the University Excellence in Teaching Award in 2001 and is author of two books: *Childhood Stress: A Handbook for Parents, Teachers and Therapists* (Whole Person Associates, 2010) and *Losing a Parent to Suicide: Using Lived Experiences to Inform Bereavement Counseling* (Routledge, 2013). Marty and his wife, Becky, are cofounders of Camp Hope, a camp for grieving children that has served as a model for similar camps around the country.

Maya Maroto is a vice president at FoodMinds where she is involved in managing strategic health professional and thought leader partnerships, developing proactive communications, and executing issues management strategies for clients. She is passionate about translating evidence-based nutrition science into understandable and actionable messages for consumers. Her background and expertise lie in federal nutrition policy, plain-language communication, consumer-focused research, and health equity. In her previous roles, Maya worked on award-winning food and nutrition outreach projects at USDA and FDA, served as a leader at a national food equity nonprofit, and spent many years in academia. Maya received her doctorate in educational leadership from Morgan State University and her master's degree in public health nutrition from the University of North Carolina at Chapel Hill. She holds a bachelor's degree in nutrition and food science from Auburn University and is also a Registered Dietitian Nutritionist (RDN).

David Stevenson serves as the President/CEO of the Central Connecticut Coast YMCA, one of the largest Ys in the United States. As part of a worldwide movement, each Y serves unique community needs with a special focus on youth development, healthy living, and social responsibility. In 2022, more than 4,000 Central Connecticut Coast Y volunteers and staff will serve over 75,000 children and families through eleven branches and seventy program sites.

Dr. Stevenson began his Y career in Ohio, and has also served at Ys in Washington, D.C.; Baltimore, MD; Pittsburgh, PA; and most recently in Connecticut. As a thirty-six-year professional in the YMCA movement, Dr. Stevenson states "With roots dating back to the 1840's, the Y continues to serve as a vital and thriving force to build spirit, mind, and body for all. And as a cause-driven movement, the Y is welcoming to all and well positioned to address the challenges of today's society."

Dr. Stevenson holds a BS in Recreation Management from Ithaca College, an MS in Health/Fitness Management from American University, and a PhD in Educational Administration from American University.

Maura Stevenson is currently an associate professor of biological sciences at Quinnipiac University in Hamden, Connecticut, where she teaches and serves as academic coordinator for anatomy and physiology. She has a BS degree from Ithaca College, an MS degree from the University of Wisconsin–LaCrosse, and her PhD was earned at American University. She was previously involved in worksite health promotion research at American University. She is a coauthor of "Using Theories and Models to Support Program Planning" in *ACSM's Worksite Health Promotion Manual: A Guide to Building and Sustaining Healthy Worksites* and "The Weight Management Triad: Dietary Intervention, Behavior Change, and Daily Activity" in *Journal of the American Association of Physician Assistants*. She has presented "Past and Future Trends of Health Promotion" at the Association for Worksite Health Promotion Conference and "Trends in School-based Health Promotion" at the Keystone Health Promotion Conference. Dr. Stevenson had previous academic appointments at Community College of Allegheny County and Robert Morris University in Pittsburgh, Pennsylvania, and at McDaniel College in Westminster, Maryland.

ABOUT THE COMPANION WEBSITE

This book is accompanied by a companion website.

www.wiley.com/go/snelling2e

This website includes:

- PowerPoint slides
- Test banks

PART ONE

THE FOUNDATION OF HEALTH PROMOTION

CHAPTER 1

HEALTH PROMOTION

An Expanding Field

Anastasia Snelling

The field of health promotion has a relatively short history compared to public health or medicine. However, it is clear that promoting health is an important component of public health and the medical field. Over the past century, US society has changed dramatically in the ways we work, live, and learn. In recent decades and as a result of the COVID-19 pandemic, these societal changes have affected individual health choices and disease patterns, and as a result, the field of health promotion has emerged as a distinct discipline to work in synergy with the fields of public health and health care. The purpose of this chapter is to familiarize students with the history of health patterns, with an emphasis on personal health behaviors, and to identify the social and environmental forces that can create a culture of health to promote a citizenry with longer, healthier lives that are free of disability and disease.

Brief Overview of Health from 1900–2020

A critical examination of the history of health issues related to death and disability in the United States provides us with an appreciation of how social and environmental factors influence disease patterns (see US Department of Health and Human Services (HHS), National Center for Health Statistics, 2019). This section briefly examines US health in the first half of the twentieth century and provides a more in-depth investigation of US health in the second half of the twentieth century.

1900–1950s

During the first half of the twentieth century (1900–1950s), the topic of health in the nation focused on developing the medical profession and establishing hospitals to treat patients. Public health departments focused on sanitation,

LEARNING OBJECTIVES

After reading this chapter, the student will be able to:

- Identify health trends related to chronic disease during the second half of the twentieth century.

- Identify the leading cause of death in the United States.

- Explain primary, secondary, and tertiary care.

- Explain modifiable and nonmodifiable risk factors.

- Explain the social determinants of health.

- Describe how the Affordable Care Act is working to improve healthy lifestyles.

Introduction to Health Promotion, Second Edition. Edited by Anastasia Snelling.
© 2024 John Wiley & Sons Inc. Published 2024 by John Wiley & Sons Inc.
Companion Website: www.wiley.com/go/snelling2e

Table 1.1   Life Expectancy at Birth, at Sixty-Five Years of Age, and at Seventy-Five Years of Age

Year	At Birth			At Sixty-Five Years			At Seventy-Five Years		
	Both Sexes	Male	Female	Both Sexes	Male	Female	Both Sexes	Male	Female
1900	47.3	46.3	48.3	11.9	11.5	12.2	*	*	*
1950	68.2	65.6	71.1	13.9	12.8	15.0	*	*	*
1960	69.7	66.6	73.1	14.3	12.8	15.8	*	*	*
1970	70.8	67.1	74.7	15.2	13.1	17.0	*	*	*
1980	73.7	70.7	77.4	16.4	14.1	18.4	10.4	8.8	11.5
1990	75.4	71.8	78.8	17.2	15.1	18.9	10.9	9.4	12.0
1995	75.8	72.5	78.9	17.4	15.6	18.9	11.0	9.7	11.9
2000	77.0	74.3	79.7	18.0	16.2	19.3	11.4	10.1	12.3
2010	78.7	76.3	81.0	19.1	17.7	20.3	12.3	11.0	12.9
2019	78.8	76.3	81.4	19.6	18.2	20.8	12.4	11.4	13.2

"*" means not available.

Source: US Department of Health and Human Services, National Center for Health Statistics (2019).

disease control, and health education. During this time, public health functions included child immunization programs, community health services, substance abuse programs, and sexually transmitted disease control.

Life Expectancy

By examining the life expectancy of men and women in the United States over time (see table 1.1), one can understand how medical and health advances have affected the health of a population. **Life expectancy** is a measure of the health status of a given population and is defined as "the average number of years a person from a specific cohort is projected to live from a given point of time" (McKenzie, Pinger, & Kotecki, 1999). At the beginning of the twentieth century, the life expectancies of men and women were 46.3 and 48.3 years, respectively. Infectious diseases such as influenza, pneumonia, tuberculosis, and gastrointestinal infections were the leading causes of death in the United States. The discovery of antibiotics and improved sanitation practices significantly contributed to increasing life expectancies by the 1950s, reaching sixty-five and seventy-one years for men and women, respectively. Life expectancy rates do vary across race and ethnicity due to several factors, including policies, health care access, and individual choices. Many health advocates have written extensively on how one's zip code predicts their life expectancy (Chetty R, Stepner M, Abraham S, et al., 2016). This correlation between life expectancy and zip code is further explored in this chapter under the social determinants of health.

Life expectancy
The average number of years that a person from a specific group is projected to live

Chronic Disease

As a result of the advances in immunizations, antibiotics, maternal and child health, and improved sanitation practices, life expectancy increased. Extending years of life was a positive advancement. However, one result of a longer life expectancy is the more signifi-cant impact that personal health choices and environmental factors have on the develop-ment of chronic conditions, sometimes referred to as **noncommunicable diseases**, which are not infectious or transferable from one person to another. **Chronic disease** is defined as a health condition or disease that lasts for a long period of time, usually longer than three months. Chronic diseases also tend to take a long period to develop. Chronic conditions such as high cholesterol have developed over years of consuming high saturated fat and cholesterol foods, which leads to high blood cholesterol levels and is a risk factor for cardio-vascular disease. These chronic conditions are usually managed with lifestyle changes, med-ication, or surgical approaches, depending on the disease.

One of the first studies conducted to measure the impact of personal health choices on cardiovascular disease was the Seven Countries Studies conducted by Ancel Keys in the 1950s (Keys et al., 1986). Keys recruited researchers in seven countries to launch the first cross-cultural comparison of heart attack risk in populations of men engaged in traditional occupations, comparing their diet and fat intake. The Seven Countries Study indicated that the risk and rates of heart attack and cardiovascular risk at the population and individual levels were directly and independently related to the level of total serum cholesterol. It demonstrated that the association between blood cholesterol level and coronary heart disease risk in the five- to forty-year follow-up was found consistently across different cultures. Cholesterol and overweight or obesity were also associated with increased mortality from cancer. The Seven Countries Study, along with other important large studies such as the Framingham Heart Study, the Nurses' Health Study, and the Women's Health Initiative, confirmed not only the importance of healthy diet but also identified weight status and regular physical activity as important factors for maintaining good general health. These studies were conducted in the mid-1950s and began to establish the influence of personal health choices on disease patterns. Since that time, hundreds of studies have been done and are now being conducted to improve our understanding of the influence of lifestyle behaviors on chronic disease (Buettner & Skemp 2016).

A more recent and ongoing project is called the Blue Zones. Buettner & Skemp (2016) sought to uncover the factors that contribute to one's longevity. Working with scientists and anthropologists, they were able to distill the evidence-based common factors that appear to increase life expectancy. These factors include diet with an emphasis on plant-based choices, physical activity, social connections, belonging, sleep, outdoor time, and spirituality. Further, they concluded that individuals need to live in environments where health is supported on a regular basis. The Seven Countries Studies focused on individual physical health choices, whereas the Blue Zones Project describes how environments need to support healthy life-styles for individuals to achieve a long and healthy life.

1960s–2020s

During the second half of the twentieth century and into the twenty-first century, a number of social and environmental changes occurred that influenced consumer health choices and behaviors. Changes in the way we live are inevitable; however, health promotion

noncommunicable diseases
not passed from one person to another, also known as chronic diseases

chronic disease
a health condition or disease that lasts for a long period of time, usually for longer than three months

professionals must examine how these changes influence health status and respond to these changes to maintain and improve health for individuals and society.

Employment

Americans were prosperous after World War II; the end of the war generated enormous advances in technology, medicine, and communications that led to new job opportunities for returning soldiers and for all citizens. Starting in the 1950s, for the first time in American history, a majority of US workers were white-collar rather than blue-collar workers (McColloch, 1983). White-collar workers tended to be involved in positions that required less physical activity than workers in blue-collar positions. People working in white-collar positions are typically sedentary for most of their day; there is a need to build physical activity back into their daily routines.

> A blue-collar worker is someone who performs manual labor. Blue-collar work may involve skilled or unskilled labor, such as in mining, mechanical, construction, or manufacturing jobs. A white-collar worker is someone who performs professional, managerial, or administrative work; examples include teachers, managers, and secretaries.

During the COVID-19 pandemic, working and learning remotely became a norm in American society. After vaccinations and boosters were available, employees and students returned to work and school. However, not everyone returned to a physical office or classroom environment and, as a result, remote work and online learning will remain part of society for the foreseeable future.

Suburbs and Cars

The housing industry boomed and shifted families into new suburban neighborhoods; the explosion of the automobile industry accompanied this shift. As people moved from urban to suburban areas, cars became more popular and necessary. Between 1945 and 1947, car production increased from 70,000 to 3.5 million (Weiner, 1992). As people moved out of the city and started owning cars, their reliance on transportation negatively influenced their daily physical activity. Chapter 6 discusses physical activity patterns in the United States and its essential role in decreasing the occurrence of chronic conditions.

Supermarkets, Food Choices, and Eating Patterns

As suburban neighborhoods were built, supermarkets and the food industry began to develop and shift to meet this new demand. In 1958, there were approximately fifteen thousand supermarkets; this number roughly doubled by the 1980s (Ellickson, 2011). In the 1960s, women began to enter the workforce, which shifted their role of preparing daily meals for the family. Then, frozen foods became more readily available at the retail level, and the fast food industry was born. In 1968, McDonalds operated approximately one thousand restaurants; by 2012, there were thirty thousand McDonalds around the world. Along with the emergence of fast food restaurants, the microwave was introduced into the family kitchen. The shift from eating what one grew during the growing season to being able to purchase large quantities of foods at any time promoted increased calorie consumption. The food environment, from the prevalence and size of supermarkets to the growth of the fast food industry, underwent significant changes during this period. The first part of the twenty-first century has brought multiple changes to the food landscape in the United States. As you will read in chapter 5, although nutrition recommendations have remained relatively stable over time, there is increased attention to the entire chain of food production from farm practices to food distribution, access, and waste.

Entertainment and Leisure Time

A shift in the physical activity patterns of adults and children also occurred. Advancing technology brought televisions into American living rooms. In 1950, less than 1% of homes had televisions. In 2012, over 83% of homes had at least one television. Between 1975 and 1985, video games such as Atari and Nintendo became available, and IBM introduced the first personal computer. People of all ages are entertained with televisions, computers, and video games, again decreasing our daily physical activity time. The emergence of social media such as text messages, Facebook, Instagram, and others does allow people to connect across different platforms and across the world; however, it also has been shown to cause detrimental effects on people's mental well-being (Naslund, Bondre, Torous, & Aschbrenner 2020).

Tobacco Use

Although Americans had been smoking throughout the entire twentieth century, by 1950, more women were smoking than ever before, and approximately 42% of all Americans smoked. Smoking was permitted everywhere: in office buildings, schools, restaurants, and airplanes. However, research started to suggest dangers associated with smoking. In 1964, the first surgeon general's report was written that clearly documented the effects of smoking on health. Early into the 1970s, concerns regarding secondhand smoke were validated, and the negative effects of smoking became clear. As a result, clean indoor air legislation and higher cigarette taxes were put into effect in an attempt to reduce the prevalence of smoking. As a nation, we continue to limit where people can smoke and require higher taxes on tobacco. Some companies and college campuses have gone smoke free. Because these actions have shown decreased rates of smoking in the United States, many advocates suggest applying similar strategies to other health behaviors. However, as you will learn in chapter 4, smoking rates have decreased yet vaping rates have increased.

By the end of 2019, life expectancy for men and women was 76.3 and 81.4 years, respectively, for all races. Advances in medicine and drug therapy for managing chronic conditions were largely responsible for the increase in life expectancy in the late twentieth century. However, much more work is needed to address systematic policies that promote health where people live, work, and learn.

Table 1.2   Leading Causes of Death in the United States and Related Risk Factors (2020)

Rank	Cause	Risk Factors
1	Heart Disease	Tobacco use, high blood pressure, elevated blood lipid levels, diet, diabetes, obesity, sedentary behavior, alcohol abuse, family history
2	Malignant neoplasms (cancer)	Tobacco use, alcohol misuse, diet, overweight, solar radiation, ionizing radiation, worksite hazards, environmental pollution, family history
3	COVID-19 pandemic	Age, lung conditions, heart disease, stroke, diabetes, weakened immune system
4	Accidents (unintentional injuries)	Alcohol misuse, tobacco use (fires), product design, home hazards, handgun availability, lack of safety restraints, excessive speed, automobile design
5	Cerebrovascular diseases (stroke)	Tobacco use, high blood pressure, elevated blood lipid levels diabetes, obesity, family history
6	Chronic lower respiratory diseases	Smoking, environmental exposure to air pollution or chemicals, dust, fumes, or secondhand smoke
7	Alzheimer's disease	Age, family history, head injury, heart health, general healthy aging
8	Diabetes mellitus	Obesity (for type 2 diabetes), diet, sedentary behavior, family history, race and ethnicity, age, blood lipid levels
9	Pneumonia and influenza	Chronic conditions such as asthma or other lung conditions, or other chronic diseases; Tobacco use, infectious agents
10	Nephritis, nephritic syndrome, and nephrosis	Associated with diseases such as diabetes or lupus, infections such as HIV, malaria, or Hepatitis B or C

Although life expectancy continued to increase, causes of death shifted from infectious diseases in the early half of the century to chronic diseases in the late 1900s and early 2000s. Lifestyle choices and environmental supports are the focus of the health promotion field today. Now, the leading causes of death in the United States are primarily chronic diseases influenced by risk factors that include personal health choices. Table 1.2 shows the leading causes of death and all related risk factors. However, note that the COVID-19 pandemic is listed as the third leading cause of death in United States and is an infectious disease.

COVID-19 Pandemic

The COVID-19 or coronavirus is a global pandemic, and many believe this virus will be worldwide for years to come. The virus killed close to seven million people worldwide, and hundreds of millions of people have contracted the virus. This global pandemic will be studied for years to come as we also learn how to prepare for and manage the next pandemic. There are many lessons that have been learned from this experience that relate to the health of individuals, communities, and society that include components of health such as physical health and social and emotional well-being. Many communities struggled to provide for the most vulnerable populations, which rely on social programs to meet basic needs such as food access and health care services. Further complicating the situation was the isolation many people experienced as they were confined to their homes to learn, work, and worship.

COVID-19 has reshaped life as we knew it prior to 2020. The changes are far-reaching and are predicted to last for years to come (Haleem, Javaid, & Vaishya, 2020). For the discipline of health promotion, practitioners have needed to revamp programs, expand offerings, and identify innovative strategies to address the myriad of issues that were exacerbated by the pandemic (Van den Broucke, 2020). It is evident that to achieve a healthy society, more entities must work toward creating healthier environments where people live, work, learn, shop, worship, or play.

Health Promotion: An Expanding Field

Health promotion, as a field of study, has a shorter history than public health and health education. The emergence of health promotion was a direct response to the changes in disease patterns in the United States, particularly the rise of chronic disease rates beginning in the mid-twentieth century. This rise is attributed primarily to two reasons: the discovery of antibiotics and vaccinations to prevent and treat infectious diseases and the adoption of lifestyle behaviors that increase risk for conditions that lead to chronic diseases.

health promotion
the process of helping people to move toward a state of optimal health through lifestyle changes

Although health promotion, public health, and health education overlap to some degree, each is a distinct field of study in and of itself. It is important to understand the distinctions among these three fields, as shown in the following definitions. According to the World Health Organization (WHO Centre for Health Development, 2004), health promotion is

> Health promotion is the process of enabling people to increase control over, and to improve, their health. It moves beyond a focus on individual behaviour towards a wide range of social and environmental interventions.
>
> As a core function of public health, health promotion supports governments, communities and individuals to cope with and address health challenges. This is accomplished by building healthy public policies, creating supportive environments, and strengthening community action and personal skills.

Dr. Michael O'Donnell (2002), a leading scholar in the field of worksite health promotion, offers this definition of health promotion:

> The art and science of helping people discover the synergies between their core passions and optimal health, enhancing their motivation to strive for optimal health, and supporting them in changing their lifestyle to move toward a state of optimal health. Optimal health is a dynamic balance of physical, emotional, social, spiritual, and intellectual health. Lifestyle change can be facilitated through a combination of learning experiences that enhance awareness, increase motivation, and build skills and, most important, through the creation of opportunities that open access to environments that make positive health practices the easiest choice. (p. 192)

Health Education

Health education is defined by the World Health Organization (WHO Centre for Health Development, 2004) as

> any combination of learning experiences designed to help individuals and communities improve their health, by increasing their knowledge or influencing their attitudes. (p. 29)

Public Health

Public health, as defined by the American Public Health Association, is: https://www.apha.org/What-is-Public-Health

Public health is the practice of preventing disease and promoting good health within groups of people, from small communities to entire countries. Public health works to track disease outbreaks, prevent injuries, and shed light on why some of us are more likely to suffer from poor health than others. The many facets of public health include speaking out for laws that promote smoke-free indoor air and seatbelts, spreading the word about ways to stay healthy, and giving science-based solutions to problems.

Discussion

These definitions clearly indicate that public health, health education, and health promotion are all working toward the common goal of improving health for individuals and society. However, distinctly different in each definition are strategies used to address health issues. Green and Kreuter (1999) suggest that

> health promotion draws on the health sciences, programs, practices, and policies that relate to the health of human populations. We must move beyond the tidy boundaries of health institutions, for much of what relates to the health of human populations happens in other sectors, such as schools, industry, social services, and welfare. (p. 2)

The essence of health promotion is to actively promote healthy living by creating a society in which a "culture of health" is evident in places where people live, work, and learn. Health promotion balances individual health behavior choices with creating environments where healthier choices become easier choices. Therefore, health promotion is broader than health education, yet health education is an important component within the field of health promotion. Further, the fields of health promotion and public health are overlapping but have different approaches to addressing the health of society. Public health, as the previous definition demonstrates, is engaged with *monitoring* the health of the public, *formulating* policies, and *ensuring* all citizens have access to health care, all of which are critical to ensuring a healthy society. Health promotion focuses primarily on chronic disease management by *monitoring* health conditions, *assisting* individuals to make healthy choices, and *formulating* policies that create healthy environments.

To illustrate an example of how professionals in the fields of health promotion and public health work together, let's consider the issue of flu vaccines. Each year, public health officials work to identify strains of flu that will be a threat to society when flu season arrives. The influenza viruses in the seasonal flu vaccine are selected each year based on surveillance-based forecasts about which viruses are most likely to cause illness in the upcoming season. This work is done primarily by public health epidemiologists and is critically important for the prevention of seasonal flu. The next step is encouraging people to obtain the flu vaccine through health communication campaigns and offering the flu vaccine in places where people frequently visit. It is in these latter steps that health promotion professionals contribute their expertise: understanding their target audience and creating health communication campaigns that trigger individuals to act on the message. In the end, both the development of the right flu vaccine and the distribution and uptake of the flu vaccine will improve the health of the society.

Social Determinants of Health

There is no one cause for the increase in behaviors related to chronic disease. We cannot point to one factor or product, such as video games, suburban neighborhoods, or soda, as the singular cause of chronic disease. Therefore, professionals need a comprehensive understanding of the social determinants of health and a broad array of strategies to approach these issues. The Department of HHS has guided the development of the determinants of health because they have been at the forefront of establishing strategic goals for the health of the United States citizenry. Since 1979, when the first surgeon general wrote *Healthy People: The Surgeon General's Report on Health Promotion and Disease Prevention*, HHS has guided the development of this overarching document on health indices and goals (US Department of Health, Education, and Welfare, 1980; US Public Health Service, 1979). Healthy People 2030 is considered a strategic document that uses identification, measurement, and tracking to reduce health disparities through a determinants-of-health approach. Chapter 9 will expand on this discussion and the state and federal approaches to addressing the social determinants of health.

The **social determinants of health** are defined as factors that significantly influence or have an impact on the health of individuals and communities. Determinants of health comprise genetic or biological factors, social and physical factors, health services, policies, and individual behaviors. The interrelationship of these factors determines the health of individuals and, collectively, the health of a population (Institute of Medicine, 2001). Understanding how each of these factors contributes to the health of an individual is important; however, the single greatest opportunity to improve health lies in personal health choices. Individual behavior choices account for almost 40% of all deaths in the United States (Mokdad, Marks, Stroup, & Gerberding, 2004).

The types of determinants of health are as follows:

social determinants of health
factors that significantly influence the health of individuals and communities, such as genetic or biological factors, social and physical factors, health services, individual behaviors, and policies

- *Biology and genetics.* These factors relate to family history because individuals can be predisposed to a condition from a parent. Other factors may relate to age; for example, as individuals age, they are predisposed to certain physical and cognitive changes.

- *Social and physical factors.* Social determinants of health include a range of issues that affect the health of people, including education, income, social support, and quality of schools. Physical factors also affect health by expanding or limiting access to healthy food and opportunities for physical activity. The physical environments where people work and live, including access to grocery stores, safe walking or biking paths, housing, worksites, and exposure to physical hazards, affect health.

Health services. Access to health services and the quality of these services affect health. Improving access to health care and preventive health services is a primary goal of the Affordable Care Act (ACA). Medical care plays a role in preventing premature deaths through early detection and management of chronic conditions; however, the role of health services in directly addressing social determinants of health is still unclear.

- *Policies.* Policies at the local, state, and national levels, as well as the workplace, affect health. Clean indoor air policies and increased taxes influence the percentage of people who smoke tobacco. School wellness policies promote healthy school environments for children, although there is little data available to assess the direct impact of these policies on childhood obesity. More recently, with the Black Lives Matter movement, much more attention is being paid to local, state, and federal policies that either promote or hinder people from achieving good health.

- *Individual behaviors.* Individual behaviors, such as food choices, physical activity, managing stress, sleep, or tobacco or vaping use, influence the development of chronic health conditions.

Each of these factors contributes to the overall health and well-being of individuals. Health promotion focuses primarily on individual behaviors and recognizes the importance of the physical and social environmental factors and policy formulation and implementation. In the first half of the twentieth century, health advances were made as a result of policies (e.g., improved sanitation practices) and medical care (e.g., discovery of antibiotics). Continued advances in medical procedures and prescription drugs have been important in improving the quality of life for those with chronic diseases. However, in the twenty-first century, to address rising health care costs and the health of people, health improvements will be derived from changes in individual health behaviors supplemented with environmental supports and policies to create a culture of health in our society.

**physical
environment**
the structures, buildings, or services that can either facilitate or hinder healthy behavior

As indicated previously, physical and social environmental factors are critical to achieving successful individual behavior change. The **physical environment** includes structures, buildings, or services that can either facilitate or hinder healthy behavior. For example, walking paths or lighted streets may encourage more walking in neighborhoods and deter crime; grocery stores may provide improved access to healthy foods and fresh fruits rather than people having to rely only on corner stores in a neighborhood, which traditionally do not stock a wide array of products. The physical environment creates the opportunity for a person to engage in the behavior, but that alone may not reach everyone.

**social
environment**
the personal relationships or networks that surround people

The **social environment** is the personal relationships or networks that surround people. Social networks establish norms of behavior, and these behaviors can facilitate or hinder healthy behavior. Back in the mid-1950s, about half of the country smoked. Smoking was a very acceptable practice, which may have influenced people to start smoking. Conversely, to help people change behaviors, social support, and networks are important for the health behavior change to be realized (Breslow, 1999). For example, if a child is overweight, it is recommended that the entire family engage in healthy eating and regular exercise to promote weight management. Worksite health promotion programs also rely on social support from employees.

Building on the determinants of health, health promotion addresses health issues in a multilayered approach using a **social-ecological model**. This model illustrates different spheres that influence individual behavior. Each individual has knowledge, beliefs, or values that will influence his or her health choices. Then there is the family unit and how the family will influence health behaviors. The next sphere is a school or workplace, and because children and adults spend six to eight hours of their day at these places, their programs and policies may influence behavior. The next sphere is the community where people live, and the last area is policy, which includes local, state, and national policies that are related to healthy environments (Sallis, Owen, & Fisher; 2008; Stokols, 1992). This model is presented in figure 1.1 and is further discussed in chapter 3 on program planning models. As you read about the different health behaviors in chapters 4 through 8, you will notice the ecological approach to improving each sphere to positively influence health behavior changes.

social-ecological model
a multilayered approach to health issues that illustrates different spheres that influence individual behavior

Important Health Promotion Concepts

Before moving into the chapters discussing the health behaviors that affect chronic disease and the resources, strategies, and models that support health promotion, this section briefly discusses concepts and terminology relevant to the field.

Risk Factors, Chronic Diseases, and Empowerment

Specific health behaviors are directly associated with chronic disease. These health behaviors are termed **risk factors**. Risk factors may be modifiable or nonmodifiable. **Modifiable risk factors** are those that an individual can change through his or her own actions, such as levels of physical activity or eating habits. **Nonmodifiable risk factors** are those that cannot be changed by the individual, such as age, gender, or family history.

risk factors
specific health behaviors that are directly associated with chronic disease

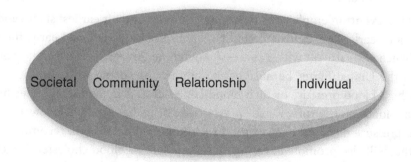

Figure 1.1   Social-ecological Model
Source: Adapted from Centers for Disease Control (2013).

modifiable risk factors

risk factors that an individual can change through his or her own actions

Health promotion focuses on the *modifiable* risk factors that individuals have the ability to change when provided with the necessary education, motivation, and a supportive environment. Approaching health from this perspective can empower people to improve their own health status and, hence, have more control over their well-being. Empowerment of individuals or communities is a key theme in the field of health promotion. When used correctly, empowerment can be a long-term strategy for making permanent changes.

nonmodifiable risk factors

risk factors that cannot be changed by the individual, such as age, gender, or family history

Health behaviors and choices occur every day in our lives. Stop and consider how many health choices you have made in the last twenty-four hours (brushing your teeth, eating breakfast, wearing a seat belt or bicycle helmet). Each of these choices may exert a strong influence on your health status, although it may be years before the effects of those choices are known. For example, smoking one cigarette will not cause lung cancer but smoking over thirty years of your life will certainly increase your chance of lung cancer.

Prevention Activities: Primary, Secondary, and Tertiary

Health prevention is an important component of managing people's health once a chronic condition develops. Individuals can actively engage in promoting their own health through regular physical activity or managing their stress, but they must also be informed about health prevention activities. Prevention activities are categorized into three levels: primary, secondary, and tertiary. Prevention activities tend to be associated with the health care system.

Primary Prevention

primary prevention

primary prevention aims to prevent the disease from occurring

Primary prevention emphasizes activities to avert illness, injury, or disease conditions. Strategies may be incorporated into an educational situation, an annual medical visit, or legislation such as no-smoking areas or the use of seat belts. For example, elementary school children may have an assembly in which information is shared to discourage them from starting to smoke tobacco, or, at the college level, there may be educational programs on the risks of drinking alcohol. During medical visits, primary prevention activities might include scheduled immunizations or appropriate cancer screenings. The ACA, described later in this chapter, prioritizes primary prevention activities.

Secondary Prevention

secondary prevention

used after the disease has occurred, but before the person notices that anything is wrong

Secondary prevention emphasizes identifying diseases at their earliest stages and treating the conditions early. Research suggests that when disease is detected early, there is a far greater chance of treatment with a successful outcome. Examples of secondary prevention abound in the United States because of the number of people with chronic conditions, including high blood pressure or high blood cholesterol. A person with either high blood pressure or blood cholesterol would be prescribed a drug that would help lower either his or her blood pressure or blood cholesterol. In addition, physicians will recommend lifestyle changes that will also promote lowering blood pressure or blood cholesterol, such as diet, weight loss, or physical activity. Managing chronic conditions by using prescription drugs is a hallmark of the health care system, which has made significant advances in treating chronic conditions.

Tertiary Prevention

Tertiary prevention relies mainly on the health care system and highlights specific medical interventions to limit advancing conditions linked to chronic diseases. If not treated, chronic conditions progress over time and cause further debilitation of the body. Tertiary prevention aims to slow the progression of the chronic condition. Rehabilitation services such as physical or occupational therapy are trademarks of this type of prevention. This type of care is usually considered the most expensive and is responsible, in part, for driving up health care costs.

tertiary prevention targets the person who already has symptoms of the disease

Discussion

Secondary and tertiary prevention activities are delivered mainly through the health care system, where the cost is considerably higher as chronic conditions advance. Unfortunately, much less attention has been given to preventing the onset of these chronic conditions (primary prevention) until recently. Since about 2000, the US Preventive Services Task Force has been established and specifically recommends that managing these conditions begins with lifestyle behavior changes (chapter 8). However, there has been a slow uptake of some of these recommendations through the medical system and personal health choices.

Health promotion activities focus on engaging individuals in primary prevention to delay or avoid the onset of chronic conditions. Recently, health promotion efforts have expanded to include policy, system, and environmental changes. However, health promotion interventions should also be part of secondary and tertiary care as well. Consider someone who is diagnosed with early stages of diabetes, is also overweight, and lives a sedentary life. This individual would benefit greatly from losing weight, eating a healthy diet, and beginning an exercise program. The health care system is remarkable at restoring health; however, the cost of this type of care is very high for those who pay the bill, including individuals, organizations, and the federal government. Therefore, the Centers for Disease Prevention and Control created and showed efficacy for a National Diabetes Prevention Program (REF; https://www.cdc.gov/diabetes/prevention/index.html). The partnership between public and private organizations works to prevent or delay the onset of type 2 diabetes through identification of those at-risk and referral to education programs to empower individuals to make lifestyle choices to prevent or delay the onset.

Health Promotion Meets the Health Care System

The United States has an employee-based health care system rather than a government-run system. This means health insurance is offered to employees through the organizations where they work. In some cases, the US government offers health insurance to special segments of the population: people over sixty-five years can enroll in Medicare, military veterans receive care through the Veterans Administration, individuals living below the poverty line, and those who are disabled are eligible for Medicaid, and the State Children's Health Insurance Program provides matching funds to states for health insurance to families with children whose incomes are modest but too high to qualify for Medicaid. There are many different health insurance programs in the United States funded by private organizations and the federal and state governments.

The US health care system, whether offered through an organization or through the federal government, has been known as a "restorative" medical system, a system that focuses primarily on treating disease rather than preventing it. The medical system has made enormous advances in detecting and treating diseases through the use of technology, surgery, and drug treatment. Because of these advances, the United States has a very expensive health care system; however, as a nation, we lag behind other countries on several key health indices, including infant mortality, life expectancy, and rates of chronic disease.

Patient Protection and Affordable Care Act

In 2010, President Barack Obama signed into law the Patient Protection and ACA, commonly referred to as the ACA (Open Congress, 2010). This monumental piece of legislation represents the most comprehensive set of health care reforms in recent US history. One significant component of the ACA was to extend health coverage to citizens in the United States by requiring individuals to have medical coverage; the goal is to have everyone contributing financially to the health care system. As a result of the ACA, it is estimated that an additional thirty-one million Americans will have access to health insurance coverage. One objective of the law is to increase by 2014 the number of quality, affordable, private health insurance plans from which more people are able to choose. By 2021, more than 35 million Americans had signed up for health care through the health care exchanges. Access to medical care is an important factor for improving health outcomes; increased access provides more opportunities to promote healthy behavior and offer age-appropriate clinical preventive services.

A second hallmark of the ACA is its emphasis on wellness, health promotion, and prevention. Two parts of the ACA are focused in this area: Title IV, Prevention of Chronic Disease and Improving Public Health, and Title V, Healthcare Workforce. Within these areas is the creation of councils to advance the priority of improving quality of health care through disease prevention and health promotion. Within Title IV, it requires the creation of the National Prevention, Health Promotion, and Public Health Council (the National Prevention Council). This council is tasked with developing the National Prevention Strategy to guide our nation in identifying the most effective and achievable means to improve health and well-being. The National Prevention Strategy envisions a prevention-oriented society in which all sectors recognize the value of health for individuals, families, and society and work together to achieve better health for all Americans (Fielding, Teutsch, & Koh, 2012; Koh & Sebelius, 2010; http://www.advancingstates.org/documentation/aca/NASUAD_materials/title_IV_analysis.pdf). Within Title V, the creation of the National Health Care Workforce Commission reviews workforce needs and makes recommendations to the federal government to ensure that national policies are aligned with consumer needs. One initiative under this title is to provide technical assistance to primary care providers about health promotion, chronic disease management, and preventive medicine. These initiatives are focused on the emphasis of health promotion and disease prevention. Both of these provisions within the ACA have had starts and stops due to the political debate of the management of healthcare services and the federal government. To date, gains have been accomplished to advance the integration of health promotion into the healthcare system.

The ACA also requires health insurance companies to cover a number of recommended preventive services, such as blood pressure or cancer screenings, without additional costs to patients. This emphasis on early detection of chronic conditions is a critical step to decreasing rates of the leading causes of death in the United States. An independent panel of medical and scientific experts serves on the US Preventive Services Task Force to identify preventive services based on the strength of the scientific evidence documenting their benefits and cost effectiveness. Chapter 8 addresses clinical preventive services and their importance to health promotion, and chapter 9 discusses the role of the federal and state governments in health activities.

Discussion

With the provisions established in the ACA, the nation is experiencing a shift in its approach to health, wellness, and the treatment of illness. One significant achievement is that the number of people who have health insurance is at an all-time high, with only 8.8% of the population without health insurance. For the first time, a greater value is being placed on health promotion and the long-term benefits of preventing disease. By viewing health through this lens, health promoters and the public health community can reframe the dialogue on many of the chronic diseases and lifestyle risk factors that plague our population. These ACA provisions underscore the value of health promotion and prevention, lending credibility to the expanding role of health promotion within the context of attaining well-being in the United States.

Positions in the Health Promotion Field

There is an enormous need and demand for the skills of health promotion professionals. Students academically trained in the field will have a scientific understanding of the body, including biology, chemistry, exercise physiology, nutrition and diet, and health psychology. Paired with this scientific knowledge, health promotion students will also possess a theoretical perspective on program planning and implementation, including assessment, methodology, and evaluation, as well as policy formulation. Chapter 10 provides an extensive discussion on a variety of settings where health promotion is occurring.

Historically, some of the first positions in the field of health promotion were responsible for managing worksite health promotion programs. With an employee-based health care system, US corporations share the overall cost of the nation's health care bill; toward the end of the twentieth century, health care costs began to rise significantly. In response to increased costs, many employers established worksite health promotion programs.

Beyond worksite health promotion programs, which continue to employ a large number of health promotion professionals, the field of health promotion has grown significantly in response to the obesity epidemic and the associated rise in the rates of chronic disease. Health promotion positions are now well established in government and nongovernmental agencies, including state and local health departments, health care providers and insurance companies, school districts, commercial gym facilities, and faith-based organizations, as well as companies that supply specialized services related to health promotion, such as social marketing campaigns, health coaching, health screenings, or health education materials.

As students explore different career options within the field of health promotion, their interests might focus on a health condition or a life stage. Health issues such as heart disease, osteoporosis, or childhood obesity can frame positions within the field. Another approach is the identification of a specific target population. Health promotion positions address individual behavior at all stages of life, from encouraging healthy prenatal behaviors during pregnancy, to early childhood growth and development, to student health in primary and secondary schools, through the life span in universities, worksites, communities, and assisted living facilities. The nation needs health promotion professionals who are trained to motivate and educate individuals to invest in healthy lifestyles and work with communities and government to build social and physical environments that support healthy living.

Summary

This chapter introduces a number of key terms and lays the foundation for the emerging field of health promotion. It briefly describes the social and physical changes to the environment from the first half of the twentieth century to the second half. It distinguishes health promotion from public health and health education. Evidence on how social, behavioral, and environmental factors have influenced our behaviors and chronic diseases is described both qualitatively and quantitatively. Understanding the forces that have brought about the changes in these factors is fundamental to the discipline of health promotion.

KEY TERMS

1. **Life expectancy:** the average number of years that a person from a specific group is projected to live

2. **Noncommunicable disease:** diseases not passed from one person to another; also known as chronic diseases

3. **Chronic disease:** a health condition or disease that lasts for a long period of time, usually for longer than three months

4. **Health promotion:** the process of helping people to move toward a state of optimal health through lifestyle changes

5. **Health education:** helping individuals and communities improve their health through learning experiences aimed at increasing knowledge or influencing attitude

6. **Public health:** organized efforts to promote the health of the community as a whole through measures such as identifying health problems, creating public policies, and ensuring access to cost-effective care

7. **Determinants of health:** factors that significantly influence the health of individuals and communities, such as genetic or biological factors, social and physical factors, health services, individual behaviors, and policies

8. **Physical environment:** the structures, buildings, or services that can either facilitate or hinder healthy behavior

9. **Social environment:** the personal relationships or networks that surround people

10. **Social-ecological model:** a multilayered approach to health issues that illustrates different spheres that influence individual behavior

11. **Risk factors:** specific health behaviors that are directly associated with chronic disease

12. **Modifiable risk factors:** risk factors that an individual can change through his or her own actions

13. **Nonmodifiable risk factors:** risk factors that cannot be changed by the individual, such as age, gender, or family history

14. **Primary prevention:** primary prevention aims to prevent the disease from occurring

15. **Secondary prevention:** used after the disease has occurred, but before the person notices that anything is wrong

16. **Tertiary prevention:** targets the person who already has symptoms of the disease

REVIEW QUESTIONS

1. What are the differences and similarities between health promotion and public health?

2. Are promoting health and preventing disease the same thing or different?

3. Why is health promotion framed as an expanding field?

4. How are the determinants of health related to the social-ecological model?

5. What is the goal of health promotion?

6. What are chronic diseases, risk factors, and levels of prevention?

7. How would you define determinants of health?

8. How would you define "a culture of health"?

9. What changes have occurred in society as a result of the COVID-19 pandemic?

STUDENT ACTIVITIES

1. Some researchers have stated that children today will have a shorter life span than their parents. Do you agree or disagree? State your reasons.

2. Draw a graphic showing the intersections of health promotion, public health, and health education.

3. Describe the social and physical environment on your college campus. What areas support health-promoting behaviors, and what areas are inconsistent with health-promoting behaviors?

4. Identify an organization that employs health promotion professionals and review the position descriptions.

5. Explain the anticipated shifts in the health care system as a result of the Affordable Care Act.

References

Breslow, L. (1999). From disease prevention to health promotion. *JAMA, 281*(11), 1030–1033.

Buettner, D. & Skemp, S. (2016). Blue zones: Lessons from the World's longest lived. *American Journal of Lifestyle Medicine, 10*(5), 318–321. doi:10.1177/1559827616637066.

Centers for Disease Control and Prevention (CDC) (2013). *A framework for prevention*. Retrieved from www.cdc.gov/violenceprevention/overview/social-ecologicalmodel.html

Chetty, R., Stepner, M., Abraham, S., Lin, S., Scuderi, B., Turner, N., . . . Cutler, D. (2016). The association between income and life expectancy in the United States, 2001–2014. *JAMA, 315*(16), 1750–1766. doi:10.1001/jama.2016.4226.

Ellickson, P. B. (2011, April 1). *The evolution of the supermarket industry: From A&P to Wal-Mart*. Simon School Working Paper Series no. FR 11–17. Retrieved from http://ssrn.com/abstract=1814166 or http://dx.doi.org/10.2139/ssrn.1814166

Fielding, J. E., Teutsch, S., & Koh, H. (2012). Health reform and healthy people initiative. *American Journal of Public Health, 102*(1), 30–33.

Green, L. W. & Kreuter, M. W. (1999). *Health promotion planning: An educational and ecological approach* (3rd ed.). Boston: McGraw-Hill.

Haleem, A., Javaid, M., & Vaishya, R. (2020). Effects of COVID-19 pandemic in daily life. *Current Medicine Research and Practice, 10*(2), 78–79. doi:10.1016/j.cmrp.2020.03.011.

Keys, A., Alessandro, M., Mariti, J. K., Blackburn, H., Buzina, R., . . . Keys, M. H. (1986). The diet and 15-year death rate in the Seven Countries Study. *American Journal of Epidemiology, 124*(6), 903–915.

Koh, H. K. & Sebelius, K. G. (2010). Promoting prevention through the Affordable Care Act. *The New England Journal of Medicine* Retrieved from www.nejm.org/doi/full/10.1056/NEJMp1008560.

Institute of Medicine (IOM) (2001). *Health and behavior: The interplay of biological, behavioral, and societal influences*. Washington, DC: Academy Press.

McColloch, M. (1983). *White collar works in transition: The boom years, 1940s–1970s*. Westport, CT: Greenwood Press.

McKenzie, J. E., Pinger, R. R., & Kotecki, J. F. (1999). *An introduction to community health*. Boston: Jones & Bartlett.

Mokdad, A. H., Marks, J. S., Stroup, D. F., & Gerberding, J. L. (2004). Actual causes of death in the United States, 2000. *JAMA*, *291*(10), 1238–1245. doi:10.1001/jama.291.10.1238.

Naslund, J. A., Bondre, A., Torous, J., & Aschbrenner, K. A. (2020). Social media and mental health: benefits, risks, and opportunities for research and practice. *Journal of Technology in Behavioral Science*, *5*, 245–257 https://doi.org/10.1007/s41347-020-00134-x.

O'Donnell, M. P. (2002). *Health promotion at the workplace* (3rd ed.). Albany, NY: Delmar.

Open Congress (2010). *H.R.3590: Patient Protection and Affordable Care Act.* Retrieved from www .opencongress.org/bill/111-h3590/show#

Sallis, J. F., Owen, N., & Fisher, E. B. (2008). Ecological models of health behavior. In K. Glanz, B. K. Rimer, & K. Viswanath (Eds.), *Health behavior and health education practice: Theory, research, and practice* (4th ed., pp. 465–485). San Francisco: Jossey-Bass.

Stokols, D. (1992). Establishing and maintaining healthy environments. Toward a social ecology of health promotion. *American Psychology*, *47*(1), 6–22.

US Department of Health, Education, and Welfare (1980). *Promoting health/preventing disease: Objective for the nation.* Washington, DC: US Government Printing Office.

US Department of Health and Human Services, National Center for Health Statistics (2019). Health, United States, 2009: With Special Feature on Medical Terminology. Hyattsville, MD. Report No. 2010–1232.

US Public Health Service (1979). *Healthy people: The surgeon general's report on health promotion and disease prevention.* Washington, DC: US Government Printing Office.

Van den Broucke, S. (2020). Why health promotion matters to the COVID-19 pandemic, and vice versa. *Health Promotion International*, *35*(2), 181–186 https://doi.org/10.1093/heapro/daaa042.

Weiner, E. (1992). *Urban transportation planning in the United States: A historical overview.* Retrieved from http://ntl.bts.gov/DOCS/UTP.html

WHO Centre for Health Development (2004). A glossary of terms for community health care and services for older persons. *Ageing and Health Technical Report*, *5* Retrieved from https://www .who.int/westernpacific/about/how-we-work/programmes/health-promotion.

CHAPTER 2

HEALTH BEHAVIOR CHANGE THEORIES AND MODELS

Understanding the Process of Behavior Change

Maura Stevenson

A primary focus of health promotion is to help people limit unhealthy behaviors and, in many cases, replace them with healthy behaviors. Health promotion professionals have long known that it is not enough to simply help people identify unhealthy behaviors in order to eliminate them. Human behavior is far too complex for that to be effective. As such, theories and models that help explain and account for the complexity of human behaviors are often used as the foundation for successful health promotion programs.

Although definitions of theories can be lengthy and complex, Cottrell, Girvan, and McKenzie (2011) offered an applied definition of a theory as it relates to health promotion: "A **theory** is a general explanation of why people act or do not act to maintain and/or promote the health of themselves, their families, organizations, and communities" (p. 100). Failure to understand theories may lead to health promotion initiatives that do not succeed because of inaccurate assumptions about participants' likelihood of successful behavior change.

Imagine an individual given the task of implementing a stop-smoking program. The individual has no knowledge of health behavior theories but establishes a plan to (1) recruit smokers and (2) convince them that smoking is harmful to their health. This individual believes that providing smokers with the knowledge that smoking is harmful to their health will cause them to quit smoking.

Although education is an important part of health behavior intervention and should not be discounted, the likelihood that these two steps alone will achieve success is very limited.

Although theories can help explain why people act or fail to act, **models** help to translate theories into a program planning framework. Models can also be used beyond the planning stage and can serve as a guide for program

LEARNING OBJECTIVES
After reading this chapter, the student will be able to:

- Define the differences between a model and theory.

- Describe the role of models and theories in changing health behavior.

- Identify the constructs in the social cognitive theory, the health belief model, the transtheoretical model of behavior change, and the theory of planned behavior.

- Discuss changes over time and how these models and theories align with changing health behaviors.

Introduction to Health Promotion, Second Edition. Edited by Anastasia Snelling.
© 2024 John Wiley & Sons Inc. Published 2024 by John Wiley & Sons Inc.
Companion Website: www.wiley.com/go/snelling2e

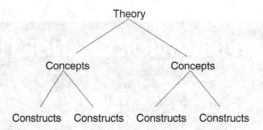

Figure 2.1   Theories, Concepts, and Constructs

theory

an explanation intended to account for the actions that people take or do not take to promote health

models

theory-based planning framework that helps guide program creation and evaluation

implementation and evaluation (Glanz & Rimer, 1995). The focus of this chapter will be on behavior change theories; planning models are discussed in chapter 3. It should be noted that two of the four theories presented here include the word *model* in their titles. Although this may be confusing, theories and models are intertwined and not always distinctly separate.

Through the study of theories, one learns that theories are subdivided into elements, generally referred to as *concepts*. Concepts in turn are described in a more concrete form referred to as *constructs*, which in their most applicable form are known as *variables* (figure 2.1). It is the variables that become the basis for assessment of a program (Cottrell, Girvan, & McKenzie, 2011).

Health Behavior Theories

Over the years, a number of theories and models related to health behavior change have been developed. In this chapter, four theories are discussed:

- Social cognitive theory (SCT)
- Transtheoretical model (TTM) of behavior change
- Health belief model (HBM)
- Theory of planned behavior (TPB)

These are the dominant theories of health behavior and health education based on the frequency of their citation within the health promotion research literature (Glanz, Rimer, & Viswanath, 2008). Each attempts to explain human behavior, motivation, and the processes of personal behavior change.

Social Cognitive Theory

Social cognitive theory (SCT)

theoretical model that frames individual behavior as a response to observational learning from the surrounding environment

Social cognitive theory (SCT), developed by Albert Bandura (1986), focuses on not just the psychology of health behavior but on social aspects as well. SCT originated as the social learning theory within a psychological domain; it expanded as concepts studied in sociology and political science were included. SCT embraces the idea that humans do not live in isolation and learn and behave not only according to their own thought processes but also in response to the environments that surround them, whether in terms of the environment of a group (workplace, for example) or the larger society as a whole (Glanz, Rimer, & Viswanath, 2008). Bandura further emphasizes that individuals are not simply products of their environments but help to create those environments. He refers to this concept as **reciprocal determinism** (Bandura, 1986).

SCT explains learning and behavior through a description of constructs (Cottrell, Girvan, & McKenzie, 2011):

- Knowledge of health risks and benefits of various health behaviors
- Perceived self-efficacy of one's ability to control one's own health behaviors
- Outcome expectations related to the consequences of particular health behaviors
- Personal health goals established by individuals
- Perceived facilitators of the desired health behaviors
- Perceived impediments to the desired health behaviors (Bandura, 2004) Each of these six constructs is described in table 2.1.

reciprocal determinism
the concept that individuals are a product of their environments and also help to create those environments

Knowledge of Health Risks and Benefits

The knowledge of health risks and benefits associated with particular behaviors serves as the precondition for change (Bandura, 2004). Although knowledge of risks and benefits is not the only factor required for behavior change, it is the obvious starting point. For example, people smoked for many years with no motivation to stop until it became known that continuing to smoke would bring risks to their health. It followed that stopping smoking would lead to health benefits.

Table 2.1 Social Change Theory and Application of Constructs

Construct	Sample Application
Knowledge of health risks and benefits	"I'm 50 pounds overweight, which puts me at increased risk for several diseases, including heart attack, stroke, and diabetes. If I lose some weight, those risks will go down."
Perceived self-efficacy	"It's realistic for me to stop eating so many calories each day and get to the gym several times a week to burn some calories."
Outcome expectations	*Physical and material:* "It will be great to fit into some of my clothes again, and I will treat myself to a new pair of jeans when I drop two sizes." *Social:* "My boyfriend will be happy if I can slim down." "I won't miss the dirty looks I get when I take a seat next to someone on the bus who thinks I take up too much room."
Personal health goals	"I'm not sure if I'll ever be able to lose fifty pounds, but I can at least try to lose ten pounds."
Perceived facilitators	"I got this great new pedometer that tracks my steps and syncs to my phone so I can make sure I get in enough activity every day." "I found this website that lets me log my food into an online journal and calculates my calorie intake." "My wife also wants to lose some weight, so we can do this together."
Perceived impediments	"It's embarrassing to go to the gym and be around all those physically fit people." "I'm going to have to take two different buses to get to the gym." "My friends are not going to want to give up nachos and beer when we go out for Friday night happy hour."

Perceived Self-Efficacy

self-efficacy

an individual's perception of his or her capability to execute a course of action necessary to achieve a goal

Perceived **self-efficacy** is referred to as the foundation of behavior change and is described as "people's judgments of their capabilities to organize and execute courses of action required to attain designated types of performances" (Bandura, 1986, p. 391). For example, a person who has come to understand the risks associated with his own state of obesity has the precondition to change behaviors that contribute to obesity, but if this individual believes "I've been overweight for all of my life and I'll always be overweight," then the likelihood that the precondition will lead to changed behavior becomes unlikely. Negative self-efficacy stalls the behavior change process in this case. Of key importance for health promotion planners and implementers is the understanding that participants must believe that they have the power to stop performing a negative behavior (smoking, for example) and perform a positive behavior (regular exercise, for example) in order to successfully achieve desired behaviors.

Outcome Expectations

The consequences associated with particular behaviors influence whether or not an individual might engage in the behavior. SCT refers to the consequences as outcome expectations. In particular, an individual may anticipate certain physical and material outcomes and social outcomes to result from changes in behaviors.

Physical and Material Outcomes   A change in an individual's behavior may be expected to result in physical outcomes and sometimes material outcomes associated with those physical outcomes. For example, a woman who enrolls in a stop-smoking program anticipates a reduction in her chronic cough and an improvement in the taste of her food. Additionally, she expects to have more money in her wallet as a result of no longer purchasing cigarettes or not having to wash her clothes as frequently as a result of no longer smoking cigarettes (Bandura, 2004).

Social Outcomes   Changes in an individual's behavior may also be expected to result in social outcomes, such as approval or disapproval from one's surrounding social groups. For example, the woman who stops smoking may desire to eliminate the disapproval of her behavior by her children that results from her smoking habit. In turn, she desires their approval if she is able to successfully stop smoking. She may also desire to eliminate the disapproval seen on the faces of her nonsmoking coworkers each time she departs the office for a smoke break (Bandura, 2004).

Personal Health Goals

Personal goals surrounding health habits set the course for behavior change. Goals can be viewed as long-term or short-term. Long-term health behavior change goals can be a challenge given that, for many people, current habits are a far cry from the desired set of habits. These individuals may be overwhelmed by the challenge, which in turn can alter their perceived self-efficacy. SCT encourages short-term goals that are less daunting than longer-term goals (Bandura, 2004). For example, an obese man may have a long-term goal to lose one hundred pounds in order to achieve a healthy body mass index. However, a one-hundred-pound weight loss is daunting; many factors can intervene over the course of the time it takes to lose one hundred pounds. A goal to begin with a ten-pound weight loss within a shorter time frame is likely to be viewed as attainable and success made more likely. Short-term successes can lead to the setting (or resetting) of new goals.

Perceived Facilitators and Perceived Impediments

Last, the perceived facilitators and impediments are important constructs in SCT and directly influence self-efficacy as well (Bandura, 2004). Smokers may perceive that their success in stopping smoking will be facilitated by the use of a nicotine substitute. As such, use of the nicotine substitute increases self-efficacy and boosts confidence in success. An impediment to the success of would-be ex-smokers might be a fear of weight gain. Moderation of the impact of such an impediment might come in the form of techniques to avoid weight gain during the stop-smoking effort. Smokers may be advised to stock their refrigerator with carrots and celery sticks as they start an effort to stop smoking so as to decrease the likelihood of snacking on less healthy, higher-calorie snacks when struck by a craving. An additional example would be a woman who embarks on a new exercise program. She may perceive that her efforts are facilitated by the accompaniment of a friend to the workout facility. An impediment may be lack of transportation to the workout facility or the loneliness of going about it without a friend.

Given the importance of self-efficacy among the constructs of SCT, Bandura (1997) describes methods for increasing self-efficacy in people who desire to change health behaviors:

- *Observational learning (social and peer modeling)*—people benefit from seeing people similar to themselves achieve successful behavior change. Testimonials from "someone who's been there" fit this category. Consider commercial advertising for stop-smoking and weight loss programs and note the frequent use of testimonials.

- *Mastery experience*—practicing a new behavior in small steps, enabling short-term success to be achieved while gradually increasing the challenge.

- *Improving physical and emotional states*—people attempting behavior change to benefit from stress reduction and being well rested, along with enhanced positive emotions about the challenge of behavior change (by avoiding negative terminology and replacing it with positive terms).

- *Verbal persuasion*—providing strong encouragement in order to boost confidence. Simply telling a person, "You can do it!" can help to improve self-efficacy.

Discussion

One can see that understanding the constructs of SCT provides valuable insight for a health promotion professional or health educator. Providing participants with knowledge of health risks and benefits of various health behaviors, enhancing their beliefs in their ability to change behaviors, helping them to establish attainable goals, and providing activities and programming that promote facilitators and limit impediments can lead to a strong foundation for successful outcomes for participants.

The literature is rich with studies of theory-based strategies, including SCT. One example is a program aimed at reducing fat intake and increasing intake of fruits and vegetables (Ammerman, Lindquist, Lohr, & Hersey, 2002). Improvements made were attributed to the constructs of goal setting, along with family and social support strategies. Other studies demonstrate an association between self-efficacy and exercise adherence in adults (Brassington, Atienza, Perczek, DiLorenzo, & King, 2002). Many community-based programs have employed SCT, including impaired driving prevention programs, efforts to prevent adolescent smoking, and heart disease prevention programs.

Transtheoretical Model of Behavior Change

transtheoretical model (TTM)
theoretical model that describes health behavior as a process characterized by stages of readiness to change

stages of change
varying levels of readiness that a person reaches while changing a health behavior

As its name implies, the **transtheoretical model (TTM)** of behavior change integrates principles and processes from several theories of behavior change. Prochaska, DiClemente, and Norcross (1992) proposed TTM after extensive work with smoking cessation and the treatment of drug and alcohol addiction. The model was subsequently adapted for use in a variety of health promotion and health behavior change settings. Using **stages of change**, TTM describes health behavior as a process and notes that at any given time individuals are at varying levels of readiness for change.

TTM differs from SCT in that it assumes that people with problem behaviors are not all beginning at the same stage of readiness to change those behaviors; in fact, one of the TTM stages of change is a stage at which people are not ready for change at all. The practical application of this model for a health promotion professional is to tailor the health promotion message according to each individual's stage of change. Applying a universal health promotion message to a group of individuals assumes that all the individuals in that group are at the same stage of readiness to make changes in their behavior. Alternatively, matching individual messages with an individual's stage of readiness may be more meaningful and thus more effective (Snelling & Stevenson, 2003).

In TTM, there are six stages of change (see figure 2.2) and ten processes of change. These stages are described in the following.

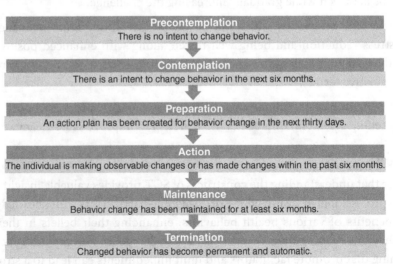

Figure 2.2   Transtheoretical Model: Stages of Change

Stages of Change

Precontemplation   During the precontemplation stage, the individual is not thinking about or intending to eliminate a problem behavior or adopt a healthy behavior in the next six months. Some planners may choose to exclude individuals in the precontemplation phase from programming efforts. However, TTM includes this stage in the model to emphasize that health promotion efforts should not exclude precontemplators. In many cases, these individuals lack awareness of the problem behavior or have regressed to this stage after an unsuccessful attempt to change the behavior (DiClemente, Schlundt, & Gemmell, 2004).

Contemplation   During the contemplation stage, an individual develops intentions to change a particular behavior within the next six months. Contemplators are aware of the positive benefits of changing their behavior but are often held back by what are perceived as negative factors influencing their actions. *Ambivalence* is often a word used to describe this stage; there is a tendency for some individuals to be chronic contemplators (Glanz, Rimer, & Viswanath, 2008). A challenge for program planners is to reduce this ambivalence in order to move contemplators to the next stage: preparation.

Preparation   During the preparation stage, the individual has clear intentions to change a problem behavior or adopt a healthy behavior in the next thirty days. Presumably, the ambivalence of the contemplation stage has been resolved to the point at which the individual believes that the benefits outweigh the negatives. Preparers may have an action plan, often as a result of a prior attempt to change the behavior (DiClemente, Schlundt, & Gemmell, 2004; Glanz, Rimer, & Viswanath, 2008). Many health promotion programs begin at levels appropriate for people in the preparation stage—participants will need to be recruited—but those in the preparation stage are ready enough to sign up for health promotion programs, such as weight-loss or smoking-cessation programs (Glanz, Rimer, & Viswanath, 2008).

Action   During the action stage, an individual is making observable changes in behavior or has made observable changes in behavior within the past six months. According to TTM, an individual in the action stage is halfway through the behavior change process (stage 4 of 6). However, it is worth noting that many other theories or models of health behavior change begin at this stage. It is well established that individuals who change behavior may be likely to relapse and spiral back to a previous stage of readiness. Those who did not experience the efforts that are part of the preparation stage as described in TTM may be particularly vulnerable to relapse due to a lack of preparation (DiClemente, Schlundt, & Gemmell, 2004). According to TTM, this is an important consideration for program planners—the early stages and preparatory steps may be key to successful behavior change.

Maintenance   During the maintenance stage, the individual has successfully changed a behavior and has maintained that change for at least six months. Individuals at this stage are at a lower risk of relapse than those in the action stage but also apply their "change processes" less frequently than those in the action stage (Glanz, Rimer, & Viswanath, 2008). In other words, the strategies employed to help change the behavior in the first place are not used as much during maintenance. For example, individuals stop going to support group meetings or journaling as they did previously. Glanz, Rimer, and Viswanath (2008) described data from the 1990 surgeon general's report that revealed that among people who had refrained from smoking for twelve consecutive months, the rate of relapse to regular smoking was 43%. When individuals abstained from smoking for five consecutive years, the rate of relapse to regular smoking was only 7%. Program planners should consider the importance of the ongoing practice of change processes for those in maintenance (as opposed to a celebration and graduation of sorts that implies that individuals are no longer at risk of relapsing).

Termination   Individuals in the termination phase have achieved a complete change in behavior with no risk of relapse. People in the termination stage are said to have 100% self-efficacy, and their behavior has become permanent and automatic (Glanz, Rimer, & Viswanath, 2008).

Processes of Change

processes of change
the covert and overt activities that people use to progress through the six stages of change

TTM also describes ten **processes of change** among its constructs. These processes are the activities used by individuals to progress through the six stages of change previously described. Each process is actually a category that includes multiple interventions, methods, and techniques. Understanding the stages of change and how behavior shifts (the processes) is a valuable tools for behavior change programs.

The ten processes are divided into two groups: (1) affective and cognitive experiential processes (thoughts and feelings) and (2) behavioral processes. Each process of change and its description are provided in table 2.2 (Glanz, Rimer, & Viswanath, 2008; Prochaska, DiClemente, & Norcross, 1992).

Additional constructs in the TTM include decision balance and self-efficacy. Decision balance simply refers to the individual's view of the pros and cons of changing a behavior. Self-efficacy in TTM is two-pronged: confidence in one's ability to sustain new behaviors across various situations and the temptations to forego new behaviors and relapse to former behaviors.

Discussion

TTM is a robust model with numerous constructs that comprise six stages of change, ten processes of change, and the additional constructs of decision balance and self-efficacy. Glanz, Rimer, and Viswanath (2008) describe several assumptions related to TTM and its application to behavior change intervention programs. Among those assumptions, and perhaps the most directly applicable to health promotion programmers, are these two:

1. A majority of at-risk populations are not prepared for action and will not be served effectively by traditional action-oriented behavior change programs.

2. Specific processes and principles of change should be matched to specific stages to maximize efficacy (DiClemente, Schlundt, & Gemmell, 2004, p. 103).

There are numerous studies examining TTM interventions. In fact, it has been described as the dominant model of behavior change (Armitage, 2009). TTM has been applied widely to numerous health behaviors, including those described in this book's part 2, "Health Behaviors."

Table 2.2 Processes of Change

Change Process	Description
Experiential Processes	
Consciousness raising	The individual seeks new information to gain understanding of the problem behavior in general and how it affects him or her personally. Actions include feedback, observation, confrontations, interpretations, bibliotherapy (selected reading), and media campaigns.
Dramatic relief	The individual experiences emotions related to behaviors and expresses feelings about the problem behavior and potential solutions. Actions include role-playing, personal testimony, and grieving.
Environmental reevaluation	The individual assesses how personal behavior affects the surrounding physical and social environment as well as the people in it. Actions include empathy training, interventions, testimonials, and public service announcements.
Self-reevaluation	The individual assesses his or her self-image, comparing the image of the self with the unhealthy behavior to an image of self without the unhealthy behavior. Actions include value clarification, imagery, and exposure to health role models.
Social liberation	The individual has access to alternative resources and assistance for behavior change. Resources may be broad, such as no-smoking zones or dining areas free of unhealthy choices, or they may be more specific for particular populations that are sometimes underserved (e.g., minority health initiatives, health promotion for homosexuals, etc.).
Behavioral Processes	
Helping relationships	The individual develops trust, acceptance, and support during attempts to change a problem behavior. Actions include building rapport, forming therapeutic alliances, and making calls to counselors or other support persons.
Self-liberation	The individual makes a commitment to change a problem behavior, including belief in their ability to change. Actions include decision-making therapy, new year's resolutions, public testimony, logotherapy (psychotherapy based on acceptance of oneself), and commitment-enhancing techniques.
Counterconditioning	The individual replaces problem behaviors with healthy behaviors. Actions include relaxation techniques, desensitization, affirmations, and other forms of positive self-talk.
Reinforcement management	The individual establishes a reward system for successes in behavior change. Actions include rewarding oneself or being rewarded by others for particular achievements in the behavior change process.
Stimulus control	The individual identifies and removes triggers for the problem behavior and replaces those with healthy or nonproblematic prompts. Actions include avoidance, rearrangement of environment, and adding prompts and techniques to cope with temptations.

It is most frequently used in the development and design of smoking-cessation programs (Glanz, Rimer, & Viswanath, 2008). Studies reveal support for and criticism of TTM, but making general conclusions is difficult. Many programs have applied only portions of TTM, with minimal consistency regarding which portions are applied. This is contrary to the concept of transtheory.

One review study of TTM (Armitage, 2009) made several conclusions. First, the stages of change may be better collapsed into two phases: motivational and volitional. Second, dividing audiences and targeting them based on which change stage they're in seems preferable to targeting people based on factors such as age or gender. Third, most criticisms of TTM are based on its stages of change; the processes of change may be the more favorable part of TTM but are less studied. Armitage (2009) examined programs that used processes of change to help smokers to quit, to encourage low-income employees to engage in more physical activity, and to influence members of the public to consume less amounts of alcohol.

Health Belief Model

health belief model (HBM)
theoretical model characterized by value-expectancy theories, which explain that behavior is influenced by values and expectations

Developed in the 1950s, the **health belief model (HBM)** was an attempt by social psychologists at the US Public Health Service to better understand a widespread reluctance of people to access disease prevention services (Snelling & Stevenson, 2003). To describe the origins of HBM, cognitive theorists often identify **value-expectancy theories**, which explain that behavior results from an individual's value of the outcome of the behavior and the expectation that a particular action or actions will lead to the outcome. When applied to health behaviors, it can be assumed that individuals value the avoidance of illness and getting well and expect particular health-related activities to lead to improved health and disease prevention (Glanz, Rimer, & Viswanath, 2008).

value-expectancy theories
theories that explain that behavior results from an individual's value of the outcome of the behavior and the expectation that a particular action or actions will lead to the outcome

There are six primary constructs of HBM, each of which is described in the following sections and in table 2.3.

Perceived Susceptibility

Perceived susceptibility refers to an individual's belief that he or she will contract a particular disease or condition. People vary in their feelings of personal vulnerability to a particular condition, depending on a variety of factors, including family history (heart disease, for example), demographics (women and breast cancer, for example), age (Alzheimer's disease, for example), and so on. People who believe they are strongly susceptible to a disease or condition may be more likely to alter behavior to prevent it, whereas those who feel they are not susceptible have little motivation to change a particular behavior (Glanz, Rimer, & Viswanath, 2008; Snelling & Stevenson, 2003).

Perceived Severity

Perceived severity refers to an individual's belief regarding the seriousness of a particular condition or disease and how it would ultimately affect that individual's life. Individuals may

Table 2.3   Constructs of the Health Belief Model

Construct	Description
Perceived susceptibility	Individual's belief that he or she will experience negative health outcomes
Perceived severity	Individual's belief about the seriousness of negative health outcomes, physically and socially
Perceived benefits	Individual's belief that behavior change will have a positive impact on health outcomes
Perceived barriers	Individual's beliefs about the negative impact of making a behavior change (cost, convenience, comfort, etc.)
Cues to action	Triggers that motivate individuals toward a change in behavior
Self-efficacy	Given all conditions and factors, individual's belief that he or she is capable of making the contemplated behavior change

consider the severity of a condition in terms of its physical consequences (for example, pain, disability, mortality, etc.) and its social consequences (impact on ability to maintain career or impact on family). An example of severity is that people consider developing cancer to be more severe than contracting the flu. Note that perceived susceptibility and severity are often referred to collectively as *perceived threat* (Glanz, Rimer, & Viswanath, 2008; Snelling & Stevenson, 2003).

Perceived Benefits

Perceived benefits refer to an individual's belief that a particular intervention is feasible and efficacious. Individuals who perceive a threat to their health and well-being may not automatically accept any and all recommended interventions; rather, they must believe that a particular action reduces the threat. Aside from personal health benefits, individuals may also consider other benefits of a changed behavior (for example, cost savings, increased approval from friends and family, etc.) (Glanz, Rimer, & Viswanath, 2008; Snelling & Stevenson, 2003).

Perceived Barriers

Perceived barriers are those actions or outcomes that the individual perceives as potentially negative aspects of a health intervention. Individuals often consider interventions in terms of cost, time commitment, convenience, side effects, and their agreeableness.

Cues to Action

Cues to action are described as the triggers that motivate individuals toward action to change behavior. Perhaps a personal health scare or that of a loved one could trigger an interest in changing a behavior associated with the health condition. Although early versions of HBM included cues to action as a construct, referring to such things as "bodily events" (Glanz, Rimer, & Viswanath, 2008, p. 49) or outside events such as a public service announcement, Glanz, Rimer, and Viswanath (2008) have noted that this construct is not well studied and is difficult to study. It remains a construct in HBM and, again, can refer to techniques to activate readiness to change.

Self-Efficacy

Self-efficacy in HBM is defined in the same way it is defined in SCT: the "conviction that one can successfully execute the behavior required to produce the outcomes," as described by Bandura (1997). In relation to other constructs of HBM, individuals may perceive a threat to their health (perceived susceptibility and severity) and must believe that a particular intervention will help them reduce the threat without unacceptable cost (benefit minus barriers). However, they must perceive that they are personally capable (self-efficacious) of overcoming identified barriers to yield the desired outcome.

Rosenstock (1974) described the first four constructs in conjunction with one another as follows: *perceived* threat (*susceptibility* and *severity*) serves as the motivation to do something, whereas the *perceived benefits* of an intervention minus the *barriers* help to guide the individual toward a particular action (see figure 2.3).

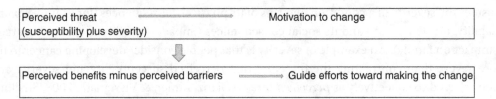

Figure 2.3   Health Belief Model in Summary

Discussion

To better understand HBM, consider the following scenarios in which some but not all of the necessary constructs are in place for an individual to change an unhealthy behavior.

- A smoker perceives a threat to his health and thinks that a smoking-cessation program will offer sufficient benefit to his health. He perceives that the barriers to participating in the program are outweighed by the benefits. However, the individual has tried to stop smoking before, potentially several times. The recall of the failed past attempts to stop smoking can jeopardize his self-efficacy in this case.

- A sedentary person has sufficient perceived threats to motivate her behavior change to become more active. Her path is to join the local YMCA at the start of the new year in order to participate in a regular exercise program. Perhaps she has underestimated the barriers; in January, it is cold and dark when she leaves work in the evening and the weather may not be conducive to making the trip to the YMCA on a regular basis, or she is going to the YMCA on her own and wonders who will miss her if she skips?

There is widespread availability of research that uses HBM to study health behaviors and examines HBM interventions to change behaviors. These studies include examinations of breast cancer screenings, colonoscopies, AIDS-related behaviors, risky sexual behaviors, eating behaviors, stop-smoking interventions, and calcium intake and exercise, to name a few (Carpenter, 2010; Glanz, Rimer, & Viswanath, 2008).

Over time, there have been proposals to increase the complexity of HBM (including cues to action and self-efficacy) and potentially improve its effectiveness in predicting successful behavior change across a wide area of health issues. Although some early reviews of the utility of HBM were supportive of its use (Glanz, Rimer, & Viswanath, 2008), more recent reviews of HBM in its simplest form (not always including cues to action and self-efficacy) have not been as supportive. The reviews, however, do make a case for increasing its complexity through the addition of self-efficacy or combining it with other models in order to improve its utility (Carpenter, 2010).

Theory of Planned Behavior

The **theory of planned behavior (TPB)** was developed from theory of reasoned action (TRA), which essentially states that behaviors result from intentions (Ajzen, 1985). In turn, a person's intention to engage in a particular behavior is a function of (1) the individual's personal attitude toward the behavior, whether it is positive or negative, and

theory of planned behavior (TPB)
theory in which an individual's intention to engage in a behavior is influenced by their personal attitude toward their behavior and their perception of subjective norms related to the behavior

(2) the individual's perception of **subjective norms** related to the behavior, the social pressures to perform or not perform a particular behavior. It follows that an individual is more likely to perform a behavior when it is viewed positively by that individual and also when the individual believes that others whom they value approve of that performance (Ajzen, 1985).

Glanz, Rimer, and Viswanath (2008) reported that TRA was effective in explaining and predicting behavior when that behavior was considered to be under volitional control of the individual. Because it was less clear that the TRA components would be similarly effective when behaviors were less volitionally controlled by an individual, Ajzen and others added the construct of *perceived control* over a behavior and, in turn, expanded TRA into TPB (Ajzen, 1985, 1991; Glanz, Rimer, & Viswanath, 2008).

TPB then has three primary constructs:

•   Personal attitude

•   Subjective norm

•   Perceived control

TPB allows that the intended behavior is a goal established by an individual but explains that there are factors beyond the control of the individual that may interfere with the goal being pursued. Each of the three described constructs has underlying factors, and the individual's beliefs about each construct are among those factors (see figure 2.4).

subjective norm
a factor of normative beliefs, that is, what valued others think about the behavior to be performed or eliminated and how motivated is the individual to seek approval from those valued others

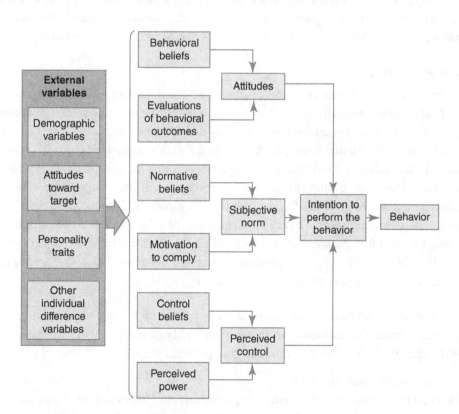

Figure 2.4   Theory of Reasoned Action and Theory of Planned Behavior

Attitude

The construct of attitude toward the behavior is a function of the individual's behavioral beliefs about the behavior and his or her evaluation of the results of performing the behavior. Individuals who believe that favorable, important outcomes will result if a behavior is performed are considered to have a positive attitude toward that behavior. A negative attitude results if an individual believes that negative valued outcomes would result from performance of the behavior (Glanz, Rimer, & Viswanath, 2008).

For example, an individual may believe that smoking is a harmful behavior. The individual evaluates the outcomes of not smoking and determines that one outcome would be weight gain. Because the individual values not being overweight, the individual may have a negative attitude toward quitting smoking in this case, which in turn affects his or her intent to stop smoking.

Subjective Norm

The construct of subjective norm is a factor of normative beliefs, that is, what do valued others think about the behavior to be performed or eliminated and how motivated is the individual to seek approval from those valued others? A positive subjective norm occurs when an individual believes that valued others approve of a particular behavior, and the individual is motivated to seek approval from those others (Glanz, Rimer, & Viswanath, 2008).

For example, a young man may consider smoking to be harmful and sees a positive outcome from quitting. However, the young man may have a parent who not only smokes but also has a view that "we are all going to die anyway, so why bother quitting?" The young man then has a negative subjective norm that influences his intention to stop smoking.

Perceived Control

perceived control refers to people's perceptions of their ability to perform a given behavior

The original TRA was based only on the described constructs of attitude and subjective norms. That theory potentially infers that performing a behavior is under volitional control. As previously described, **perceived control** was added as a construct to TRA as it developed into TPB (Ajzen, 1985; Glanz, Rimer, & Viswanath, 2008). The perceived control construct is influenced by the individual's control beliefs, those beliefs that facilitate or inhibit factors that exist related to the behavior and the individual's perception of the power of these factors to facilitate the behavior or impose a barrier to it (Glanz, Rimer, & Viswanath, 2008).

Volitional control represents a very important part of TPB in that it is the construct that sets it apart from TRA. As such, it is important to consider the factors that influence an individual's volitional control over a particular intended behavior. Those factors are classified as either internal factors or external factors.

internal factors perceived possession of personal characteristics that influence an individual's ability to control his or her behavior

Internal Factors   **Internal factors** include the very general perceived possession of personal characteristics that influence an individual's ability to control his or her behavior, as well as the specific factors listed in the following (Ajzen, 1985):

Information, Skills, and Abilities

- A woman may intend to participate in regular exercise. However, if she lacks knowledge about resources, safe ways to begin an exercise program, how to strength train, and so on, then volitional control is reduced.

Willpower

• A man may intend to abstain from tobacco use but is unable to say no when his best buddies, who are smokers, insist that he join them for a tailgate party at which a significant amount of smoking will take place.

Emotions

• A recently divorced woman intends to abstain from alcohol use but finds herself extremely sad on her first Christmas Eve alone. Overwhelmed by her emotions, she may turn to the very behavior she seeks to avoid.

External Factors   There are two major categories of **external factors**, as described in the following (Ajzen, 1985).

external factors
situational and environmental factors that influence an individual's ability to control his or her behavior, including opportunity, time, and dependence on others

---

OPPORTUNITY AND TIME

A woman signs up for a week-long weight loss camp at a location that requires her to travel via plane. If a hurricane takes place and the flight is canceled, none of the other factors of her intention to lose weight are changed, but the opportunity to engage in weight loss behaviors is affected by circumstances beyond her control. Alternatively, perhaps her job situation has changed such that she no longer has the time to go to the camp as she had intended. In either case, the likelihood that she still intends to lose weight is great, and the behavior may occur with a different opportunity or more time.

DEPENDENCE ON OTHERS

The more any behavior depends on other people, the less there is volitional control for the individual. For example, two college roommates sign up for a safe sex workshop hosted by their campus health center. If one roommate decides she is unable to go, the other is unlikely to go. If the instructor of the workshop cancels the session, neither roommate will go.

For time, opportunity, and dependence on others, such barriers may result in only temporary changes in the intentions of individuals to engage in particular behaviors. In the best case, performance of the behavior may be only delayed. However, if factors beyond an individual's control are numerous and repeated, it can ultimately result in more permanent changes in intentions (Ajzen, 1985).

TPB describes a structure for interventions to improve health behaviors for target populations. Through the identification of behavioral beliefs, normative beliefs, and control beliefs, interventions are designed to adjust those beliefs in turn to adjust attitude, subject norms, and perceived control in such a way that individuals' intentions to perform healthy behaviors are favorably oriented (Glanz, Rimer, & Viswanath, 2008).

There is evidence that TPB has been successfully used in health promotion settings in which smoking, exercise, mammography, and sexually transmitted disease prevention were the targets (Glanz, Rimer, & Viswanath, 2008). Glanz, Rimer, and Viswanath (2008) noted the strength of perceived behavioral control, in particular, as a predictor of behavior change and have recommended its consideration during the design of health promotion interventions.

Historical Perspective

In the 1980s, the health science community initiated a concerted effort to identify interventions that might help people alter behaviors associated with particular diseases (Institute of Medicine, 1982). The early interventions were largely in the form of public education campaigns and targeted at individuals. Numerous publications referred to HBM and TRA-TPB as the foundation of such efforts (Glanz, Rimer, & Viswanath, 2008).

In 1964, the US surgeon general released America's first report on smoking and health. Many health education campaigns ensued, and many people stopped smoking. Eventually, these came to be considered initial gains. The focus of HBM and TRA-TPB on raising awareness about risks of unhealthy behaviors and benefits of changing those behaviors seemed to require additional constructs to better reach larger numbers of people and affect a wider variety of health behaviors. To be sure, the role of health knowledge in shaping attitudes and beliefs was necessary, but perhaps not sufficient to make initial gains into lasting behavior changes (Orleans & Cassidy, 2008).

Bandura's SCT (1986) identified knowledge of health risks as a construct, similar to HBM and TPB, but added external determinants of behavior and offered perceived facilitators and perceived impediments as constructs. Described as the dominant behavior change theory or model even today, SCT helped shift the focus from *why to* change unhealthy behaviors toward *how* to change those unhealthy behaviors and replace them with healthy ones. With this expanded focus came suggestions for modifying one's surrounding environments so as to reduce temptation and relapse, improving self-efficacy for behavior change.

A similar shift also took place with regard to the target of behavior change interventions. Early efforts targeted individuals. Later models targeted populations. The stages of change model served as a way to avoid a one-size-fits-all approach that inevitably results when targeting populations. The model's recognition that behavior change is a process with recognizable steps enabled tailoring of interventions; it is said to have had a significant impact on how health behavior intervention programs are designed and implemented (Orleans & Cassidy, 2008). As noted previously in this chapter, the tendency of some programs to begin at the action stage, assuming that all participants are indeed ready to change behaviors, can be problematic, particularly in the case of individuals who relapse into problem behaviors. Those individuals would not have had the benefit of completing preparation for behavior change and thus would not necessarily re-prepare for another attempt, understanding that relapses are not necessarily failures, but part of the behavior change process.

Summary

This chapter provided an introduction to four theories of behavior, along with evidence of the application of those theories in health behavior change settings. A visual of the constructs associated with these theories is found in table 2.4. Some aspects of the theories are

Table 2.4   Presented Theories and Their Constructs

SCT	TTM	HBM	TPB
Knowledge of health risks and benefits	Stages of change:	Perceived susceptibility	Perceived attitude
Perceived self-efficacy	• Precontemplation	Perceived severity	Subjective norms
Outcome expectations	• Contemplation	Perceived benefits	Perceived control
Personal health goals	• Preparation	Perceived barriers	Internal:
Perceived facilitators	• Action	Cues to action	• Information, skills, and abilities
Perceived impediments	• Maintenance	Self-efficacy	• Willpower
	• Termination		• Emotions
	Processes of change:		External:
	• Consciousness raising		• Opportunity and time
	• Dramatic relief		• Dependence on others
	• Environmental reevaluation		
	• Self-reevaluation		
	• Social liberation		
	• Helping relationships		
	• Self-liberation		
	• Counterconditioning		
	• Reinforcement management		
	• Stimulus control		
	• Decision balance (pros and cons)		
	• Self-efficacy		

similar, and others are unique. Additional theories also exist; however, the four described are considered the dominant theories in the field at this time.

Perhaps the most significant construct that stretches across the four dominant theories is self-efficacy—a person's belief in his or her own ability to be successful in a given situation. It would follow that interventions targeting people with strong senses of self-efficacy are more likely to succeed than those targeting people with weak senses of self-efficacy. As such, behavior change theories include various other constructs designed to help planners of interventions boost the self-efficacy of people involved in behavior change interventions.

Knowledge and understanding of behavior change theories is the first step in the program planning process in a health promotion setting. A health promotion program planner must decide which theory or theories are most applicable to a particular setting. Glanz,

Rimer, and Viswanath (2008) asserted that the strength of health promotion interventions will be enhanced through the application of multiple theories but warned that health promoters should take care to avoid redundancy, overlap, and difficulty in interpretation.

Although chapter 3 describes program planning based on theory, it should be emphasized that prior to targeting program participants and customizing health behavior interventions, understanding the contributing factors of behavior and the impact of the environment are critical.

KEY TERMS

1. **Theory:** an explanation intended to account for the actions that people take or do not take to promote health

2. **Models:** theory-based planning framework that helps guide program creation and evaluation

3. **Social cognitive theory (SCT):** theoretical model that frames individual behavior as a response to observational learning from the surrounding environment

4. **Reciprocal determinism:** the concept that individuals are a product of their environments and also help to create those environments

5. **Self-efficacy:** an individual's perception of his or her capability to execute a course of action necessary to achieve a goal

6. **Transtheoretical model of behavior change (TTM):** theoretical model that describes health behavior as a process characterized by stages of readiness to change

7. **Stages of change:** varying levels of readiness that a person reaches while changing a health behavior

8. **Processes of change:** the covert and overt activities that people use to progress through the six stages of change

9. **Health belief model (HBM):** theoretical model characterized by value-expectancy theories, which explain that behavior is influenced by values and expectations

10. **Value-expectancy theories:** theories that explain that behavior results from an individual's value of the outcome of the behavior and the expectation that a particular action or actions will lead to the outcome

11. **Theory of planned behavior (TPB):** theory in which an individual's intention to engage in a behavior is influenced by personal attitude toward the behavior and the individual's perception of subjective norms related to the behavior

12. **Subjective norm:** a factor of normative beliefs, that is, what valued others think about the behavior to be performed or eliminated and how motivated is the individual to seek approval from those valued others

13. **Perceived control:** refers to people's perceptions of their ability to perform a given behavior.

14. **Internal factors:** perceived possession of personal characteristics that influence an individual's ability to control his or her behavior

15. **External factors:** situational and environmental factors that influence an individual's ability to control his or her behavior, including opportunity, time, and dependence on others

REVIEW QUESTIONS

1. Why do we need to study health behavior theories?

2. What are the different theories and models described in the chapter, and how do you identify their differences?

3. How are these theories applied to behavior change programs?

STUDENT ACTIVITIES

1. For each of the stages within the stages of change construct, what type of information would be part of a behavior change program? For example, in the precontemplation stage, you might consider a social marketing campaign that uses an emotional appeal.

2. For each of the processes of change within the transtheoretical model, translate each change process into a short phrase, for example, consciousness raising—just get people thinking about the behavior.

3. Identify one or two constructs that appear in each of the theories or models for behavior change.

4. Which of the approaches to behavior change resonates with you and why?

References

Ajzen, I. (1985). From intentions to actions: A theory of planned behavior. In: *Action-control: From cognition to behavior* (ed. J. Kuhl and J. Beckman), 11–39. Heidelberg, Germany: Springer.

Ajzen, I. (1991). The theory of planned behavior. *Organization Behavior and Human Decision Processes 50*: 179–211.

Ammerman, A.S., Lindquist, C.H., Lohr, K.N., and Hersey, J. (2002). The efficacy of behavioral interventions to modify dietary fat and fruit and vegetable intake: A review of the evidence. *Preventive Medicine 35* (1): 25–41.

Armitage, C.J.I. (2009). Is there utility in the transtheoretical model? *British Journal of Health Psychology 14*: 195–210.

Bandura, A. (1986). *Social foundations of thought and action: A social cognitive theory*. Englewood Cliffs, NJ: Prentice-Hall.

Bandura, A. (1997). *Self-efficacy: The exercise of control*. New York: W. H. Freeman.

Bandura, A. (2004). Health promotion by social cognitive means. *Health Education & Behavior* 31 (2): 143–164.

Brassington, G.S., Atienza, A.A., Perczek, R.E. et al. (2002). Intervention-related cognitive versus social mediator of exercise adherence in the elderly. *American Journal of Preventive Medicine 23* (2 Supplement): 80–86.

Carpenter, C.J. (2010). A meta-analysis of the effectiveness of health belief model variables in predicting behavior. *Health Communication 25*: 661–669.

Cottrell, R., Girvan, J.T., and McKenzie, J. (2011). *Principles and foundations of health promotion and education*, 5e. Upper Saddle River, NJ: Benjamin Cummings.

DiClemente, C.C., Schlundt, D., and Gemmell, L. (2004). Readiness and stages of change in addiction treatment. *American Journal on Addictions 13* (2): 103–119.

Glanz, K. and Rimer, B.K. (1995). Theory at a glance: A guide for health promotion. In: *Health education: Creating strategies for school and community health education* (ed. G.G. Gilbert and R.G. Sawyer), 79–81. Boston: Jones & Bartlett.

Glanz, K., Rimer, B.K., and Viswanath, K. (ed.) (2008). *Health behavior and health education: Theory, research and practice*. San Francisco: Jossey Bass.

Institute of Medicine (1982). *Health and behavior: Frontiers of research in the biobehavioral sciences* (ed. D.A. Hamburg, G.R. Elliott, and D.L. Parron). Washington, DC: National Academies Press.

Orleans, C.T. and Cassidy, E.F. (2008). Health-related behavior. In: *Health care delivery in the United States*, 9e (ed. A.R. Kovner and J.R. Knickman), 267–297. New York: Springer.

Prochaska, J.O., DiClemente, C.C., and Norcross, J.C. (1992). In search of how people change: Applications to addictive behaviors. *American Psychiatrist 47*: 1102–1114.

Rosenstock, I.M. (1974). The health belief model and preventive health behavior. *Health Education Monographs* 2 (4): 354–386.

Snelling, A.M. and Stevenson, M.O. (2003). Using theories and models to support program planning. In: *ACSM's worksite health promotion manual: A guide to building and sustaining healthy worksites*. Columbus, MO: Human Kinetics.

CHAPTER 3

PROGRAM PLANNING MODELS

Anastasia Snelling

Health promotion programs that initiate and sustain health behavior change do not happen by chance but are a result of a systematic approach to understanding the factors that influence change in individuals and groups. To develop effective programs, program planners must use a framework or model that ensures that the intended results will be achieved. This chapter presents the most recognized and respected program planning model, the PRECEDE–PROCEED model, as well as four other program planning models. Two of these models are based on the social-ecological theory of planning, two are considered consumer-based planning models, and the fifth is considered a community-level program planning model.

These health promotion program models share many of the same elements, but the steps may be different, or the models may emphasize different aspects of the planning process. Regardless of which planning model is selected as the basis of a health promotion program, the use of a model is critical. The use of an established model prompts program planners to consider all phases of program planning and ensures a comprehensive, well-designed program. More advanced practitioners may successfully identify the model that best meets the needs of a specific program, population, or setting through review of prior experiences.

Effective Health Promotion Planning

The goal of health promotion program planning is to "intervene" to improve the health of individuals or communities. Hence, program planning centers on gathering assessment information and designing an intervention that will improve the health of populations or decrease the risk of illness, disability, or death.

LEARNING OBJECTIVES
After reading this chapter, the student will be able to:

- Describe the purpose of program planning models.

- Explain the social-ecological model and how it relates to program planning.

- Identify key elements of the PRECEDE–PROCEED model.

- Discuss key elements of the MATCH model.

- Define the elements of health communication planning models.

- Explain the similarities and differences between program planning models and health communication models.

- Summarize why these models are an important step to successful health promotion programs.

Introduction to Health Promotion, Second Edition. Edited by Anastasia Snelling.
© 2024 John Wiley & Sons Inc. Published 2024 by John Wiley & Sons Inc.
Companion Website: www.wiley.com/go/snelling2e

Different from the health behavior change theories presented in chapter 2 that focus on why and how people make health behavior changes, program planning models serve to guide the development, implementation, and evaluation of a specific health promotion program. A **planning model** is a blueprint for building and improving programs (Crosby & Noar, 2011). Ultimately, in order to address a target behavior and population, program planners must incorporate behavior change theories into program planning models when designing and implementing the intervention.

Effective planning ensures that practitioners can accomplish the following:

- Understand the health issue the program will be addressing

- Identify the population the program will target

- Identify the policy and educational approaches necessary to bring about or support the desired changes

- Establish a logical program development process

- Set priorities and goals

- Establish objectives to achieve goals

- Assess progress

- Measure impact and outcomes

Often in organizations, time is limited; under the pressure of deadlines and demands, there may be a tendency to skip the planning stage. However, following a program planning model process saves health promotion practitioners time in the long run. There may not be one perfect model; however, effective models should be sequential, adaptable to different populations, and ultimately lead to the intended outcomes of improved health (Glanz, Rimer, & Viswanath, 2008).

Social-ecological Model

The twenty-first century has brought a shift from individual-oriented programs to those that encompass environmental strategies. As noted in chapter 1, the determinants of health have expanded our understanding of how and why people make health behavior choices. Health promotion professionals recognize that by making the healthy choice the easy choice in the places people live, work, and learn, people will be more likely to live healthier lives. Further, by extending health promotion programs beyond the individual approach, there is an opportunity to reach a larger population, especially those individuals who are in the pre-contemplation stage of behavior change. The program planning models included in this chapter reflect a shift from an individual-focused approach to an environment- and community-oriented approach. Chapter 2 presented the social cognitive theory, emphasizing the role of environment and behavior change. An ecological approach is one that considers the role of the environment on the target audience, along with their health status, behavior, and skills.

The **social-ecological model of planning** is based on the interrelationships of human beings and their environments (Stokols, 1996), recognizing that within the environment

planning model
serves to guide the development, implementation, and evaluation of a specific health promotion program; a blueprint for building and improving programs

there are physical, social, economic, and cultural forces that have the potential to alter health outcomes. The environment is important, but not to the exclusion of the individual. This theory includes individual attributes such as genetics, behaviors, and knowledge. Other social and environmental factors are also acknowledged in the theory, such as environmental settings, sectors of influence, and norms and cultures within society (figure 3.1). The social-ecological model has made an important contribution to the field of health promotion, particularly with regard to the design of interventions to improve health behaviors. No longer are programs designed only with the individual in mind; they must assess other factors that may either hinder or facilitate the behavior change process.

Figure 3.1 provides a graphic representation of an ecological model for physical activity and healthy eating designed for the United States Department of Agriculture's Dietary Guidelines for Americans. The social-ecological model is evident in the PRECEDE–PROCEED model as well as all of the other models presented in this chapter.

social-ecological model of planning
a planning model based on the interrelationships of human beings and their environments, recognizing that within the environment there are physical, social, economic, and cultural forces that have the potential to alter health outcomes

PRECEDE–PROCEED Model

The **PRECEDE–PROCEED model** is considered the most popular and well-respected model in the field of health promotion program planning. The model was designed in the 1970s and has been widely used by planners and practitioners to guide program design, implementation, and evaluation for a variety of diverse health promotion programs. This model uses an ecological approach to program planning and is considered by many to be the gold standard in health promotion planning due to the extensive assessments that are required prior to any program development being initiated.

PRECEDE–PROCEED model
a nine-phase logic model, using an ecological approach, applied in health promotion program planning

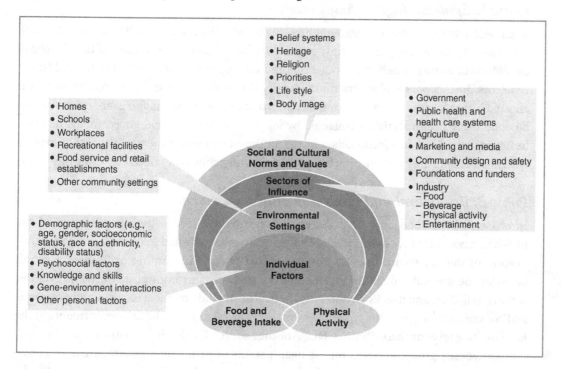

Figure 3.1   A Social-Ecological Framework for Nutrition and Physical Activity Decisions
Source: US Department of Agriculture and US Department of Health and Human Services (2010).

There is a strong emphasis on gaining a thorough understanding of the health issue, the target audience, and the environment prior to implementing a policy or program. In addition, the model encourages community involvement to ensure community buy-in and support, which are essential for sustaining behavior change. Thousands of research studies have examined PRECEDE–PROCEED and numerous articles have been published regarding the model, its applications, and professional commentaries.

The nine-phase logic model is subdivided into two phases: PRECEDE and PROCEED. PRECEDE is an acronym for **p**redisposing, **r**einforcing, and **e**nabling **c**auses in **e**ducational **d**iagnosis and **e**valuation (phases 1 through 4). PROCEED is an acronym for **p**olicy, **r**egulatory, and **o**rganizational **c**onstructs in **e**ducational and **e**nvironmental **d**evelopment (phases 5 through 9).

Phase 1: Social Assessment

In phase 1, social assessment involves an investigation into the quality of life of the target population to accurately understand it. This is best accomplished by involving community members. General quality-of-life information regarding measurable social factors such as unemployment rates, poverty, crime, and population density can be obtained through government offices or other sources. Beyond these statistics, it is critical to engage community members to voice their needs, wants, and desires. Using a combination of statistical data and community voices and opinions results in a more comprehensive and complementary approach to understanding the social factors of a community.

Phase 2: Epidemiological Assessment

epidemiology
the study of the distribution and determinants of health-related conditions or events in defined populations and the application of findings to control health problems

In phase 2, epidemiological assessment involves the identification of health issues and associated goals. **Epidemiology** is the study of the distribution and determinants of health-related conditions or events in defined populations and the application of findings to control health problems. In this phase, planners must identify the health issue and the population that is affected by the health issue. Gathering this information and answering relevant questions can be done using health statistics collected by local, state, and national governments or other health organizations. In addition, data from community members themselves, as they explore what health issues are most pressing for their community, should be collected during this phase.

Phase 3: Behavioral and Environmental Assessment

In phase 3, behavioral and environmental assessment includes the identification of the health behaviors that are associated with the health issue selected in phase 2 and the identification of the key environmental influences that may be promoting or hindering health behavior. Behavioral indicators include factors such as consumption patterns, preventive actions, self-care, and use. Environmental indicators include medical services and economic and community gauges. This type of information can be found in health departments at the local or state level or through the CDC. Another source for this information could be nonprofit advocacy groups focused on the health status of people in a general area. The environmental indicator data may be available at local or state health offices, or reports may be available at advocacy organizations.

Phase 4: Educational and Ecological Assessment

In phase 4, educational and ecological assessment occurs to identify the factors that will facilitate changes in individual behavior and the environmental context. These types of factors are called *predisposing, enabling,* and *reinforcing.*

- *Predisposing factors* occur at the cognitive level and include knowledge, self-efficacy, attitudes, skills, and beliefs. These antecedents to behavior provide the motivation for the behavior.

- *Enabling factors* help individuals act on their motivation to change behavior. Examples include the presence of walking paths, skills to cook healthy foods, community resources, and laws.

- *Reinforcing factors* are the continuing rewards or incentives to repeat the behavior.

These factors can be concrete or abstract and may come from self, family, coworkers, or peers. These factors can help health promotion planners identify and better understand health-compromising and health-enhancing behaviors.

Phase 5: Administrative and Policy Assessment

In phase 5, administrative and policy assessment involves the identification of organizational and administrative opportunities and barriers for developing and implementing a program. Opportunities might include local community sentiment or organizational support, financial support, or available staff to support the program. Policy assessment involves identifying existing policies and regulations that either support or discourage the behavior changes that are being advanced. Policies can be found in organizations, local communities, schools, or government. Regardless of where the program is being implemented, it is critical to review the regulations and policies that govern that setting to clearly understand how they will influence the program.

Phase 6: Program Implementation

In phase 6, the program is implemented based on the assessment and planning processes identified in phases 1 through 5. Program implementation can vary based on the results of the assessments and the desires of the target audience. In the early days of health promotion, educational programs were the intervention of choice. Now, interventions might include a citywide policy to limit secondhand smoke, a social marketing campaign to encourage physical activity, or a text message program to limit drunk driving. It is in this stage that understanding best practices for behavior change meets creative and innovative thinking.

Phases 7, 8, and 9: Evaluation Phases

Phases 7, 8, and 9 are the evaluation phases that comprise three types of evaluation: process, impact, and outcome.

- *Process evaluation* (phase 7) collects information regarding program implementation. Is the program being implemented according to the developed protocol? Were changes to initial plans made, and why? Is the program having the reach that was originally antici-pated? Process evaluation is valuable for program improvement and replication pur-poses but does not examine any resulting behavioral changes.

- *Impact evaluation* (phase 8) measures the impact of the program. Specifically, what are the measurable changes in predisposing (knowledge, skills, or attitudes), enabling (physical environment or policies), and reinforcing (positive or negative feed-back) factors?

- *Outcome evaluation* (phase 9) measures the actual change in health and social benefits or the quality of life for the target participants. This evaluation determines the effect the program had on the community and if the program reached its intended goals.

See table 3.1 for a description of the PRECEDE–PROCEED model components and figure 3.2 for a graphical representation.

Table 3.1   PRECEDE–PROCEED Model

Phase	Title	Description
1	Social assessment	Assessment in both objective and subjective terms of high-priority problems for the common good, defined for a population by economic and social indicators and by individuals in terms of their quality of life.
2	Epidemiological assessment	Identification of the extent, distribution, and causes of a health problem in a defined population.
3	Behavioral and environmental	Identification of the specific health-related actions that will most likely cause a health outcome. A systematic assessment of the factors in the social and physical environment that interact with behavior to produce health effects or quality-of-life outcomes.
4	Educational and ecological assessment	Assessment of the factors that predispose, enable, and reinforce a specific behavior. A predisposing factor is any characteristic of a person or population that motivates behavior prior to the occurrence of the behavior. An enabling factor is any characteristic of the environment that facilitates action and any skill or resource required to attain a specific behavior. A reinforcing behavior is any reward or punishment that follows or is anticipated as a consequence of a behavior, serving to strengthen the motivation for or against the behavior.
5	Administrative and policy	An analysis of the policies, resources, and circumstances prevailing in an organization to facilitate or hinder the development of the health promotion program.
6	Implementation	The act of converting program objectives into actions through policy changes, regulation, and organization.
7	Process evaluation	Assessment of the program, including number of individuals reached by the program or the feedback on the program from participants.
8	Impact evaluation	Assessment of program effects including changes in predisposing, enabling, and reinforcing factors, as well as behavioral and environmental changes.
9	Outcome evaluation	Assessment of the effect of a program, including changes in health and social benefits or quality of life.

Source: Adapted from Green and Kreuter (2005).

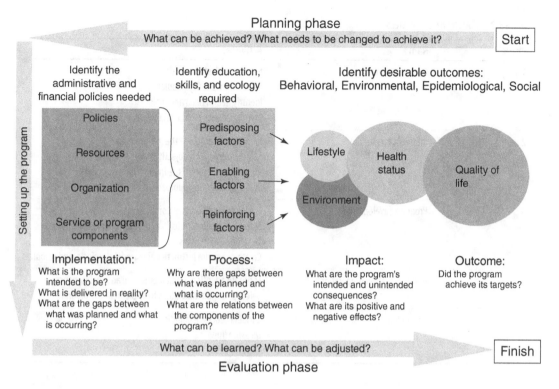

Figure 3.2 PRECEDE–PROCEED Model
Source: Green (2009)/Anton & Lily.

Multilevel Approach to Community Health (MATCH)

The **multilevel approach to community health (MATCH) model**, similar to PRECEDE–PROCEED, is considered an ecological model of program planning. The MATCH framework focuses on assessing population health and working with communities to help them identify opportunities for improving community health and to find and implement evidence-based programs and policies to address the identified health issues. As may be seen from the phases identified in table 3.2, less time is dedicated to assessment compared to the PRECEDE–PROCEED model. The emphasis of this model is on program implementation, with more time devoted to intervention planning, program development, and program implementation. Understanding the population and health issues may help health promotion planners decide which of these two models is more appropriate to guide the planned intervention. Figure 3.3 provides a graphic representation of the MATCH model.

Consumer-based Planning Models for Health Communication

Health communication and social marketing campaigns have become key components of health promotion for a number of reasons. **Consumer-based planning models** focus on the consumer or intended audience, borrowing concepts from the business marketing field and applying those concepts to health promotion. Understanding behavior change through a business marketing approach recognizes that consumers have choices to make when

multilevel approach to community health (MATCH) model an ecological model of program planning focusing on assessing population health and working with communities to help them identify opportunities for improving community health and to find and implement evidence-based programs and policies that address the identified health issues

Table 3.2   MATCH Phases and Steps

Phase	Name	Activities
1	Goal selection	Select health status goals Select high-priority population(s) Identify health behavior goals Identify environmental factor goals
2	Intervention planning	Identify the targets of the intervention Select intervention objectives Identify mediators of the intervention objectives Select intervention approaches
3	Program development	Create program units or components Select or develop curricula and create intervention guides Develop session plans Create or acquire instructional materials, projects, and resources
4	Implementation preparations	Facilitate adoption, implementation, and maintenance Select and train individuals to implement the program
5	Evaluation	Conduct process evaluation Measure impact Monitor outcomes

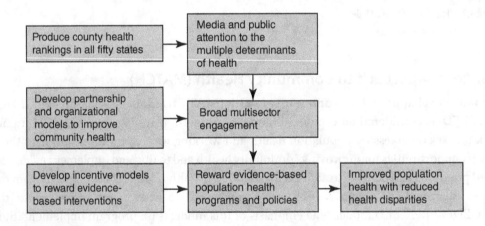

Figure 3.3   MATCH Model

Source: Kindig, Booske, and Remington (2010)/US Department of Health and Human Services/Public Domain.

consumer-based planning models
models that focus on the consumer or intended audience, borrowing concepts from the business marketing field, and applying those concepts to health promotion

selecting health behaviors. If a health promotion program is to achieve success, program planners need to consider their "competition" and apply applicable business marketing concepts to promote, or "sell," health behavior change. In business marketing, there is a financial exchange for the customer between money and a product; in health marketing, the "product" is a health behavior and improved health outcomes, and the "cost" to the customer is time, effort, and motivation for a change.

Effective communications campaigns raise awareness of and share information about health issues with large audiences and are usually considered the first step in the behavior change process. Also, effective campaigns may motivate individuals to act. Consistent messaging over a period of time sustains the message for the target audience. As technology and communication tools develop and change, health promotion messages can be more diverse and targeted to broader or more specific audiences. With the recent, significant increase in social marketing to promote healthy behavior among populations, health communication campaigns have become an important strategy in health promotion activities.

Health promotion messages are communicated through numerous methods that can be categorized by the following:

- Mass media (e.g., television, radio, billboards)

- Small media (e.g., brochures, posters)

- Social media (e.g., Facebook, Twitter, Weblogs)

- Interpersonal communication (e.g., one-on-one or group education)

The Community Preventive Services Task Force (www.communityguide.org) is an independent, nonfederal, unpaid body, appointed by the director of the CDC. It is composed of sixteen members who represent a broad range of research, practice, and policy expertise in community preventive services, public health, health promotion, and disease prevention. The task force was established in 1996 by the US Department of Health and Human Services to provide evidence-based recommendations regarding community preventive services, programs, and policies that are effective in saving lives, increasing longevity, and improving Americans' quality of life. This group recommends health communication campaigns that use multiple channels to facilitate adoption and maintenance of health-promoting behaviors (e.g., increased physical activity through pedometer distribution combined with walking campaigns).

The two most prominent health communication models are CDCynergy, developed by the CDC, and *Making Health Communication Programs Work*, developed by the National Cancer Institute (NCI). These models are similar to one another and are described in the following sections.

CDCynergy

CDCynergy (www.cdc.gov/healthcommunication/CDCynergy) was developed by the Office of Communication at the CDC. The steps or phases of this model closely resemble those of the PRECEDE–PROCEED model, although CDCynergy clearly emphasizes marketing and business communication concepts that include population feedback, segmentation principles, and targeted communication strategies.

The CDCynergy model emphasizes a process that involves the following actions:

- Using research to describe and determine the causes of the health issue

- Describing the audience affected by the health issue

- Exploring a range of strategies to address the issue or problem

CDCynergy
a planning model developed by the CDC that emphasizes marketing and business communication concepts that include population feedback, segmentation principles, and target communication strategies

- Developing a comprehensive communication plan that includes audience research, pretesting, production, and launch
- Planning for and conducting evaluation activities throughout the entire process

Phase 1: Understanding the Problem

Phase 1 is identifying and fully understanding the problem, determining who is being affected by the problem, and assessing the factors that will affect the direction of the project. During this phase, health promotion planners use descriptive epidemiological data and conduct a strengths, weaknesses, opportunities, and threats (SWOT) analysis.

Phase 2: Problem Analysis

Phase 2 involves problem analysis to identify the factors that contribute to the health problem, the population groups affected by it, and a list of potential partners. During this phase, goals are written to guide the strategy. Phase 2 relies on analytic epidemiologic methods to delineate the causes of the problem identified in the previous phase. Based on this analysis, program planners then identify and select intervention activities that strike at the root of the problem determinants. Also in phase 2, it is recommended that program planners solidify partners and consider the program budget.

Phase 3: Communication Planning

Phase 3 is communication program planning, the center of CDCynergy. During this phase, communication planning begins in earnest. Health promotion planners decide whether communication will be used as a dominant intervention or to support other intervention activities. Based on this determination, audiences are identified and segmented, communication goals and objectives are formulated, and formative research is conducted. Formative evaluation is a method of judging the components of program while it is being developed. The results of the formative research in this phase will be used to develop a creative brief. The creative brief is used to inform the development of messages and the testing and selection of settings, channel-specific activities, and materials that will be used to disseminate the messages to intended audiences.

CHANNEL-SPECIFIC ACTIVITIES INCLUDE THE FOLLOWING:

- Interpersonal channels (e.g., physicians, friends, family members, counselors, parents, clergy, and coaches of the intended audiences)
- Group channels (e.g., brown bag lunches at work, classroom activities, neighborhood gatherings, and club meetings)
- Organizations and community groups (e.g., advocacy groups)
- Mass media channels (e.g., radio, network and cable television, magazines, direct mail, billboards, transit cards, newspapers)
- Interactive digital media channels (e.g., Internet websites, bulletin boards, newsgroups, chat rooms, CD-ROMs, kiosks)

Phase 4: Program and Evaluation Development

Phase 4 focuses on program and evaluation development and involves pretesting the communication concepts, messages, and materials that were developed in phase 3. Ideally, pretesting is done by engaging a sample of the target audience to assess how they respond to the selected strategy. In this phase, planners use the brief developed in the previous phase to guide the process of testing and selecting concepts, messages, settings, channel-specific activities, and materials. The decisions made during these activities culminate in a communication plan that lays out who will do what, when, where, and how often in executing health promotion communication activities.

Phase 5: Program Implementation and Management

Phase 5 is described as program implementation and management. The purpose of this phase is to provide guidance on how to systematically conceptualize, plan, execute, and provide meaningful and timely feedback on an evaluation.

Phase 6: Evaluation

Phase 6 is the overall feedback or evaluation phase for the program planners to identify key findings that resulted from the program. During this phase, program practitioners evaluate the communication plan, modify the program based on feedback, and disseminate lessons learned.

Making Health Communication Programs Work

Originally printed in 1989, **Making Health Communication Programs Work** is a guide to communication program planning developed by the Office of Cancer Communications (OCC, now the Office of Communications) of the NCI. During the twenty-five years that NCI has been involved in health communication, ongoing evaluation of its communication programs has affirmed the value of using specific communication strategies to promote health and prevent disease (Parvanta & Freimuth, 2000). The *Making Health Communications Programs Work* model is considered a practical guide for planning and implementing a health promotion effort. The Health Communication Program Cycle (see figure 3.4) is supported by the NCI and can be accessed on their website, called *Making Health Communication Programs Work* (www.cancer.gov/cancertopics/cancerlibrary/pinkbook/page1).

Making Health Communication Programs Work a guide to communication program planning developed by the National Cancer Institute

As displayed in figure 3.4, this model identifies a four-step process to effective health communication planning. The stages constitute a circular process in which the last stage feeds back to the first as health promoters work through a continuous loop of planning, implementation, assessment, and improvement. Similar to the CDCynergy model, this model focuses on consumers, engaging them in the assessment of the health issue and the design of the communication plan or intervention to address the health issue. Table 3.3 describes activities for each of the CDCynergy model phases.

Health Promotion Planning Model for Community-Level Programs

As the need for increased health promotion activities and programs at the community level has grown since the new millennium, new models have been developed to focus on the

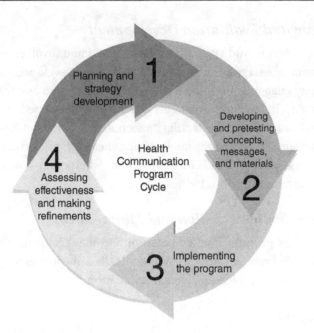

Figure 3.4   Health Communication Program Cycle
Source: U.S. Department of Health and Human Services.

Table 3.3   CDCynergy Program Planning Model

Phase	Title	Activities
1	Planning and strategy development	Identify how the organization can use communication to effectively address a health issue. Identify the intended audiences; use consumer research to craft a communication strategy. Design an evaluation plan.
2	Developing and pretesting concepts, messages, and materials	Develop relevant messages. Draft messages. Pretest messages with intended audiences.
3	Implementing the program	Communicate with partners and clarify involvement. Activate communication and distribution. Document procedures and compare progress to timelines. Refine the program continuously.
4	Assessing effectiveness and making refinements	Assess the degree to which the target population is receiving the program. Assess the immediate impact on the target population and refine the programs as necessary. Ensure that program delivery is consistent with protocol. Analyze changes in the target population.

unique nature of community-level health intervention programs. Although the PRECEDE–PROCEED and MATCH models are applicable to community-level programs, the mobilizing for action through planning and partnerships (MAPP) model was designed with the inter-relationships of communities in mind.

The MAPP model emphasizes the importance of successful partnerships in the development of activities and solutions to address health issues. For example, as communities begin to address rising obesity rates, the issue of access to healthy food has been identified as a potential barrier to combating obesity. This community-level model is very useful in communities that want to address the issue of food deserts and the reliance on corner stores, providing the right steps for a community to address the issue of access to healthy foods for its residents.

Mobilizing for Action through Planning and Partnerships (MAPP)

The **MAPP model** was created by the National Association for County and City Health Officials (NACCHO) to assist local health departments and local health coalitions with program planning that specifically targets community health issues. MAPP is a community-driven strategic planning process for improving community health. Using an interactive process, the framework helps communities apply strategic thinking to prioritize public health issues and identify resources to address them (Kindig, Booske, & Remington, 2010; Minkler & Wallerstein, 2005).

mobilizing for action through planning and partnerships (MAPP) model a planning model developed by the National Association of County and City Health Officials to assist local health departments and local health coalitions with program planning that specifically targets community health issues

Phase 1: Organizing for Success and Partnership Development

This first phase centers on two critical and interrelated activities: organizing the planning process and developing partnerships. The purpose of this phase is to structure a planning process that builds commitment, engages participants as active partners, uses participants' time well, and results in a plan that can be realistically implemented.

Phase 2: Visioning

This phase provides focus, purpose, and direction to the MAPP process so that participants collectively achieve a shared vision for the future. A shared community vision provides an overarching goal for the community.

Phase 3: Assessments

This phase focuses on conducting four assessments: (1) community themes and strengths, (2) the capacity of the local public health system, (3) the community health status based on epidemiological data, and (4) the focus of where change needs to or should occur. These assessments provide important information, unique to that community, for improving community health outcomes.

Phase 4: Identify Strategic Issues

During the fourth phase, planning participants work together to prioritize the most important issues facing the community. Once these issues are recognized, strategic solutions are identified or developed by exploring the results of the previous assessments and determining how those issues affect the achievement of the shared vision.

Phase 5: Formulate Goals and Strategies

This phase builds on the strategic issues that were identified and involve the formulation of goal statements related to those issues. Planning participants then pinpoint strategies for addressing issues and achieving goals related to the community's vision.

Phase 6: The Action Cycle

During this phase, planning, implementing, and evaluation occur. The local public health system or other health promotion coalition develops and implements an action plan for addressing priority goals and objectives. Further evaluation is emphasized to identify what activities are having the most impact on changing the targeted health issue.

MAP-IT

When Healthy People 2020 was launched, the Department of Health and Human Services also launched MAP-IT, a framework for creating, implementing, and evaluating programs. The acronym MAP-IT stands for mobilize, assess, plan, implement, and track.

This framework is similar to the steps identified in other program planning models. What makes this framework different is that it is on the Healthy People 2020 website. Healthy People 2020 is the strategic plan for health improvement of Americans and is discussed in chapter 9. The MAPIT framework helps all types of health professionals create programs to promote healthy communities. Table 3.4 presents some key questions to use for each stage of the MAP-IT framework.

Connecting Health Behavior Theories to Program Planning Models

Chapter 2 and this chapter contain the building blocks for creating programs that will sustain behavior change. The constructs, theories, phases, and models are a health promotion professional's tools of the trade, and, when used correctly, programs will more likely create success for individuals, organizations, and communities. Knowing and applying these theories and models will distinguish your skill set from other professionals and, most importantly, will demonstrate that practice-based evidence is a key to helping health-promoting change to reverse the behaviors linked to chronic disease.

The next five chapters discuss behaviors that promote healthy living. As you read and discuss the chapters, keep in mind the content of these first two chapters and begin to apply the constructs of how people change behaviors and how programs must collect and use data on the target audience to design a program specifically tailored for that population.

Table 3.4   Key Questions for Each Stage of MAP-IT

Mobilize	Assess	Plan	Implement	Track
What are the vision and mission of the coalition?	Who is affected and how?	What is our goal? What do we need to do to reach our goal?	Are we following our plan? What can we do better?	Are we evaluating our work? Did we follow the plan?
Why do I want to bring people together?	What resources do we have?	Who will do it?		What did we change?
Who should be represented?	What resources do we need?	How will we know when we have reached our goal?		Did we reach our goal?
Who are the potential partners (organizations and businesses) in my community?				

Summary

This chapter introduced the process by which program planners develop, implement, and evaluate health promotion programs. To ensure that a program achieves the intended results, the identification and use of a program planning model are an important first step. This chapter describes two ecological models, two health communication models, and one community model. Although these models are most commonly accepted in the health promotion field, there are many other program planning models available to health promotion practitioners. The most important factor is to identify a model that is appropriate for the project and use that model as a guide for program development. Program planning may seem "instinctual" to some, but using a model that provides a step-by-step guide ensures that a thorough assessment and planning process guides the implementation of the program.

KEY TERMS

1. **Planning model:** serves to guide the development, implementation, and evaluation of a specific health promotion program; a blueprint for building and improving programs

2. **Social-ecological model of planning:** a planning model based on the interrelationships of human beings and their environments, recognizing that within the environment there are physical, social, economic, and cultural forces that have the potential to alter health outcomes

3. **PRECEDE–PROCEED model:** a nine-phase logic model, using an ecological approach, applied in health promotion program planning

4. **Epidemiology:** the study of the distribution and determinants of health-related conditions or events in defined populations and the application of findings to control health problems

5. **Multilevel approach to community health (MATCH) model:** an ecological model of program planning focusing on assessing population health and working with communities to help them identify opportunities for improving community health and to find and implement evidence-based programs and policies that address the identified health issues

6. **Consumer-based planning models:** models that focus on the consumer or intended audience, borrowing concepts from the business marketing field and applying those concepts to health promotion

7. **CDCynergy:** a planning model developed by the CDC that emphasizes marketing and business communication concepts that include population feedback, segmentation principles, and target communication strategies

8. **Making Health Communication Programs Work:** a guide to communication program planning developed by the NCI

9. **Mobilizing for action through planning partnerships (MAPP) model:** a planning model developed by the National Association of County and City Health Officials to assist local health departments and local health coalitions with program planning that specifically targets community health issues

REVIEW QUESTIONS

1. At which stage in the program planning model will you use the theories of behavior change?

2. How will using a program planning model save time in the long run?

3. How are the models similar and how are they different?

4. What issues might arise if you do not use a program planning model?

5. The PRECEDE–PROCEED model has five assessment phases. What sources could you use to obtain the data for each phase?

STUDENT ACTIVITIES

1. Many health promotion practitioners enjoy the implementation phase of program planning. Identify key reasons why the assessment and evaluation phases are critical to the success of any program.

2. Identify a social marketing campaign, its message, the target audience, what behavior change theory it is employing, and what recommendations you would suggest to improve it and why.

3. Identify one article in the literature that exemplifies each of the program planning models.

4. Describe the ecological model and relate it to program planning.

References

Crosby, R. and Noar, S.M. (2011). What is a planning model? An introduction to PRECEDE-PROCEED. *Journal of Public Health Dentistry 71*: S7–S15.

Glanz, K., Rimer, B.K., and Viswanath, K. (ed.) (2008). *Health behavior and health education: Theory, research and practice*, 4e. San Francisco: Jossey-Bass.

Green, L. W. (2009). *PRECEDE-PROCEED model*. Retrieved from www.lgreen.net/precede.htm

Green, L.W. and Kreuter, M.W. (2005). *Health program planning: An educational and ecological approach*, 4e. Boston: McGraw-Hill.

Kindig, D.A., Booske, B.C., and Remington, P.L. (2010). Mobilizing action toward community health (MATCH): Metrics, incentives, and partnerships for population health. *Preventing Chronic Disease 7* (4): A68. Retrieved from www.cdc.gov/pcd/issues/2010/jul/10_0019.htm.

Minkler, M. and Wallerstein, N. (2005). Improving health through community organization and community building: A health education perspective. In: *Community organizing and community building for health*, 2e (ed. M. Minkler), 26–50. New Brunswick, NJ: Rutgers University Press.

Parvanta, C.F. and Freimuth, V. (2000). Health communication at the Centers for Disease Control and Prevention. *American Journal of Health Behaviors 24* (1): 18–25.

Stokols, D. (1996). Translating social ecological theory into guidelines for community health promotion. *American Journal of Health Promotion 10* (4): 282–298.

US Department of Agriculture and US Department of Health and Human Services (2010). Helping Americans make healthy choices. In: *Dietary guidelines for Americans 2010*, 56. Washington, DC: US Government Printing Office.

PART TWO

HEALTH BEHAVIORS

CHAPTER 4

TOBACCO USE

Trends, Health Consequences, Cessation, and Policies

Laurie DiRosa

Since 1964, when Surgeon General Luther L. Terry first published the definitive report that smoking caused lung cancer in men, the culture of smoking has dramatically changed for the better (US Department of Health and Human Services, 2014). We see the impact of these changes daily as smokers huddle in obscurely located "smoking areas" outside of office buildings, malls, hospitals, and other public establishments. As of October 1, 2022, 28 states had enacted comprehensive smoke-free laws banning smoking in all workplaces, restaurants, and bars. This equals 66.7% of the US population currently living under a ban on smoking (American Nonsmokers' Rights Foundation, 2022). However, according to the Centers for Disease Control (CDC), progress has stalled since 2011, with 58 million Americans still exposed to secondhand smoke (2018).

This culture is much different from the one sixty years ago, when smoking was permitted everywhere, including on airplanes and in doctors' offices. Before conclusive evidence linked smoking to lung cancer, approximately 42% of the US population smoked. Today, 12.5% of U.S. adults aged 18 years or older are current cigarette smokers (CDC, 2022a). Government bans on smoking did not begin until the 1990s; in 1995, California became the first state to enact a statewide smoking ban, and in 1998, the US Department of Transportation banned smoking on all commercial passenger flights (CDC, 2012a). Although smoking rates have much improved, the United States is still short of the Healthy People 2030 goal of only 6.1% of the US population smoking (Healthy People, 2022). Smoking is not only hazardous to our health but it also affects our culture and economy; government policies have been established to control the spread of its addictive capacity.

Just as smoking has a pervasive effect on the organs and cells throughout our body, it also has a pervasive effect on our society. Those in the health

LEARNING OBJECTIVES
After reading this chapter, the student will be able to:

- Describe the trends of tobacco use over the past several decades.

- Discuss the effects tobacco has on the human body.

- Identify the barriers to tobacco cessation programs.

- Summarize best practices for tobacco cessation.

- Restate the policies that have been enacted to limit tobacco use.

- Explain the impact that clean indoor air has had on smoking rates.

promotion field continue to work to encourage current smokers to quit and to discourage adolescents and others from starting the habit. This chapter discusses general tobacco-related statistics, the chronic diseases related to smoking, smoking trends and changes in the United States related to smoking, and effective cessation programs.

Tobacco Use

Tobacco use remains the single most preventable cause of death and disease in the United States (CDC, 2022b). Despite ongoing efforts by health promotion professionals, people continue to smoke, putting their bodies at risk for cancer, cardiovascular disease (CVD), pulmonary disease, and reproductive and developmental effects. Despite a decrease in cigarette smoking in general, additional tobacco products are now flooding the market (e.g., e-cigarettes). Figure 4.1 identifies many different cancers and chronic diseases that are causally linked to mainstream smoking and also identifies additional illnesses and cancers that occur through secondhand smoke exposure.

Tobacco Use Statistics

Data from 2020 indicate that 19% of United States reported using any commercial tobacco product (cigarettes, e-cigarettes, cigars, smokeless tobacco, and pipes); overall, the current cigarette smoking rate is 12.6% (National Center for Health Statistics, 2022). Of those who smoke, almost 80% smoke every day. The proportion of those who smoke more than 30 cigarettes per day is 6.4%, whereas the proportion of those who smoke one to nine cigarettes per day is 25% (CDC, 2022a).

The person most likely to smoke is male, between fifteen and forty-four years old, living below the poverty level, and of low education (GED or no high school diploma). The ethnic group with the highest rate of smoking is American Indians at 27.1% (CDC, 2022a). It is more common for those with a disability to smoke compared to individuals without disabilities (19.8% versus 11.8%) (CDC, 2022a).

Adolescents

In 2012, the surgeon general published a report specifically focused on adolescent tobacco use (US Department of Health and Human Services, 2012). This is a vulnerable population that deserves special attention when it comes to smoking because they are more susceptible to tobacco marketing and are also easily influenced by peers and social pressure to experiment with smoking. Research indicates that 80% of adult smokers begin by age 18, and 99% of all first-time tobacco use occurs before age 26—this is alarming, yet provides hope. Health promotion professionals can significantly reduce the number of smokers overall if they can successfully prevent their first use at a young age. The health risks of beginning to smoke at a young age are particularly high; becoming addicted to nicotine as a minor promotes longer lifetime use and greater chances of heart and lung damage (US Department of Health and Human Services, 2012). Research shows the presence of atherosclerosis in young smokers, which can lead to reduced lung growth and function in later years (US Department of Health and Human Services, 2012).

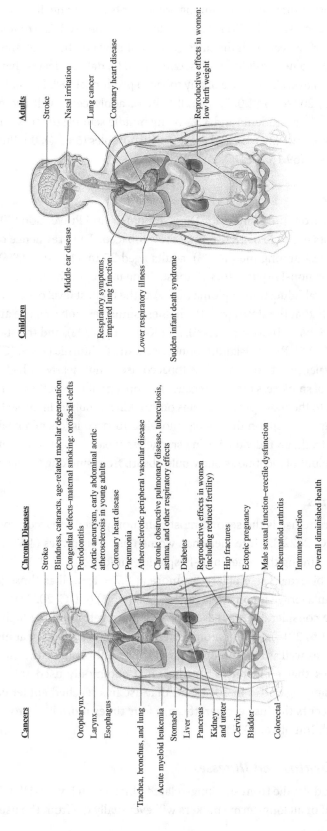

Cancers

Oropharynx
Larynx
Esophagus
Trachea, bronchus, and lung
Acute myeloid leukemia
Stomach
Liver
Pancreas
Kidney
and ureter
Cervix
Bladder
Colorectal

Chronic Diseases

Stroke
Blindness, cataracts, age-related macular degeneration
Congenital defects—maternal smoking: orofacial clefts
Periodontitis
Aortic aneurysm, early abdominal aortic
atherosclerosis in young adults
Coronary heart disease
Pneumonia
Atherosclerotic peripheral vascular disease
Chronic obstructive pulmonary disease, tuberculosis,
asthma, and other respiratory effects
Diabetes
Reproductive effects in women
(including reduced fertility)
Hip fractures
Ectopic pregnancy
Male sexual function—erectile dysfunction
Rheumatoid arthritis
Immune function
Overall diminished health

Adults

Stroke
Nasal irritation
Lung cancer
Coronary heart disease
Reproductive effects in women:
low birth weight

Children

Middle ear disease
Respiratory symptoms,
impaired lung function
Lower respiratory illness
Sudden infant death syndrome

Figure 4.1 The Health Consequences Causally Linked to Smoking and Exposure to Secondhand Smoke

Note: The condition in gray is a new disease that has been causally linked to smoking in this report.
Source: US Department of Health and Human Services (2004, 2006, 2012).

A focus on preventing first-time use among adolescents among health promotion professionals has proven successful—in 2011, 19% of adolescents smoked. Currently, as of 2021, 1.5% smoke cigarettes. However, with the introduction of new combustible, smokeless, and e-products, this is posing a new risk for adolescents. In 2021, data indicates that 19.4% have used an e-cigarette, with overall ever-use of any tobacco product at 28% for middle and high school students (CDC, 2022c). In 2022, overall 9.4% of adolescents will use e-cigarettes, with 14.1% being high school students and 3.3% being middle school students. Most of these students use e-cigarettes daily (27.6%), and most use disposables (55.3%), the Puff Bar brand (29.7%), and a fruit flavor (69.1%) (CDC, 2022d).

Smokeless Tobacco

According to 2020 data from the Centers for Disease Control and Prevention (2022), an estimated 2.3% of US adults over age of 18 use smokeless tobacco. The prevalence of smokeless tobacco use is the highest among men (4.8%), adults aged 25 to 44 years (2.8%), American Indian or Alaska Native, non-Hispanic (6.8%), those living in the south (2.7%), in a rural area (5.9%), and have a General Education Diploma (GED) as the highest level of education (3.8%). Data from 2018 indicate that the states with the highest smokeless tobacco use are Wyoming (8.8%), West Virginia (8.3%), Mississippi (7.4%), and Kentucky (7.0%), and the states with the lowest are New Jersey (1.4%), Rhode Island, Connecticut, and California (1.8%) (CDC, 2022e).

Although the prevalence rate of smokeless tobacco use is not nearly as high as cigarette smoking levels, the use of smokeless tobacco is cause for concern. It is hypothesized that continued use may be related to the more prevalent bans on smoking in public, increased excise taxes on cigarettes, and the misconception that using smokeless tobacco is less of a health risk than smoking cigarettes. In truth, an individual using smokeless tobacco eight to ten times a day is absorbing the same amount of nicotine as one would absorb from smoking 60 cigarettes a day.

Electronic Cigarettes

Among adults, e-cigarette use is the second most commonly used tobacco product behind cigarettes at 3.7% (CDC, 2022a). More men than women use e-cigarettes (4.6% versus 2.8%), with the highest usage among the other, non-Hispanic ethnic group (7.8%). Those identifying as lesbian, gay, or bisexual use e-cigarettes more at 8.7%, as well as those single/never married (6.2%), with an average income of over $75,000 (4.5%) (CDC, 2022a).

In response to the considerable increase in use of e-cigarettes among high school students (900% from 2011 to 2015), the Surgeon General published a report that highlights the use and dangers of use, as well as recommendations for prevention and education strategies. In this report, it states that e-cigarettes are the most commonly used tobacco product among youth, surpassing cigarettes in 2014, and that use has reached epidemic levels (US DHHS, 2016). Adolescents that use e-cigarettes are four times more likely to smoke traditional cigarettes (Truth Initiative, 2021)

Smoking-related Deaths and Illnesses

A total of 480,000 US adults die from smoking-related illnesses each year (US DHHS, 2014). It is predicted that half of all long-term smokers will eventually die from the use of tobacco.

For every eight smokers who die from tobacco use, one nonsmoker will die from passive smoking. For every person who dies from tobacco use, 20 more people suffer from at least one serious tobacco-related illness. It is estimated that secondhand smoke exposure causes approximately 3,000 deaths from lung cancer, 46,000 deaths from heart disease, and 430 newborn deaths from sudden infant death syndrome (SIDS) annually (US Department of Health and Human Services, 2006). Most significantly, smoking could kill eight million people each year by 2030 worldwide if prevalence rates remain constant (World Health Organization, 2012).

As shown in figure 4.1, cigarette smoking has been causally linked to cancer of the larynx, esophagus, trachea, bronchus, lungs, blood, stomach, pancreas, kidney, bladder, ureter, and cervix. Additionally, the chronic diseases of coronary artery disease, vascular disease, periodontitis, blindness, pneumonia, chronic obstructive pulmonary disease (COPD), asthma, reduced fertility, and incidences of stroke and aneurysms are also causally linked to smoking. Smokeless tobacco use leads to nicotine addiction as often as cigarette smoking does and has been linked to cancer of the mouth and gums, periodontitis, and tooth loss. Studies also suggest a relationship between smokeless tobacco use and precancerous oral lesions, oral cancer, and cancers of the kidney, pancreas, and digestive system, as well as death from cardiovascular and cerebrovascular disease (US Department of Health and Human Services, 2010). An estimated eight thousand people die each year because of smokeless tobacco use (CDC, 2012c).

Tobacco-related Costs

The economic burden of tobacco use is calculated through direct and indirect costs. **Direct costs** include health care expenditures required to address smoking-related illnesses. **Indirect costs** include lost earnings due to premature death (mostly due to lung cancer, ischemic heart disease, and COPD). Experts calculate that in 2018, cigarette smoking cost the United States $612 billion, with $240 billion in direct costs and $372 billion indirectly through losses in productivity from illness and premature death (Xu, Shrestha, Trivers, Linda, Armour, & King 2021; Shrestha et al., 2022; US DHHS, 2014). According to newly published research, annual healthcare expenditures attributable to all current e-cigarette use were $15.1 billion (Wang, Sung, Lightwood, Yao, & Max 2022).

direct costs
in managed care, the costs of labor, supplies, and equipment to provide direct patient care services

indirect costs
resources forgone as a result of a health condition

Smoking Tobacco and Chronic Disease

There is no risk-free level of exposure to tobacco smoke. When tobacco smoke is inhaled, the toxic compounds in the smoke are transferred from the lungs to the bloodstream. This enables the toxins to travel throughout the body, affecting nearly every organ. As noted previously in this chapter, there is clear evidence linking smoking to cancer, CVD, pulmonary disease, and reproductive and developmental effects. In fact, smoking is the cause of 30% of all cancer deaths and nearly 80% of all deaths from COPD. This section will review the biological basis of how smoking causes these diseases.

Cancer

The National Cancer Institute defines **cancer** as uncontrolled cell growth in any part of the body. Depending on where in the body the cell growth occurs, these cells can form tumors and affect the tissues surrounding them. Normally, DNA produces genes that keep cell growth under control. However, sometimes DNA becomes damaged and creates mutated genes that no longer control cell growth and natural cell death.

Carcinogens are toxic compounds that can damage DNA and lead to the cancerous growth of cells. Cigarette smoke contains the potent carcinogens polycyclic aromatic hydrocarbons, N-nitrosamines, aromatic amines, 1,3-butadiene, benzene, aldehydes, and ethylene oxide. These particular carcinogens are proven to have a significant role in changing cellular pathways and the genetic processes that foster the growth and development of cancer (Hecht, 1998). As shown in figure 4.2, these carcinogens can cause cancer through three different pathways. The most common pathway of cancer formation is when carcinogens are not detoxified but rather activated, damaging DNA and the coding process. The miscoded DNA produces mutated genes that are not able to control cell growth, resulting in cancerous cell growth. Alternatively, co-carcinogens and tumor promoters are activated through regular cigarette smoking, which stimulate cell growth and at the same time silence tumor suppressor genes. Third, nicotine and nitrosamines can bind to receptors, activating proteins that are important in cell growth and transformation. All of these pathways lead to uncontrolled cell growth and cancer.

Of course, not everyone who smokes will get cancer, although the risk for cancer among smokers is higher than among nonsmokers. Cancer occurrence varies based on each individual's ability to detoxify carcinogens, repair damaged DNA, and, if need be, kill damaged cells.

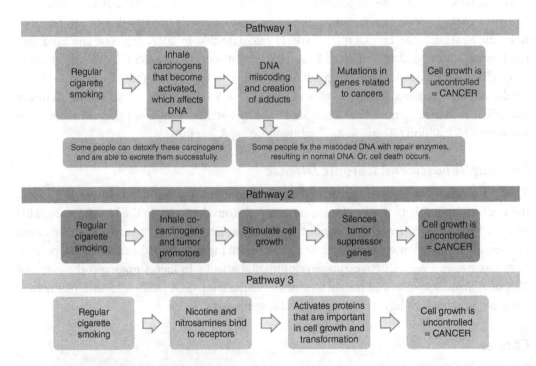

Figure 4.2 How Cigarette Smoking Causes Cancer
Source: US Department of Health and Human Services (2010), chapter 5.

Cardiovascular Disease

A primary risk factor for **CVD** is smoking. In the United States, more than one-third of all deaths from CVD can be attributed to smoking. In addition to being an independent risk factor for CVD, smoking also has a significant effect on other CVD risk factors, specifically high blood pressure, diabetes mellitus, and high blood lipids. The surgeon general warns that a smoker who also presents with two additional risk factors will have eight times the risk of CVD as compared to a nonsmoker with no other risk factors. There is no safe level of smoke exposure. CVD risk occurs at low levels of use, including infrequent smoking and exposure to secondhand smoke. Therefore, smoking fewer cigarettes each day does not reduce the risk of CVD; only smoking cessation reduces the risk of CVD.

> **cardiovascular disease (CVD)** refers to conditions that involve narrowed or blocked blood vessels that can lead to a heart attack, chest pain (angina), or stroke

The cardiovascular system moves blood and lymph throughout the body to deliver oxygen and nutrients to the cells and pick up cellular waste. This circulation of materials relies on healthy, flexible, and strong arteries and veins to properly move these fluids through the system. CVD occurs when arteries that deliver blood to the heart become clogged, the valves of the heart are damaged, or the heart does not pump effectively. Also, arteries can become clogged, harden, and weaken, or blood clots can form that stop the flow of blood to the heart or brain, causing death.

Cigarette smoke causes CVD through various mechanisms; nicotine, carbon monoxide, and oxidizing chemicals are most responsible for damage to the cardiovascular system. Nicotine is a drug that continually stimulates the nervous system, increasing the resting heart rate, which is a possible risk for CVD. Carbon monoxide binds with hemoglobin the same way that oxygen does; however, it is more powerful at doing so. Therefore, smokers are left with less oxygen released to cells. In the long term, in order to compensate for the loss of hemoglobin to carbon monoxide, the body produces more red blood cells to deliver oxygen. The negative effect is thicker blood, which is not as easy to pump through the arteries and veins.

The presence of oxidizing chemicals (e.g., free radicals) in cigarette smoke reduces the amount of antioxidants found in the body naturally. Fewer antioxidants available to combat toxins, specifically the antioxidant vitamin C, leads to inflammation, the inner linings of blood vessels not functioning properly, oxidation of low-density lipoproteins, and the activation of platelets. This cascade of ill effects ultimately leads to blood clots, which can cause death if they lodge in the heart or lungs.

In summary, cigarette smoking causes damage to the interior linings of arteries, increases heart rate, increases blood pressure, reduces oxygen and nutrients to the heart, and reduces blood flow to the heart. These conditions may cause stroke, aortic aneurysm, peripheral arterial disease, coronary heart disease (CHD), or sudden death due to a heart attack.

Pulmonary Disease

In a typically functioning **lung**, when a person inhales, **oxygen** travels down the trachea to tubes that eventually branch off into smaller tubes called bronchioles. At the end of these bronchioles, gas exchange occurs as oxygen is absorbed and carbon dioxide is released in

lung

one of the usually paired compound saccular thoracic organs that constitute the basic respiratory organ of air-breathing vertebrates; the lungs remove carbon dioxide from and bring oxygen to the blood and consist essentially of an inverted tree of intricately branched bronchioles communicating with thin-walled terminal alveoli swathed in a network of delicate capillaries where the actual gaseous exchange of respiration takes place

oxygen

the odorless gas that is present in the air and necessary to maintain life; patients with lung disease or damage may need to use portable oxygen devices on a temporary or permanent basis

the tiny air sacs called alveoli. The bronchioles and alveoli are elastic and increase and decrease in size with every inhalation and exhalation.

Each day, adults inhale approximately ten thousand liters of air. This necessitates a system for removing inhaled particles (such as pollen and road dust) and repairing damage to the lungs due to the particles. Some of the respiratory system's mechanisms for removing potentially damaging particles include creating mucous, coughing, sneezing, blocking with nasal hair, and using alveolar macrophages to destroy carcinogens.

When a smoker inhales a cigarette, the smoke travels the same path as oxygen does from the mouth, through the trachea, to the upper lungs, and ultimately to the alveoli, where gas exchange occurs. Along this path, the carcinogens present in cigarette smoke damage the respiratory system. Although there are mechanisms to repair the damage, the large volume and large size of the toxic particles present in cigarette smoke cause repairs to fall behind, ultimately leading to pulmonary disease.

Acrolein, formaldehyde, nitrogen oxides, cadmium, and hydrogen cyanide found in cigarette smoke damage the lungs. Together, these carcinogens damage the cilia in the lungs, impair lung defenses, irritate the membranes, and create oxidative stress. Research indicates that with chronic cigarette smoking, nearly 60% of the inhaled particles from cigarette smoke are not removed and remain in the lower lung. Additionally, up to 20 mg of tar per day is deposited in the lungs per cigarette smoked. The presence of these particles and tar creates inflammation, which in turn creates oxidative stress from an immune response to the carcinogens. This inflammation and response are the hallmarks of pulmonary disease. The diseases specifically caused by the carcinogens in smoke are COPD and asthma.

> COPD is a progressive condition that includes the diseases of chronic bronchitis and emphysema. With COPD, airflow is diminished due to either alveoli losing their elasticity, the walls between alveoli being destroyed, airway walls becoming thick and inflamed, or excess mucous being created and clogging airways.

Chronic bronchitis is defined as a specific set of symptoms—that of a productive cough for three months in each of two successive years where other causes of productive chronic cough have been excluded. Emphysema is a condition defined by a certain pattern of lung damage in which the lung's elasticity is damaged and airspaces are permanently enlarged. This does not allow the lungs to properly inflate and deflate with air, making victims feel as if they are always out of breath.

Asthma is a chronic inflammatory disease of the airways that is characterized by airflow obstruction; symptoms include wheezing, breathlessness, chest tightness, and coughing in response to a stimulus, in this case, cigarette smoke. Immediate treatment is necessary to remove the symptoms and increase airflow.

Reproductive and Developmental Effects

The female and male reproductive systems rely on healthy blood flow, appropriate hormone levels, and undamaged DNA to create new human life and for women to carry the fetus to full-term delivery. The toxic compounds found in smoke, specifically carbon monoxide, nicotine, cadmium, lead, mercury, and polycyclic aromatic hydrocarbons, are associated with adverse reproductive outcomes, such as infertility, miscarriage, and congenital abnormalities.

Among women, research indicates that 13% of infertility may be attributed to smoking. Follicle-stimulating hormones (necessary for ovulation), as well as estrogen and progesterone (necessary for normal menstruation), are adversely affected by the toxins in cigarette smoke and nicotine. Additionally, carcinogens can diminish oviduct functioning, making fertilization difficult when the egg is not able to travel to the uterus to be fertilized by sperm. Among men, evidence links smoking to chromosome changes and DNA damage in sperm, which affects pregnancy viability and may cause anomalies in offspring.

Smoking prior to conception and throughout pregnancy can have damaging effects on the fetus, including congenital abnormalities and miscarriage. Damage to the fetus is primarily due to the presence of carbon monoxide, which binds to hemoglobin and decreases oxygen flow to the fetus. Additionally, placental abnormalities are also possible, leading to fetal loss, preterm delivery, or low birth weight.

Smokeless Tobacco and Chronic Disease

Smokeless tobacco is a tobacco product that is not smoked but rather placed directly in the mouth, cheek, or lip to be sucked or chewed; the saliva is either swallowed or spit out and is commonly referred to in the United States as *dip, snuff, snus, or chew.*

In addition to traditional loose tobacco that has been on the market for many years, "snus," is also readily available. Snus is particularly popular among adolescents because it does not require the user to spit and can therefore be concealed from parents and teachers. Similar to chewing tobacco, this form of moist tobacco is placed between the upper gum and lip—the difference is that it is sold in a small packet rather than loose tobacco (Boon, 2012).

Another new smokeless tobacco product, dissolvable tobacco, hit the test market in 2011 (Figure 4.3). This is sold as pellets, flat strips, or sticks, and is designed to look like nontobacco products. For example, the pellet shape resembles Tic Tacs, the flat sheets look similar to breath strips, and the sticks look like toothpicks. The user ingests this tobacco orally; spitting is not required for the use of the product.

Other, less popular smokeless tobacco products available in the United States include loose-leaf chewing tobacco, which is sold in small strips of leaves and flavored with sugar or licorice, plug chewing tobacco, which is sold in oblong blocks and sweetened, and nasal snuff, which is sold as a fine tobacco powder that is sniffed through the nostrils by the user.

In addition to these more traditional smokeless tobacco products, e-cigarettes are now the most popular smokeless tobacco product. **E-cigarettes** were introduced in 2008 and are also referred to as vapes, vape pens, mods, and tanks. "JUULing" is a common verb used for the use of an e-cigarette and is named after the most popular brand (Truth Initiative, 2021). They are devices that vaporize a mixture of water, propylene glycol, nicotine, and flavorings into an aerosol. They are battery-powered and cost anywhere from $70 to $90 for a starter pack that includes the device, chargers, and nicotine cartridges. Each cartridge costs

smokeless tobacco
a tobacco product that is not smoked but rather placed directly in the mouth, cheek, or lip to be sucked or chewed; the saliva is either swallowed or spit out and is commonly referred to in the United States as *dip, snuff, snus, or chew*

e-cigarettes
devices that vaporize a mixture of water, propylene glycol, nicotine, and flavorings; battery powered and cost anywhere from $70 to $90 for a starter pack that includes the device, chargers, and nicotine cartridges. Can also be called e-cigs, vapes, vape pens, mods, and tanks.

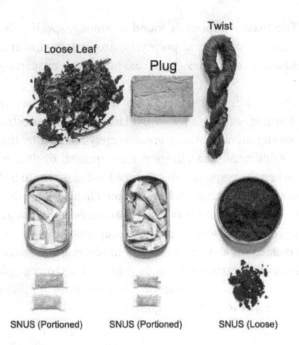

Figure 4.3   Smokeless Tobacco Products
Source: US Food and Drug Administration (2022)

approximately $2 and equals a pack of cigarettes in terms of "puffs." The cartridge can look like a cigarette, cigar, pipe, pen, or a USB flash drive, and users inhale on it just as they would a cigarette through a mouthpiece. Studies have shown that the amount of nicotine provided per e-cigarette is highly variable, with some exceeding levels of cigarettes. In 2018, three-quarters of e-cigarettes contained at least 4% nicotine, with JUUL containing 5% (59 mg/ml) and competitors at 7%. There are currently no restrictions on the concentration of nicotine (Truth Initiative, 2021).

The Food and Drug Administration (FDA) has not successfully regulated e-cigarettes as of this writing. In May 2016, the FDA asserted that e-cigarettes meet the definition of a tobacco product and therefore can be regulated under the Tobacco Control Act (US FDA, 2016). The FDA pushed back compliance submissions to August of 2022; currently, only a handful of select products (e.g., Solo, VERVE, Vapeleaf, and NJOY Daily) have been granted market authorization. The most popular brand, JUUL, has been denied a marketing order but has since sued the FDA and currently has a court-ordered stay on the order (Public Health Law Center, 2022).

Health promotion professionals are particularly concerned about smokeless tobacco and e-cigarettes. Because users no longer need to spit out tobacco-filled saliva, smokeless tobacco use can easily be concealed, deterring cessation and prevention efforts among adolescents. Youth may be more inclined to experiment with this type of tobacco because the risk of being seen is reduced. Additionally, smokeless tobacco and e-cigarettes are often marketed toward adult smokers trying to quit as a safer, healthier alternative; however, they have fruit and candy flavors, making them very appealing to youth. Although adults may switch to these products instead of quitting, this further enables their nicotine addiction rather than curtailing use.

Harm Reduction

Nicotine is the primary ingredient in smokeless tobacco and is a highly addictive drug. However, nicotine itself is not the primary cause of diseases related to cigarette smoking. This has created a very heated scientific debate over whether or not smokeless tobacco is as harmful as previously reported (Grimsrud, Gallefoss, & Løchen, 2012). Discussions regarding whether or not health professionals should promote the use of smokeless tobacco to those who are unwilling or unable to quit smoking are starting to occur. This strategy of "harm reduction" has gained popularity in other countries, such as the United Kingdom (Rodu, 2011). However, the United States does not endorse this strategy. Although it is clear that compared to the health effects of cigarette use, the health risks of smokeless tobacco use are significantly less, they still exist (Scientific Committee on Emerging and Newly-Identified Health Risks, 2008). According to the US Surgeon General, there is presently inadequate evidence to conclude that e-cigarettes, in general, increase smoking cessation (US DHHS, 2020).

Therefore, it remains the recommendation to abstain from all tobacco use. Chronic diseases associated with smokeless tobacco use are described in the following sections.

nicotine
a colorless, poisonous alkaloid derived from the tobacco plant and used as an insecticide; the substance in tobacco to which smokers can become addicted

Cancer

There are 28 known carcinogens in smokeless tobacco, including N-nitrosamino acids, volatile N-nitrosamines, polycyclic aromatic hydrocarbons, volatile aldehydes, hydrazine, metals, and radioactive polonium. Tobacco-specific nitrosamines (TSNAs) are carcinogens considered to be the most important because of their abundance in smokeless tobacco. Although TSNAs are also found in products not related to smoking (such as food and beer), there are one hundred to one thousand times higher levels in smokeless tobacco products. Studies indicate that these TSNAs are the main cause of oral cancer in smokeless tobacco users. The specific aspects of the mechanism remain unclear; however, in general, the metabolic activation of TSNAs (specifically NNK and NNN) leads to the formation of DNA adducts, which leads to uncontrolled cell growth and cell death (Boffetta, Hecht, Gray, Gupta, & Straif 2008).

In 2007, a monograph published by the World Health Organization and the International Agency for Research on Cancer Working Group on the Evaluation of Carcinogenic Risks to Humans stated that smokeless tobacco use is carcinogenic to humans, causing oral and pancreatic cancer. More recently, additional meta-analyses completed in 2008, 2009, and 2011 have shown that there is no increased risk for pancreatic cancer (Bertuccio et al., 2011; Lee & Hamling, 2009; Sponsiello-Wang, Weitkunat, & Lee, 2008). The risk for oral cancer remains, as previously documented.

Cardiovascular Disease

The amount of nicotine that a smokeless tobacco user will take in is similar to that of a cigarette smoker, although the nicotine from smokeless tobacco is absorbed at a much slower rate than from a cigarette. Nicotine affects receptors in the brain that activate the release of epinephrine, a hormone that increases heart rate and blood pressure. Nicotine also constricts coronary arteries and other blood vessels. The additives found in smokeless tobacco (such as licorice and sodium) also increase the blood pressure of the user. Therefore, smoke-less tobacco use results in a chronic state of increased heart rate and blood pressure.

According to some studies, the long-term effects of smokeless tobacco can include greater risk of fatal heart attack and fatal stroke because users have a reduced chance of survival after such events. In 2010, the American Heart Association (AHA) released a policy statement, based on data from two large studies in the United States and Sweden, that smokeless tobacco use did not increase the incidence or prevalence of high blood pressure, the risk of nonfatal or fatal heart attack, or biochemical risk factors for CVD (Heidenreich et al., 2011). However, the statement indicated that the use of smokeless tobacco results in an elevated risk of death from stroke. The AHA does not endorse the use of smokeless tobacco, despite the results of the report, but firmly recommends abstaining from its use.

Pregnancy

Similar to smoking cigarettes, using smokeless tobacco poses serious risks to the developing fetus. Research indicates that the nicotine in smokeless tobacco increases the risk of still-birth, premature delivery, and possibly preeclampsia, which is a dangerous state of high blood pressure, among other symptoms. The only way to cure preeclampsia is to deliver the baby, even if it is very early in the pregnancy. Mothers who use smokeless tobacco have a higher risk of giving birth to a low-birth-weight baby, putting the baby at risk for many com-plications such as problems fighting infection, difficulty eating and gaining weight, breath-ing problems, bleeding in the brain, intestinal diseases, and SIDS.

Oral Complications

According to the CDC, smokeless tobacco is linked to cancer of the mouth and gums, gum disease (periodontal disease and gingivitis), and tooth loss. The constituents of smokeless tobacco cause the cells of the mouth to not grow properly, creating tumors. These tumors can either remain in the mouth, or the cancer cells can dislodge and travel to other parts of the body. They can attach to lymph nodes and other organs, causing metastatic cancer that is only treatable through chemotherapy, radiation, and surgery. Oral cancer is associated with a high death rate; the five-year survival rate is only 50% and much lower in minority populations.

Smokeless tobacco also causes gum disease, which is when the gums pull away from the teeth and form pockets that become infected with bacteria. The body recognizes this infec-tion and attempts to remove the infected area, but this results in destroying the bone and tissue that hold the teeth in place. This results in painful chewing and eventual tooth loss.

Secondhand Smoke Exposure and Chronic Disease

secondhand smoke

the mixture of the smoke produced by a lit cigarette and smoke exhaled by the smoker; more than fifty carcinogens are present in secondhand smoke

Secondhand smoke is the mixture of the smoke produced by a lit cigarette and smoke exhaled by the smoker. The smoke of a lit cigarette, termed sidestream smoke, tends to have higher concentrations of the carcinogens than cigarette smoke inhaled by the smoker. More than fifty carcinogens are present in secondhand smoke. Research indicates that second-hand smoke, also called involuntary smoking, can result in premature death and disease in children and adults, primarily through the same mechanisms by which smoking causes disease in smokers.

Exposure to secondhand smoke has decreased by about half since the late 1980s. Previously, 88% of those greater than four years old were exposed to tobacco smoke. Today, that number has decreased to 43% (US Department of Health and Human Services, 2006). Most of this exposure occurs in the home and the workplace, despite the trend toward banning smoking in public places. Lower-income children are more likely to be exposed to smoke in their homes compared to other populations. In 2019, about 25% of middle and high school students reported breathing secondhand smoke in their homes and 23% reported it in their vehicles, with a larger percentage of non-Hispanic black and non-Hispanic white being exposed than Hispanic students (Walton et al., 2020). As stated previously, it is estimated that secondhand smoke exposure causes approximately three thousand deaths from lung cancer and forty-six thousand deaths from heart disease.

The 2006 surgeon general's report, *The Health Consequences of Involuntary Exposure to Tobacco Smoke* (US Department of Health and Human Services, 2006), concluded that secondhand smoke causes the following:

1. *Immediate adverse effects on the cardiovascular system and coronary heart disease.* Secondhand smoke causes platelet and endothelial dysfunction, which leads to 25–35% increase in CHD. There is an increased risk of stroke; however, there is no causal relationship established to date. One thousand seventeen hundred excess deaths of nonsmokers from CHD can be attributed to secondhand smoke due to exposure in the workplace.

2. *Lung cancer.* Similar to the causal effect of smoking on lung cancer, secondhand smoke exposure causes genetic changes that lead to lung cancer (see figure 4.2). Studies show a 20–30% increase in the risk of lung cancer for those living with someone who smokes regularly. More than fifty studies have addressed the association between exposure and lung cancer among a diversity of populations (more than 20 countries are represented); all but eight studies indicate causal effects.

3. *Increased risk for SIDS, acute respiratory infections, ear problems, and more severe asthma in children.* Although the biological basis for all SIDS cases is still unclear, research is sufficient to associate SIDS with exposure to secondhand smoke. The smoke that the infant breathes in affects the brain's ability to regulate breathing and to properly respond to hypoxia. Nerve cell development and function are also affected by the presence of the carcinogens in the smoke. Approximately 10% of all SIDS cases can be attributed to exposure. It is also estimated that annually, because of secondhand smoke exposure, between 24,300 and 71,900 low birth weight–preterm babies are born, 202,300 asthma cases are diagnosed, and 789,700 ear infections are reported.

4. *Slowed lung growth and respiratory symptoms in children who live with parents who smoke.* Adverse effects on the lungs begin with exposure of the fetus to secondhand smoke from the mother and other smokers in the house. The components in secondhand smoke reduce airway size and change lung properties (e.g., reduces elasticity) by affecting the hormones that speed lung maturation but inhibit their growth. As the child grows into late adolescence, coughing and wheezing occur in response to the nerves that control reflex response in the lungs being stimulated and irritated.

Political and Cultural History of Tobacco Use

Significant changes have occurred in US culture and government policy with regards to smoking, which may have seemed unimaginable fifty years ago. During the second half of the twentieth century, US culture went from accepting smoking to avoiding it. This change in attitude, which was heavily influenced at the beginning by the 1964 surgeon general's report that showed smoking caused lung cancer in men, was then continuously influenced by the large volumes of research disseminated in the following years on the wide spectrum of ill effects of smoking, and resulted in policy changes at the state and federal levels to reduce the incidence of secondhand smoke and protect citizens from big tobacco advertising schemes. These policy changes started in the 1990s, when California passed the first Clean Indoor Air Act and the Master Settlement Agreement (MSA) was signed. Subsequently, state and federal policies, such as the Family Smoking Prevention and Tobacco Control Act of 2009, began to further change the culture of smoking.

Historically, records indicate that as early as 1914 local governments may have acted to limit or control tobacco use. That year, Houston, Missouri, prohibited the sale of tobacco to minors, and in 1936, Milwaukee, Wisconsin, prohibited smoking on buses.

Most of the changes we are familiar with today started to take place around 1970 and reached their height in 1998 with the MSA.

Warning Labels

In 1966, the United States began to require warning labels on cigarettes. The message was simple and cautionary: "Cigarette Smoking May be Hazardous to Your Health." From 1970 to 1985, with evidence supporting its statement, the message became a warning: "The Surgeon General Has Determined that Cigarette Smoking is Dangerous to Your Health." The warning labels that we are familiar with today were required beginning in 1985. One of the following four labels is required to be on a cigarette pack:

- Smoking Causes Lung Cancer, Heart Disease, Emphysema, And May Complicate Pregnancy

- Quitting Smoking Now Greatly Reduces Serious Risks to Your Health

- Smoking By Pregnant Women May Result in Fetal Injury, Premature Birth, And Low Birth Weight

- Cigarette Smoke Contains Carbon Monoxide

In March 2020, the US FDA changed the warnings for cigarette packages and advertisements—the first change since 1985. The 11 warnings are both textual and photo-based and are required to appear prominently on cigarette packages and in advertisements, occupying the top 50% of the area of the front and rear panels of cigarette packages and at least 20% of the area at the top of cigarette advertisements. The new warnings must be randomly and equally displayed and distributed on cigarette packages and rotated quarterly in cigarette advertisements. The effective date of these warning labels is November 6, 2023 (US FDA, 2021a). The 11 warning labels are:

- Tobacco smoke can harm your children.
- Tobacco smoke causes fatal lung disease in nonsmokers.
- Smoking causes head and neck cancer.
- Smoking causes bladder cancer, which can lead to bloody urine.
- Smoking during pregnancy stunts fetal growth.
- Smoking can cause heart disease and strokes by clogging arteries.
- Smoking causes COPD, a lung disease that can be fatal.
- Smoking reduces blood flow, which can cause erectile dysfunction.
- Smoking reduces blood flow to the limbs, which can require amputation.
- Smoking causes type 2 diabetes, which raises blood sugar.
- Smoking causes cataracts, which can lead to blindness.

Starting in 2010, as part of the **2009 Tobacco Control Act**, smokeless tobacco products were required to show a warning label. One of the following four labels is required to be on the two principal sides of the package and cover at least 30% of each side:

- This product can cause mouth cancer.
- This product can cause gum disease and tooth loss.
- This product is not a safe alternative to cigarettes.
- Smokeless tobacco is addictive.

2009 Tobacco Control Act includes more than 20 provisions, rules, and regulations; targeting adolescents, there are specific provisions that restrict the sale of cigarettes and smokeless tobacco and restrict tobacco product advertising and marketing

Purchasing Restrictions

Age restrictions on who can purchase cigarettes have existed in the United States since 1992. In December 2019, Congress passed a federal law called "Tobacco 21" raising the tobacco age from 18 to 21 nationwide with no exemptions to any retail establishments or persons (US FDA, 2021b). This restriction includes cigarettes, cigars, and e-cigarettes (US FDA, 2021a). However, there is no state or federal law that prohibits the *use* of tobacco, just the purchase of tobacco products. In other words, there is no penalty for smoking tobacco if you are younger than twenty-one years of age.

Taxation

Tobacco has a long history of taxation in the United States. In 1862, the federal government instituted the first tobacco tax. By 1969, all states and the District of Columbia had instituted additional state tobacco taxes. The largest federal tobacco tax increase occurred in 2009, when the tax was increased by 62 cents to $1.01 per pack. This particular increase in tax may have resulted in the 8.3% decrease in cigarette sales in 2009. There has not been another federal tax increase since then, although a 100% increase to

$2.02 was proposed (but removed) in the 2021 congressional session in a budget reconciliation bill.

Increasing tobacco taxes is an important step in decreasing the number of tobacco users in the United States. Research indicates that for every 10% increase in price, youth smoking decreases by 7%, and overall smoking decreases by approximately 4%. Epidemiologic estimates predict that increasing the cost of cigarettes could lead to the prevention of two million adolescents from starting to smoke, help one million adults quit, prevent 900,000 smoking-caused deaths, and save $44.5 billion in long-term health care costs.

Each state has the ability to set its own tax rate in regard to cigarette sales. As of March 2021, the average state cigarette tax is $1.91 per pack. There is a significant gap between levels of taxation in tobacco states (states that grow tobacco) and nontobacco states. Tobacco states impose average taxes of 48.5 cents, whereas nontobacco states impose taxes averaging $1.61. The District of Columbia has the highest tax rate of $4.50 per pack; Georgia has the lowest at 0.37 cents. It is estimated that for each pack sold, $17.26 is spent on health care related to smoking. Therefore, even the highest tax rate does not cover the direct costs of smoking.

1998 Master Settlement Agreement

Master Settlement Agreement (MSA) a joint lawsuit that was settled by forty-six states in November 1998; during the mid-1990s, the attorneys general of forty-six states sued Philip Morris, Inc., R. J. Reynolds, Brown & Williamson, and Lorillard, commonly referred to as the four "big tobacco" companies, for damages and health care costs to states that resulted from tobacco use by state residents; the settlement payout is $246 billion over twenty-five years; each state is awarded a yearly payment

The **MSA** is a joint lawsuit that was settled by forty-six states in November 1998 (National Association of Attorneys General, 1998). During the mid-1990s, the attorney generals of forty-six states sued Philip Morris, Inc., R. J. Reynolds, Brown & Williamson, and Lorillard, commonly referred to as the four "big tobacco" companies, for damages and health care costs to states that resulted from tobacco use by state residents. The settlement payout is $246 billion over twenty-five years; each state is awarded a yearly payment. There are more specific provisions of the agreement, with a number that specifically affect public health by moving "big tobacco" away from an industry that freely advertised to youth using cartoons and promotions to one that is restricted in its advertising markets and no longer permitted to obscure or dilute the health risks of tobacco use. Practically speaking, as a student reading this text, you may not have experienced the days when "Joe Camel" was more recognized by children than Mickey Mouse, when smokers redeemed their "Marlboro Miles" for free products with Marlboro logos (lighters, hats, shirts, and various household items), or when sporting events sponsored by big tobacco were household names (e.g., "Winston Cup" NASCAR premier race). The MSA is responsible for establishing this new antitobacco culture and may have played a key role in the 21% decrease in cigarette sales since the settlement was announced. Table 4.1 lists the specific provisions of the MSA.

Recent Efforts to Reduce Tobacco Use

In general, US public opinion regarding smoking has changed. According to the 2018 Gallup poll on smoking bans, a majority of Americans (59%) are still in favor of a smoking ban and clean indoor air for all (McCarthy, 2018). This has not changed from the 2011 poll, when a similar 59% were in favor of a smoking ban.

Table 4.1 Provisions of the Master Settlement Agreement

• Prohibition of youth targeting	• Limitations on lobbying
• Limitation of tobacco brand name sponsorship	• Restrictions on advocacy concerning settlement proceeds
• Elimination of outdoor advertising and transit advertising	• Dissolution of the Tobacco Institute, Inc., the Council for Tobacco Research—USA, Inc., and the Center for Indoor Air Research, Inc.
• Prohibition of tobacco payments related to tobacco products and media	• Regulation and oversight of new tobacco-related trade associations
• Ban on tobacco brand-name merchandise	• Prohibitions on agreements to suppress research
• Ban on youth access to free samples	• Prohibition on material misrepresentations
• Ban on gifts to underage persons based on proof of purchase	• Granting public access to documents
• Limitation of third-party use of brand names	• Establishing tobacco control and underage use laws
• Ban on tobacco brand names	• Establishment of a national foundation (Legacy—responsible for the Truth campaign)
• Minimum pack size of 20 cigarettes	
• Corporate culture commitments related to youth access and consumption	

As public opinion has shifted since the new millennium, major federal, state, and local initiatives have further discouraged smoking in the United States. These initiatives include the expansion of the authority of the FDA to regulate the sales, advertising, and ingredient content of all tobacco products, an increase in the federal tobacco excise tax to $1.01 per pack, and the passage of comprehensive statewide smoke-free laws in 28 states, as well as Washington D.C., the Navajo Nation, Puerto Rico, and the U.S. Virgin Islands. In addition, workplace and school policies and community programs have been effective in discouraging smoking among adults and adolescents.

National Policy

Federal antitobacco policies and laws have been enacted since the 1990s to discourage smoking, protect citizens from big tobacco advertising schemes, protect citizens from secondhand smoke, and prevent adolescent tobacco use. It is a federal law that all domestic and international flights departing from the United States be smoke-free. Also, federal law inhibits smoking in agencies that receive federal funding to serve youth (e.g., schools). In 1998, an executive order was passed stating that all buildings owned, rented, or leased by the federal government must be smoke-free. Effective as of 2018, the US Department of Housing and Development passed a rule that all public housing be smoke-free, impacting more than 940,000 housing units. A historic federal law that was passed is the Family Smoking Prevention and Tobacco Control Act of 2009. The most recent federal law passed is "Tobacco 21," making it illegal for retailers to sell tobacco products to anyone under the age of 21.

Family Smoking Prevention and Tobacco Control Act of 2009

In June 2009, President Barack Obama signed into law the Family Smoking Prevention and Tobacco Control Act (Tobacco Control Act). The main goal of this law is to prevent and reduce tobacco use by adolescents under the age of 18. It is well established that most first-time use of tobacco occurs at a young age; only 1% of the smoking population reports first cigarette use after the age of 26, with 88% initiating before the age of 18. The law gives the FDA the authority to regulate the marketing, sales, and development of all tobacco products, new and old. It is appropriate to grant the FDA this regulatory authority because the agency's purpose is to protect the public's health by ensuring the safety and security of consumable products—including but not limited to the food supply, human drugs and medical devices, cosmetics, and dietary supplements. In order to oversee full implementation of the Tobacco Control Act, the FDA established the Center for Tobacco Products and the Tobacco Products Scientific Advisory Committee.

The Tobacco Control Act includes more than 20 provisions, rules, and regulations. Targeting adolescents, it has specific provisions that restrict the sale of cigarettes and smokeless tobacco, and restricts tobacco product advertising and marketing. For example, proof of age (over 18) is required to purchase cigarettes and smokeless tobacco, and face-to-face sales (no vending machines) are required unless in certain adult-only facilities. Also, tobacco companies are not permitted to sponsor sporting or entertainment events or distribute free samples of cigarettes and brand-name promotional items (e.g., Marlboro gym bags). The Tobacco Control Act prohibits the use of reduced harm claims such as "light," "low," or "mild" unless approved by the FDA, requires the tobacco industry to submit marketing documents for FDA approval, and requires certain standards for tobacco products. Marketing orders (permission from FDA to market the new product) are now also required for new products and those that are claiming the product "reduces harm" compared to cigarette smoking (e.g., e-cigarettes and smokeless tobacco) (US Food and Drug Administration, 2012).

Also under the Tobacco Control Act, the tobacco industry is required to disclose research findings regarding the health effects of tobacco use and information about the ingredients and constituents in tobacco products. There are more than seven thousand chemicals in tobacco and tobacco smoke, termed harmful and potentially harmful constituents (HPHCs). HPHCs are chemicals or chemical compounds that cause or may cause health problems. The FDA created a list of 20 HPHCs that are easy to test for their presence in tobacco products and are representative of the full list of seven thousand HPHCs. The list of the amount of HPHCs in specific products is available on the FDA website (www.fda.gov/TobaccoProducts/GuidanceComplianceRegulatoryInformation/ucm297786.htm). However, the ingredient list will not be labeled on the box. Consumers will need to access the list via the Internet or through printed documents. For the list of HPHCs required to be disclosed in cigarettes and smokeless tobacco, see table 4.2.

RECENT EFFORTS TO REDUCE TOBACCO USE

Table 4.2 List of Harmful and Potentially Harmful Constituents (HPHCs) in Cigarette Smoke and Smokeless Tobacco

Cigarette Smoke	Smokeless Tobacco
Acetaldehyde	Acetaldehyde
Acrolein	Arsenic
Acrylonitrile	Benzo[a]pyrene
4-Aminobiphenyl	Cadmium
1-Aminonaphthalene	Crotonaldehyde
2-Aminonaphthalene	Formaldehyde
Ammonia	Nicotine (total and free)
Benzene	4-(methylnitrosamino)-1-(3-pyridyl)-1-butanone
Benzo[*a*]pyrene	*N*-nitrosonornicotine
1,3-Butadiene	
Carbon monoxide	
Crotonaldehyde	
Formaldehyde	
Isoprene	
Nicotine (total)	
4-(methylnitrosamino)-1-(3-pyridyl)-1-butanone	
N-nitrosonornicotine	
Toluene	

The Tobacco Control Act also requires more prominent warning labels for cigarettes and smokeless tobacco products. As discussed previously, the labeling requirements will be in full effect in November 2023 (see figure 4.4).

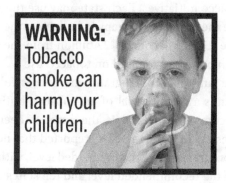

Figure 4.4 Example of one of the 11 required images.

Source: US Food and Drug Administration FDA/Public Domain

State Policy

State antitobacco policies and programs focus primarily on restricting smoking in public places and preventing adolescent smoking initiation.

Smoking Bans

Many states have implemented the Clean Indoor Air Act by banning smoking in certain locations and under certain circumstances, with varying provisions. The Clean Indoor Air Act typically prohibits smoking in enclosed public places, including bars and restaurants. They do not typically prohibit smoking in private workplaces; however, many workplaces are voluntarily going smoke-free. Some states allow exemptions for certain facilities, such as tobacconists, cigar bars, casinos, and private clubs. Violations are typically enforced by the health department and are considered civil infractions. Multiple violations may result in multiple fines or business license suspensions.

According to the American Nonsmokers' Rights Foundation (2022), as of April 2022, 62.3% of the US population is protected by a 100% smoke-free workplace, restaurant, and bar law. Twenty-seven states and two U.S. territories have these comprehensive laws. The states with no 100% smoke-free state law are Virginia, West Virginia, Montana, Kentucky, Tennessee, Alabama, Georgia, Oklahoma, Texas, Wyoming, Mississippi, South Carolina, and Alaska.

Smoke-free bans in casinos continue to be a hot topic and progress has been made post-COVID-19 pandemic. As of July 2022, approximately 1,000 casinos and gaming properties have 100% smoke-free indoor air policies, and this includes 157 Indian gaming facilities that found no decrease in revenue when they were smoke-free during the pandemic. However, at least 90% of casino workers are still exposed to secondhand smoke as several states exempt casinos from their statewide smoking ban - Indiana, Louisiana, Mississippi, Missouri, Nevada, New Jersey, and Pennsylvania (American Nonsmokers Rights Foundation, 2022a).

Master Settlement Agreement State Initiatives

The MSA is now approaching its twenty-fifth year of being implemented, with research showing that the states continue to underfund tobacco prevention and cessation programs. One of the downsides of the agreement is that states are not required to use the annual settlement money for antitobacco initiatives. Each state may use the money at its own discretion; states consistently use the money to fill gaps in budgets rather than to address tobacco use. In Fiscal Year 2022, the states will collect $27 billion from the settlement and taxes but will only spend 2.7% of it on programs focused on tobacco use.

Research suggests that antitobacco programs are successful at increasing cessation rates. The CDC recommends a certain level of antitobacco initiative spending based on state populations. The recommended level is the amount deemed necessary to affect changes in tobacco use rates. As of 2022, the CDC reported that not a single state currently funds tobacco prevention programs at the recommended level, with only Oregon and Alaska spending three-quarters of the recommended level and ten states at half the recommended amount. Connecticut spent zero of its settlement money on tobacco initiatives in 2022. The top three states in actual spending (California, Florida, and NY) currently spend a total of

$365 million, which is more than the other 47 states combined (Campaign for Tobacco-Free Kids, 2022).

Local Policy

Most successful statewide smoking bans started with grassroots efforts of local municipalities implementing smoke-free legislation. In order to be considered 100% smoke-free, municipalities must ban smoking in all workplaces (including offices, factories, and warehouses) and all restaurants and bars (no separate smoking section or ventilated room is allowed). According to the American Nonsmokers' Rights Foundation, as of October 2022, there will be 1,158 local municipalities that are 100% smoke-free, which equals 62.5% of the US population protected from secondhand smoke. Common restrictions include bans on smoking in outdoor areas, near (15 to 20 feet) entrances and windows of enclosed places, and public outdoor places such as beaches and parks, outdoor stadiums, and other sports and entertainment venues. Although not required or typically covered under a municipal policy, approximately 2,605 universities and colleges have implemented a voluntary smoke-free campus policy. Municipalities are now also starting to act on banning the use of e-cigarettes, with 1,006 restricting use in 100% smoke-free venues. Colleges and universities are also banning e-cigarettes, with 2,254 prohibiting use. While progress is being made, the US still has 37.5% of the population exposed to secondhand smoke on the job (American Nonsmokers' Rights Foundation, 2022b).

Effective Programs That Discourage Tobacco Use

In order to further decrease the percentage of people smoking, effective tobacco control programs need to be implemented by employers, in communities, in schools, and for individuals. As stated previously, the proportion of adult smokers has decreased from 42.4% in 1965 to 12.6% of the population in 2021. However, despite this victory, the United States is still short of its Healthy People 2030 goal of 6.1%.

Healthy People 2030

Healthy People is a federal interagency work group that sets ten-year agendas for improving the health of Americans. These agendas are used by health promotion professionals to guide decisions regarding what types of programs should be provided and to whom. The Healthy People 2030 tobacco-related goal is to reduce illness, disability, and death related to tobacco use and secondhand smoke exposure. There are 27 specific objectives to meet to attain this goal, which fall under six categories: (1) General Tobacco Use, (2) Adolescents, (3) Cancer, (4) Health Care, (5) Health Policy, and (6) Pregnancy and Childbirth. For a full list of these objectives, see table 4.3. Chapter 9 explores other state and federal government activities.

According to the most recent Surgeon General's report on smoking cessation (2020), 55.4% of smokers have made a past-year quit attempt, demonstrating interest in quitting. More than three out of five adults have successfully quit smoking. Strategies for quitting vary, with counseling and medication use increasing; however, more than two-thirds of smokers who tried to quit did not use an evidence-based treatment approach but instead

Table 4.3   Healthy People 2030 Objectives Related to Tobacco Use

Category	Objective
Tobacco use - general	Reduce current tobacco use by adults
	Reduce current cigarette, cigar, and pipe smoking in adults
	Increase past-year attempts to quit smoking in adults
	Increase successful quit attempts in adults who smoke
	Increase the proportion of worksites with policies that ban indoor smoking
	Reduce current cigarette smoking in adults
	Increase Medicaid coverage of evidence-based treatment to help people quit using tobacco
	Increase the proportion of smoke-free homes
	Increase the number of states, territories, and DC that prohibit smoking in worksites, restaurants, and bars
Adolescents	Reduce current cigarette smoking in adolescents
	Reduce current use of smokeless tobacco products among adolescents
	Reduce current cigar smoking in adolescents
	Eliminate cigarette smoking initiation in adolescents and young adults
	Reduce current e-cigarette use in adolescents
	Reduce the proportion of adolescents exposed to tobacco marketing
	Reduce current tobacco use in adolescents
	Reduce current use of flavored tobacco products in adolescents who use tobacco
	Reduce the proportion of people who do not smoke but are exposed to secondhand smoke
Cancer	Reduce the lung cancer death rate
Health Care	Increase the proportion of adults who get advice to quit smoking from a health care provider
	Increased use of smoking cessation counseling and medication in adults who smoke
Health Policy	Increase the number of states, territories, and DC that raise the minimum age for tobacco sales to 21 years
	Increase the national average tax on cigarettes
	Eliminate policies in states, territories, and DC that preempt local tobacco control policies
	Increase the number of states, territories, and DC that prohibit smoking in multiunit housing
Pregnancy and Childbirth	Increased abstinence from cigarette smoking among pregnant women
	Increase successful quit attempts in pregnant women who smoke

chose a different modality—such as switching to other tobacco products. Smokers who quit successfully are more likely to remain smoke-free if they use an evidence-based approach. There are a variety of effective programs available to help smokers quit (US Department of HHS, 2020).

Population-based Strategies

Population-based strategies have been shown to be effective in helping smokers quit. According to the Surgeon General's report on smoking cessation (2020), there is sufficient evidence to support the following population-based strategies as effective—quit lines, increasing the price of tobacco products, smoke-free policies, mass media campaigns, comprehensive state tobacco control programs, and large pictorial health warnings.

Effective Examples of Population-based Strategies

Multimedia interventions are most likely to be successful in reducing smoking rates if they are part of a complex set of interventions, for example, one component of a state tobacco control program. In a systematic review of multimedia interventions, over half of the studies reported an increase in abstinence from smoking (Secker-Walker, Gnichn, Platt, & Lancaster, 2002). The campaigns with longer duration, more intense advertising, and part of a larger comprehensive tobacco control plan were most likely to be successful. A few examples of effective campaigns are provided in the following sections.

Truth Initiative

One provision of the 1998 MSA was the establishment of a national foundation, the Legacy Foundation (now known as Truth Initiative), focused on antitobacco messaging and preventing adolescents from initiating tobacco use. Funded by the MSA, the Truth Initiative has implemented multimedia campaigns and programs to meet this goal. They ran the first national adult cessation campaign since 1967, called EX, targeted at adult smokers who were open to quitting but did not know how to successfully quit. From March 2008 to September 2008, advertisements ran on cable TV, with 68% of the ads running in the first three months of the campaign. The message was simple and relayed in an empathic voice from smoker to smoker: relearn life without cigarettes. The ads prompted viewers to go to their website for support (www.becomeanEX.org). Research showed that the campaign was effective in increasing quit attempts (Vallone, Duke, Cullen, McCausland, & Allen 2011). Although the campaign is no longer running, the website is active with virtual online support, customized quit plans, text message support for quitting vaping and smoking, and virtual support groups.

The truth® campaign is another successful Truth Initiative population-based intervention. It is the longest-running campaign and is aimed at empowering youth to decide not to smoke. It is an ongoing publicity campaign that connects with youth online and in-person, through videos, digital and social channels, branded merchandise, and presence at music and sporting events. They expose the truth about smoking, vaping, and nicotine, offering facts about the health effects of tobacco use as well as the marketing tactics of the tobacco industry (Truth Initiative, 2022)

An example of one of their successful advertising initiatives was "The Sunny Side of Truth," which in 2008 used sarcasm in a Broadway-style theme to promote the truth of the hazards of smoking. Research suggested that 22% of the overall decline in youth smoking was attributable to the truth® campaign, resulting in 300,000 fewer youth smokers after the campaign ran (Matthew et al., 2005). Additionally, exposure to the campaign resulted in more accurate perceptions of peer smoking, which has been shown to deter initiation (Davis, Nonnemaker, & Farrelly, 2007).

Currently, truth® is running the "Breath of Stress Air" campaign with videos, interactive educational webpages, quizzes, and a text-to-quit vaping program called "This is Quitting." To date, approximately 250,000 are quitting vaping with the program. Research is currently being conducted on the effectiveness of this new campaign.

Tips from Former Smokers

"Tips" was the first federally funded mass media campaign to reduce smoking rates. It is a $54 million campaign funded through the Prevention and Public Health Fund of the Patient Protection and Affordable Care Act (ACA). The CDC ran the campaign for twelve weeks starting in March 2012. It consisted of thirty-second radio and TV ads, print media, billboards, videos on YouTube, and Facebook and Twitter posts. The target audience was aged 18 to 44, and the short-term goal was to prompt people to quit and raise awareness of free government resources to help smokers quit. The ads ran in English and Spanish and featured real people telling stories of how it feels to have a tobacco-related disease and how they finally quit for good. The diseases featured include Buerger's disease (blocking of blood vessels, which leads to infection in the limbs and results in multiple amputations), heart disease and stroke, cancer, and asthma due to secondhand smoke. The campaign successfully raised awareness (reached 80% of smokers), as shown by tripled hits to the website and double the amount of calls to the quit line (Rigotti & Wakefield, 2012). Long-term results of the campaign indicate that there was a 12% increase in quit attempts during the campaign, with 1.6 million additional smokers making a quit attempt. It is estimated that 100,000 smokers remained smoke-free at the end of the campaign, and at least one hundred thousand of these will stay smoke-free long term. Based on these estimates, the CDC reports that this will add one-third to a half a million quality-adjusted life years to the US population (McAfee, Davis, Alexander, Pechacek, & Bunnell, 2013).

Every Try Counts

The FDA launched its first campaign for adult smokers in 2018 called "Every Try Counts." The goal was to reach smokers ages 25–54 who have attempted to quit in the last year but were not successful in 25 specific US counties with high adult smoking rates. The campaign encouraged them to continue to try to quit, even after failing previously, as quitting is a process and takes several tries to quit completely. Two years into the campaign, there was a national shift to reach a broader audience, resulting in 45 million adult smokers receiving messages. The campaign delivered tailored digital messaging around retail establishments where tobacco products were sold. Ads also were sent to smokers open to quitting – and shared resources. Although the campaign is no longer active, through a partnership with the National Institute of Health's National Cancer Institute, resources are still available through the webpage (everytrycounts.org) and include text message programs, a mobile quitting app, trained cessation counselors available online or by phone, and information about FDA-approved cessation medications (US FDA, 2022a). Research on the effectiveness of the campaign is currently underway through a multi-year outcome evaluation study on tobacco-related knowledge, attitudes and beliefs, and changes in motivation to quit smoking (US FDA, 2017).

Worksite Initiatives

An employer can expect to save nearly $6000 annually for each employee who successfully quits using tobacco. The savings are derived from decreased health care costs of $2,050 and increased productivity of $3,760 (Berman, Crane, Seiber, & Munur, 2014). Compared to nonsmoking employees, smokers are 33% more likely to miss work and be absent an average of 2.7 more days per year (Weng, Ali, & Leonardi-Bee, 2013).

The primary objectives of worksite smoking programs are to decrease the number of smokers and reduce employee exposure to secondhand smoke. A workplace smoking ban is the most effective strategy to achieve these objectives. Research indicates that bans can reduce exposure by an average of 72%. At minimum, it is recommended that a workplace smoking ban prohibit smoking in the building and within fifteen to 20 feet of all entrances, windows, and ventilation intakes. Companies can take it a step further and deem their property a smoke-free campus, which would require employees to leave company property to smoke (discouraging smoke breaks) (CDC, 2012b). Companies should also ensure that health insurance covers smoking cessation counseling and medications fully, without barriers to access, by offering them at the worksite and/or financial incentives to employees who quit and abstain for at least six months (Adams, 2020).

Some employers offer **smoking cessation programs** for employees. These programs include counseling and quit lines and are most effective when offered on-site for easy employee access. Companies that are large enough may hire a health educator or a tobacco cessation counselor to provide individual or group counseling. It is recommended that employees participate in more than four sessions lasting more than ten minutes with a counselor. Implementing a workplace smoking ban with referral services to smoking cessation programs is ideal. It is well established that a combination of intensive counseling, over-the-counter (OTC) nicotine replacement therapy (nicotine patch, gum, or lozenge), and prescription medications (bupropion SR, varenicline tartrate, nicotine spray, or inhaler) is the most effective individual treatment. Employee health benefits should provide full coverage of these treatments. A combination of all these strategies provides a comprehensive tobacco cessation program that is more effective than any single program alone (US Office of Personnel Management, 2013).

smoking cessation programs interventions, such as counseling and quit lines, are designed to help individuals quit smoking

Practical Examples of Worksite Initiatives
Quest Diagnostics

Quest Diagnostics provides diagnostic testing services to 151 million patients annually. They employ approximately forty-nine thousand employees and are located worldwide. Their in-house health promotion program, called HealthyQuest, is focused on improving the health of their employees as well as creating an overall culture of health. Their smoking cessation program is part of HealthyQuest and is provided by an outside vendor. In-house, however, Quest has more than 600 employees who volunteer to be leaders on the health promotion team. Most of the leaders are either former smokers or those trying to quit.

The duties of the leaders are to educate employees on the long-term health effects of smoking on themselves as well as the effects on those around them. They also champion corporate smoking events (such as the Great American Smokeout) and support tobacco-free corporate guidelines by implementing them in their business units. They encourage their fellow employees to join the smoking cessation program that is provided free of charge and serve as mentors and as resource persons.

After implementation of HealthyQuest, the quit rate was 35%, and the overall prevalence of smoking decreased by 2% (Partnership for Prevention, 2008). The company reported the following tips for large corporations interested in adding a smoking cessation program: (1) do not be judgmental, (2) be sure the health promotion teams are compassionate and committed, (3) encourage employee testimonials, because this will drive others to join, (4) create program specific to the corporate culture, not one that is cookie cutter, (5) and collect objective data to inform leadership on the effectiveness of the program as well as resource allocation needs.

Union Pacific Railroad

Union Pacific Railroad is the largest railroad serving 23 states west of the Mississippi, with fifty thousand employees. It has been in business for more than 150 years and has a large percentage of fifth-generation employees. Its health promotion program, HealthTrack, has a tobacco program wrapped into it titled Butt Out and Breathe. For the program, employees are asked to assess their stage of change (readiness to quit) and, based on their stage, are given a tailored intervention. The interventions range from covered pharmacologic treatment (including OTC nicotine replacement therapy), individual health coaching, and online services, to self-help guides. Employees are given progress reports every three, six, and twelve months as well as multi-year progress reports if applicable.

Union Pacific Railroad has successfully created a culture that is reflective of a tobacco-free environment. The key initiatives the company has undertaken are: (1) integrating non-smoking as a safety rule within its safety structure, because it found that smoking is a risk for getting injured on the job, (2) a hiring policy that does not hire job candidates who smoke (in the states where it is legal to ask the question), (3) advocating for the city of Omaha to be smoke-free, and (4) writing into managers' job agreements the provision that they will support the smoke-free initiatives of the company. The success of the program has been dramatic—in the early 1990s, its smoking rate was 40%; after the program, it was 17%.

School Initiatives

Various methods have been used in schools to prevent smoking initiation among adolescents. Information-giving curricula teach students about the prevalence, incidence, and risks of tobacco use. Social competence programs teach students cognitive behavioral skills and self-management personal and social skills to resist media and interpersonal influences to initiate smoking. Social influence programs teach students refusal skills; increase awareness of media, peer, and family influences and encourage public commitments not to smoke. All three of these methods may also be used in combination, enabling a more comprehensive approach. Some multimodal programs combine curricular programs with community-based initiatives and policy changes on the taxation, sale, and availability of tobacco.

In a review of ninety-four randomized controlled trials that used one or more of the previously mentioned interventions, results indicated that information given alone is less effective or no different from other models. Social competence interventions had some positive short-term results, as did so social influence programs, although neither did in the long term (Thomas & Perera, 2006). Programs that combine social competence and influence showed success in the short term; however, there is insufficient evidence to make a definitive determination if a combined model is more effective than social influence programs alone. Last, of four studies that tested the impact of social influence and competence programs in the context of larger community initiatives, three showed positive results. In sum, information-only programs have not been shown to be effective, social influence programs can be effective in the short term, and adding components such as community involvement may improve effectiveness.

The CDC's guideline on school health programs, developed by numerous agencies and based on existing research and practice, lists seven recommendations to prevent tobacco use among school-aged students. These comprise: (1) school policies that ban smoking and tobacco advertising on school grounds, (2) requiring instruction on avoiding tobacco use, (3) providing K–12 tobacco prevention education, (4) teacher training, (5) involving parents and families, (6) providing cessation programs for students and staff, and (7) regularly evaluating the program for effectiveness (CDC, 2008).

Practical Examples of School Initiatives

West Virginia Schools

In collaboration with state and community agencies and using the strategies discussed previously, West Virginia was successful in reducing its high school smoking rate from 28% to 22% in two years. Its efforts were widespread, starting with a state mandate that all students receive instruction on tobacco and potential health hazards from tobacco use in grades K–12. It also developed a Regional Tobacco Prevention Specialist Network, which resulted in tobacco prevention initiatives in all fifty-five school districts in the state. At the school level, the state developed a teen smoking cessation program titled Not-On-Tobacco (N-O-T) that is conducted in all West Virginia secondary schools. In collaboration with the American Lung Association of West Virginia, the state also created an antitobacco youth movement called Raze, which involves more than seven thousand students (CDC, 2011b).

Raze is comprised of youth aged 11–18 and through events, social media campaigns, and "commotions" (educational opportunities through crowd awareness), they tell the truth about Big Tobacco. They have recently taken on e-cigarettes and vaping, with commotions such as "No Vape November" where students pledge to not vape for 30 days, and "Clouded by Lies" where students create cloud-shaped speech bubbles with lies about vaping and share them on social media (Raze, 2022).

South Carolina Schools

In a collaborative effort among school boards and state agencies, South Carolina was successful in increasing the number of school districts adopting its model, comprehensive, tobacco-free school policy from 22% to 35% two years later. Its success was due to the implementation of the community roundtable model to promote and train school administrators on the comprehensive program and the employment of a school health policy coordinator. The program includes policies regarding use of tobacco on school property, procedures for enforcement, education for tobacco prevention, cessation programs, and information about tobacco industry advertising (CDC, 2011b).

Community Initiatives

community

"encompasses a diverse set of entities, including voluntary health agencies; civic, social, and recreational organizations; businesses and business associations; city and county governments; public health organizations; labor groups; health care systems and providers; health care professionals' societies; schools and universities; faith communities; and organizations for racial and ethnic minority groups" (CDC)

According to the CDC (2014, p. 22), a **community** "encompasses a diverse set of entities, including voluntary health agencies; civic, social, and recreational organizations; businesses and business associations; city and county governments; public health organizations; labor groups; health care systems and providers; health care professionals' societies; schools and universities; faith communities; and organizations for racial and ethnic minority groups." In a review of the current literature on effective community-based interventions, the CDC developed a best practices guideline for health promotion professionals at the state and community levels to implement effective treatment and cessation programs. In summary, community-based interventions should focus on changing social norms related to smoking by advocating and initiating policy changes at the state level (US Department of Health and Human Services, 2007). For example, communities may offer educational programs or quit line support that is advertised through mass media campaigns run by the state encouraging adults to quit smoking. The main goal is to have state and community agencies work together in order to increase the reach of smaller, individual-based clinical and educational interventions.

These recommendations are based on the evidence that community-based interventions alone do not affect prevalence of smoking. A systematic review of 37 studies showed that although programs were successful in increasing the knowledge of health risks, changing attitudes toward smoking, increasing quit attempts, and providing better environmental and social support for quitting, community-level smoking rates did not decrease. In the best-designed trial, the US COMMIT study, there was disappointingly no difference in prevalence. However, the authors point out that the studies that were included in the systematic review had measurement issues; therefore, health promotion professionals should make greater efforts to use sound methodologies to evaluate their programs. Also, they should consider the following:

- Use community members to staff coalitions and task forces and supervise implementation.
- Allow several years to realize the results of interventions and provide readily available resources throughout the community.
- Use mass media to change social norms.
- Provide referral services to health professionals specifically trained in tobacco cessation techniques.
- Provide nicotine replacement therapy and prescription medications at little or no cost.

Individual Programs

The individual-based treatments that have been shown to be effective in helping people quit smoking cigarettes are: brief clinical interventions from a doctor; individual, group, or telephone counseling; behavioral counseling; intensive one-on-one counseling; OTC and prescription medications; proactive quit line counseling, short text message services (particularly if they are interactive and tailored), and internet-based interventions (particularly if they are interactive and contain behavior change techniques) (AHRQ, 2008, US DHHS, 2020). OTC medications include nicotine replacement products such as the nicotine patch, gum, and lozenges. Prescription medications include nicotine inhalers, nasal spray, bupropion SR (Zyban), and varenicline tartrate (Chantix). Research indicates that successful, sustained quitting results from a combination of intensive counseling and some sort of medication, be it OTC or prescription (or a combination of both) (US HHSS, 2008; US DHHS, 2020).

For smokeless tobacco cessation, a systematic review of 25 randomized controlled trials revealed that the best intervention is behavioral intervention, followed by telephone counseling and oral examination with feedback on effects of smokeless tobacco use. Prescription drugs such as bupropion SR (Wellbutrin) and OTC nicotine replacement products are not shown to be effective (Ebbert, Montori, Erwin, & Stead, 2011). Varenicline (Chantix) is effective in increasing abstinence among snus users, according to a single study.

Challenges to Reducing Smoking

Significant health promotion challenges to reducing smoking are discussed in this section.

Access to Treatment

Getting access to treatment methods and support is the first step to quitting smoking. According to Healthy People 2030, 19 states have comprehensive Medicaid insurance coverage for evidence-based tobacco treatment. Given that 21.7% of those enrolled in Medicaid and other public health plans are smokers (significantly more than the general population), this creates a challenge for this demographic to obtain much needed tobacco cessation services (CDC, 2004; National Center for Health Statistics, 2022a). The Tobacco Use and Dependence Guideline Panel (2008) recommends a systems approach to identifying and treating patients who use the health care system. However, data show that only 20% of visits to office- and hospital-based ambulatory care settings offer tobacco cessation services or order treatments, and baseline data from Healthy People 2030 shows that in 2015, 57% of adults got advice to quit from their healthcare provider. The Healthy People 2030 revised objective is to increase the proportion to 66%.

In response to the overwhelming evidence that tobacco cessation treatment is effective and cost-saving, managed care plan coverage of comprehensive tobacco treatment has increased significantly to 90%. However, employers, who are purchasers of insurance coverage, are still not offering tobacco cessation programs to their employees. Research shows that only 20% of employers offer these services free of charge through their insurance coverage—even though employers rank the impact and value of tobacco cessation services as very high. Additionally, of these 20%, only 4% offer optimal services (Bondi, Harris, Atkins, French, & Umland, 2006), which should include brief advice from a physician, three hundred minutes of behavioral counseling from a multidisciplinary team over eight sessions, and at least one form of medication. This type of program costs about $1,500 per smoker, a cost that employers may not be willing to pay, even though the return on investment can be up to $5.45 per dollar spent (O'Donnell & Roizen, 2011).

When Medicaid expanded eligibility due to the ACA, 32 states were able to increase cessation coverage for adult enrollees. Although all of these states cover some cessation treatments, only 19 covers all seven FDA-approved cessation medications. All states also imposed one or more barriers to accessing at least one cessation treatment (CDC, 2016). There is opportunity for more Medicaid expansion in additional states. Research indicates that when smokers do not have to pay for treatment, there is an increase in the number of smokers attempting to quit, use of evidence-based treatments, and success in quitting (Reda, Kotz, Evers, & van Schayck, 2012).

Addictive Property of Nicotine

According to the *International Classification of Diseases*, tenth revision (ICD-10) (CDC, 1999), a person is considered to be dependent on a substance if he or she exhibits any of the following three criteria in a twelve-month period:

- Increased tolerance
- Physical withdrawal at times
- Strong desire to take drug
- Difficulty controlling use
- Persistent use despite harmful consequences
- Higher priority is given to drug use than to other activities and obligations

It is clear that tobacco users display these behaviors on a regular basis due to the presence of the drug nicotine in tobacco leaves. It has been reported that nicotine causes addiction much the same as heroin and cocaine, making cessation difficult. Nicotine affects the body by affecting the ventral tegmental area of the brain and dopamine neurotransmitters. Dopamine levels are increased by nicotine because it directly stimulates and excites several nicotinic acetylcholine receptors (nAChRs). These nAChRs are present in several systems, but the most extensively researched are the dopamine, glutamate (an excitatory neurotransmitter), and GABA (an inhibitory neurotransmitter) systems. When dopamine is increased through these systems, the tobacco user feels good and thus becomes addicted to the substance.

The addictive property of nicotine is a unique challenge. Unlike changing other health behaviors, such as increasing physical activity or using sunscreen, quitting smoking involves overcoming physical withdrawal symptoms. These symptoms can be painful and are easily cured by smoking a cigarette or chewing tobacco. Health promotion professionals should be mindful of this when assisting someone in the quitting process and should encourage the use of OTC and prescription nicotine replacement therapies to lessen the withdrawal symptoms.

Common withdrawal symptoms can include feeling depressed, irritable, anxious, restless, hungry; having trouble thinking clearly; difficulty concentrating; sleep issues; and a slower heart rate.

Tobacco Industry Practices

The tobacco industry is well aware of the addictive properties of their products and understands the difficulty of quitting. They understand that by getting adolescents addicted, they have a lifetime consumer. They also know that chronic use of their product will end with the death of the customer, so they need to consistently attract new, young lifetime users. In order to accomplish this task in the wake of the MSA, which limits direct marketing to adolescents, the tobacco industry has several practices in place. They regularly lobby against tobacco tax increases, the implementation of local and state Clean Indoor Air acts, graphic cigarette warning labels, and restrictions on selling to adolescents. The evidence is clear that these types of initiatives decrease the number of adult and adolescent smokers. They also develop new products that are specifically geared to attract adolescent users—such as e-cigarettes that are flavored with common candy and fruit flavors. In some areas, adolescents can use these products in places where cigarettes are not allowed, giving them full access to the addictive product. They also appeal to adolescents' fascination with new technology and electronics, reducing the focus of the product as a cigarette per se and more as an innovative electronic device.

Summary

This chapter reviewed the general statistics related to tobacco use in the United States; discussed the chronic diseases related to tobacco use and their biological basis; considered the social, political, and economic changes in the United States, along with how the culture, policies, and environment changed in relation to tobacco use. Further, it provided a discussion on the evidence-based and practice-based prevention and cessation programs for general and specific populations. Tobacco use has a profound influence on the health of Americans. Health promotion professionals need to be aware of the information provided herein in order to develop and implement effective programs to decrease the number of tobacco users in this country.

KEY TERMS

1. **Direct costs:** in managed care, the costs of labor, supplies, and equipment to provide direct patient care services

2. **Indirect costs:** resources forgone as a result of a health condition

3. **Cancer:** a term used for diseases in which abnormal cells divide without control and are able to invade other tissues

4. **Carcinogens:** a cancer-causing substance or agent

5. **Cardiovascular disease (CVD):** refers to conditions that involve narrowed or blocked blood vessels that can lead to a heart attack, chest pain (angina), or stroke

6. **Lung:** one of the usually paired compound saccular thoracic organs that constitute the basic respiratory organ of air-breathing vertebrates; the lungs remove carbon dioxide from and bring oxygen to the blood and consist essentially of an inverted tree of intricately branched bronchioles communicating with thin-walled terminal alveoli swathed in a network of delicate capillaries where the actual gaseous exchange of respiration takes place

7. **Oxygen:** the odorless gas that is present in the air and necessary to maintain life; patients with lung disease or damage may need to use portable oxygen devices on a temporary or permanent basis

8. **Smokeless tobacco:** a tobacco product that is not smoked but rather placed directly in the mouth, cheek, or lip to be sucked or chewed; the saliva is either swallowed or spit out and is commonly referred to in the United States as *dip, snuff, snus, or chew*

9. **E-cigarettes:** devices that vaporize a mixture of water, propylene glycol, nicotine, and flavorings; battery-powered and cost anywhere from $70 to $90 for a starter pack that includes the device, chargers, and nicotine cartridges

10. **Nicotine:** a colorless, poisonous alkaloid derived from the tobacco plant and used as an insecticide; the substance in tobacco to which smokers can become addicted

11. **Secondhand smoke:** the mixture of the smoke produced by a lit cigarette and smoke exhaled by the smoker; more than fifty carcinogens are present in secondhand smoke

12. **2009 Tobacco Control Act:** includes more than 20 provisions, rules, and regulations; targeting adolescents, there are specific provisions that restrict the sale of cigarettes and smokeless tobacco and restrict tobacco product advertising and marketing

13. **Master Settlement Agreement (MSA):** a joint lawsuit that was settled by forty-six states in November 1998; during the mid-1990s, the attorneys general of forty-six states sued Philip Morris, Inc., R. J. Reynolds, Brown & Williamson, and Lorillard, commonly referred to as the four "big tobacco" companies, for damages and health care costs to states that resulted from tobacco use by state residents; the settlement payout is $246 billion over twenty-five years; each state is awarded a yearly payment

14. **Smoking cessation programs:** interventions, such as counseling and quit lines, designed to help individuals quit smoking

15. **Community:** According to the CDC, "encompasses a diverse set of entities, including voluntary health agencies; civic, social, and recreational organizations; businesses and business associations; city and county governments; public health organizations; labor groups; health care systems and providers; health care professionals' societies; schools and universities; faith communities; and organizations for racial and ethnic minority groups"

REVIEW QUESTIONS

1. What are the health concerns with smoking tobacco and using smokeless tobacco?

2. What are the definitions of direct and indirect costs associated with smoking?

3. What are the three pathways by which smoking can cause cancer?

4. What is the prevalence of smoking now versus fifty years ago? What do you think had the most influence in changing the prevalence?

5. What is the prevalence of including e-cigarette use among the adolescent population?

6. What are the new tobacco products on the market today? What effect do you think these new products will have on adolescent use?

7. What does the term *secondhand smoke* mean, and what are the associated health risks?

8. What is the Master Settlement Agreement (MSA)? What are the provisions of the MSA? What effect do you feel the agreement had on the way smoking is viewed today?

9. Identify the warnings currently used on cigarette packs. Do you feel that the new graphic warnings will be more effective than the past text-only warnings? If they are more effective, in what way would they be—to deter new users or to stop current users?

10. What are current local, state, and federal policies on smoking?

11. Do you think the e-cigarette should be considered part of Clean Indoor Air acts? Why or why not?

12. What are the implications of tobacco industry's practices to develop new products that are specifically geared toward adolescents?

STUDENT ACTIVITIES

1. Create a social marketing campaign for the following groups:

    a. African American high school students in the precontemplation stage

    b. New parents in the contemplation stage

    c. Nursing or medical students in the preparation stage

2. Conduct a literature search on the cost of a pack of cigarettes in two states: one in a tobacco producing state, and one in a state that does not produce tobacco. If the cost is different, discuss who and what contributes to the pricing of a pack of cigarettes.

3. Debate whether a company should be allowed to hire or not hire smokers.

References

Adams, J. (2020). Good for health, good for business: The business case for reducing tobacco use. *Public Health Report, 135*(1), 3–5.

Agency for Healthcare Research and Quality. (2008). *Treating Tobacco Use and Dependence.* Retrieved from www.ahrq.gov/prevention/guidelines/tobacco/clinicians/update/index.html

American Nonsmokers' Rights Foundation (2022). *Percent of population covered by 100% smokefree non-hospitality workplace, restaurant, and bar laws in effect as of October 1, 2022.* Retrieved from https://no-smoke.org/wp-content/uploads/pdf/WRBPercentMap.pdf

American Nonsmokers' Rights Foundation (2022a). *Bridging the gap: Status of smokefree air in the United States, 2022.* Retrieved from https://no-smoke.org/wp-content/uploads/pdf/BridgingtheGap-ExecutiveSummary.pdf

American Nonsmokers' Rights Foundation (2022b). *Overview list- Number of smokefree and tobacco related laws as of October 1, 2022.* Retrieved from https://no-smoke.org/wp-content/uploads/pdf/mediaordlist.pdf

Berman, M., Crane, R., Seiber, E., & Munur, M. (2014). Estimating the cost of a smoking employee. *Tobacco Control, 23*(5), 428–433.

Bertuccio, P., La Vecchia, C., Silverman, D. T., Petersen, G. M., Bracci, P. M., Negri, E., . . . Boffetta, P. (2011). Cigar and pipe smoking, smokeless tobacco use and pancreatic cancer: An analysis from the International Pancreatic Cancer Case-Control Consortium (PanC4). *Annals of Oncology.* doi:10.1093/annonc/mdq613.

Boffetta, P., Hecht, S., Gray, N., Gupta, P., & Straif, K. (2008). Smokeless tobacco and cancer. *Lancet Oncology, 9,* 667–675.

Bondi, M. A., Harris, J. R., Atkins, D., French, M. E., & Umland, B. (2006). Employer coverage of clinical preventive services in the United States. *American Journal of Health Promotion, 20*(3), 214–222.

Boon, A. (2012, June 15). *Smokeless tobacco in the United States.* Retrieved from www.tobaccofreekids.org/research/factsheets/pdf/0231.pdf

Campaign for Tobacco Free Kids (2022, January 13). *Broken promises to our children: A state-by-state look at the 1998 Tobacco Settlement 23 years later.* Retrieved from https://www.tobaccofreekids.org/what-we-do/us/statereport/

Centers for Disease Control and Prevention (1999). *International classification of diseases.* Retrieved from www.cdc.gov/nchs/icd/icd10cm.htm

Centers for Disease Control and Prevention (2004). State Medicaid coverage for tobacco-dependence treatments—United States, 1994–2002. *Morbidity and Mortality Weekly Report, 53*(03), 54–57.

Centers for Disease Control and Prevention (2008). *School health guidelines to prevent tobacco use, addiction, and exposure to secondhand smoke.* Atlanta: Centers for Disease Control and Prevention.

Centers for Disease Control and Prevention (2012a, July 24). *History of the surgeon general's reports on smoking and health.* Retrieved from www.cdc.gov/tobacco/data_statistics/sgr/history/index.htm

Centers for Disease Control and Prevention (2012b, August 30). *Workplace health promotion: Tobacco-use cessation.* Retrieved from www.cdc.gov/workplacehealthpromotion/implementation/topics/tobacco-use.html

Centers for Disease Control and Prevention (2012c, December 18). *Smokeless tobacco facts.* Retrieved from www.cdc.gov/tobacco/data_statistics/fact_sheets /smokeless/betel_quid/index.htm

Centers for Disease Control and Prevention (2016). State Medicaid expansion tobacco cessation coverage and number of adult smokers enrolled in expansion coverage – United States, 2016. *Morbidity and Mortality Weekly Report, 65*(48), 1364–1369.

Centers for Disease Control and Prevention (2018). Exposure to secondhand smoke among non-smokers – United States, 1988-2014. *Morbidity and Mortality Weekly Report, 67*(48), 1342–1346.

Centers for Disease Control and Prevention (2022a). Tobacco product use among adults – United States, 2020. *Morbidity and Mortality Weekly Report, 71*(11), 397–405.

Centers for Disease Control and Prevention (2022b). *Smoking and cigarettes.* Retrieved from https://www.cdc.gov/tobacco/data_statistics/fact_sheets/fast_facts/index.htm

Centers for Disease Control and Prevention (2022c). Tobacco product use and associated factors among middle and high school students — National youth tobacco survey, United States, 2021. *Morbidity and Mortality Weekly Report, 71*(5), 1–29.

Centers for Disease Control and Prevention (2022d). Notes from the field: E-cigarette use among middle and high school students — United States, 2022. *Morbidity and Mortality Weekly Report, 71*(40), 1283–1285.

Centers for Disease Control and Prevention (2022e). *Smokeless Tobacco Product Use in the United States.* Retrieved from https://www.cdc.gov/tobacco/data_statistics/fact_sheets/smokeless/use_us/index.htm

Davis, K., Nonnemaker, J., & Farrelly, M. (2007). Association between national smoking prevention campaigns and perceived smoking prevalence among youth in the United States. *Journal of Adolescent Health, 41*(5), 430–436.

Ebbert, J., Montori, V., Erwin, P., & Stead, L. (2011). Interventions for smokeless tobacco use cessation. *Cochrane Database of Systematic Reviews, 2*, CD004306. doi:10.1002/14651858 .CD004306.pub4.

Grimsrud, T., Gallefoss, F., & Løchen, M.-L. (2012). At odds with science? *Nicotine & Tobacco Research, 15*(1), 302–303.

Healthy People 2030. (2022, November 26). *Reduce current cigarette smoking in adults – TU-02.* Retrieved from https://health.gov/healthypeople/objectives-and-data/browse-objectives/tobacco-use/reduce-current-cigarette-smoking-adults-tu-02

Hecht, S. (1998). Biochemistry, biology, and carcinogenicity of tobacco-specific *N*-nitrosamines. *Chemical Research in Toxicology, 11*(6), 559–603.

Heidenreich, P. A., Trogdon, J. G., Khavjou, O. A., Butler, J., Dracup, K., Ezekowitz, M. D., . . . Woo, Y. J. (2011). Forecasting the future of cardiovascular disease in the United States; a policy statement from the American Heart Association. *Circulation, 123*(8), 933–944.

Lee, P. & Hamling, J. (2009). Systematic review of the relation between smokeless tobacco and cancer in Europe and North America. *BMC Medicine, 7*, 36.

Matthew, C., Farrelly, K., Davis, M., Haviland, L., Messeri, P., & Healton, C. (2005). Evidence of a dose–response relationship between "truth" antismoking ads and youth smoking prevalence. *American Journal of Public Health, 95*(3), 425–431.

McAfee, T., Davis, K., Alexander, R., Pechacek, T., & Bunnell, R. (2013). Effect of the first federally funded US antismoking national media campaign. *Lancet.* doi:10.1016/S0140–6736(13)61686–4.

McCarthy, J. (2018). *One in four Americans support total smoking ban.* Retrieved from https://news .gallup.com/poll/237767/one-four-americans-support-total-smoking-ban.aspx

National Association of Attorneys General (1998). *The master settlement agreement.* Retrieved from www.naag.org/backpages/naag/tobacco/msa/msa-pdf

National Center for Health Statistics (2022a). *Cigarette smoking and electronic cigarette use.* Retrieved from https://www.cdc.gov/nchs/fastats/smoking.htm

National Center for Health Statistics (2022b). *Early release of selected estimates based on data from the 2021 National Health Interview Survey.* Retrieved from https://www.cdc.gov/nchs/data/nhis/earlyrelease/earlyrelease202204.pdf

O'Donnell, M. & Roizen, M. (2011). The SmokingPaST framework: Illustrating the impact of quit attempts, quit methods, and new smokers on smoking prevalence, years of life saved, medical costs saved, programming costs, cost effectiveness, and return on investment. *American Journal of Health Promotion, 1*(26), e11–e23.

Partnership for Prevention (2008). *Advanced care management: Diabetes, obesity, weight management and smoking cessation programs.* Washington, DC: Third Employer Health & Human Capital Congress.

Public Health Law Center (2022). *2022 FDA updates – E-cigarettes, synthetic nicotine and flavors.* Retrieved from https://www.publichealthlawcenter.org/commentary/220825/8/25/22-2022-fda-updates-e-cigarettes-synthetic-nicotine-flavors

Raze West Virginia (2022). *Raze: Tear down tobacco lies.* Retrieved from https://razewv.com/about-raze

Reda, A., Kotz, D., Evers, S., & van Schayck, C. (2012). Healthcare financing systems for increasing the use of tobacco dependence treatment. *Cochrane Database of Systematic Review, 6,* CD004305. doi:10.1002/14651858.CD004305.pub4.

Rigotti, N. & Wakefield, M. (2012). Real people, real stories: A new mass media campaign that could help smokers quit. *Annals of Internal Medicine, 156*(12), 907–910.

Rodu, B. (2011). The scientific foundation for tobacco harm reduction, 2006–2011. *Harm Reduction Journal, 8*(19), 1–22.

Scientific Committee on Emerging and Newly-Identified Health Risks (SCENIHR) (2008). *Scientific opinion on the health effects of smokeless tobacco products.* Brussels, Belgium: Health & Consumer Protection DG, European Commission Retrieved from http://ec.europa.eu/health/archive/ph_risk/committees/04_scenihr/docs/scenihr_o_013.pdf.

Secker-Walker, R., Gnichn, W., Platt, S., & Lancaster, T. (2002). Community interventions for reducing smoking among adults. *Cochrane Database of Systematic Reviews, 2,* CD001745. doi:10.1002/14651858.CD001745.

Shrestha, S. S., Ghimire, R., Wang, X., Trivers, K. F., Homa, D. M., & Armour, B. S. (2022). Cost of cigarette smoking attributable productivity losses, United States, 2018. *American Journal of Preventative Medicine, 63*(4), 478–485.

Sponsiello-Wang, Z., Weitkunat, R., & Lee, P. (2008). Systematic review of the relation between smokeless tobacco and cancer of the pancreas in Europe and North America. *BMC Cancer, 8,* 356.

Thomas, R. & Perera, R. (2006). School-based programmes for preventing smoking. *Cochrane Database of Systematic Reviews, 3,* CD001293. doi:10.1002/14651858.CD001293.pub2.

Tobacco Use and Dependence Guideline Panel (2008). *Treating tobacco use and dependence: 2008 update.* Rockville, MD: US Department of Health and Human Services Retrieved from www.ncbi.nlm.nih.gov/books/NBK63952.

Truth Initiative (2021). *Action needed: E-cigarettes.* Retrieved from https://truthinitiative.org/sites/default/files/media/files/2022/03/Truth_E-Cigarette_Factsheet_update_May_2021.pdf

Truth Initiative (2022). *Youth smoking and vaping prevention.* Retrieved from https://truthinitiative.org/what-we-do/youth-smoking-prevention-education

US Department of Health and Human Services (2004). *The health consequences of smoking: A report of the surgeon general.* Atlanta: US Department of Health and Human Services, Centers for Disease Control and Prevention, National Center for Chronic Disease Prevention and Health Promotion, Office on Smoking and Health.

US Department of Health and Human Services (2006). *The health consequences of involuntary exposure to tobacco smoke: A report of the surgeon general—Executive summary.* Atlanta: US Department of Health and Human Services, Centers for Disease Control and Prevention,

Coordinating Center for Health Promotion, National Center for Chronic Disease Prevention and Health Promotion, Office on Smoking and Health.

US Department of Health and Human Services (2007). *Best practices for comprehensive tobacco control programs—2007*. Atlanta: US Department of Health and Human Services, Centers for Disease Control and Prevention, National Center for Chronic Disease Prevention and Health Promotion, Office on Smoking and Health.

US Department of Health and Human Services (2008). *Treating tobacco use and dependence: 2008 update—clinical practice guidelines*. Rockville, MD: US Department of Health and Human Services, Public Health Service, Agency for Healthcare Research and Quality.

US Department of Health and Human Services (2010). *How tobacco smoke causes disease: The biology and behavioral basis for smoking-attributable disease; a report of the surgeon general*. Atlanta: US Department of Health and Human Services, Centers for Disease Control and Prevention, National Center for Chronic Disease Prevention and Health Promotion, Office on Smoking and Health.

US Department of Health and Human Services (2012). *Preventing tobacco use among youth and young adults: A report of the surgeon general*. Atlanta: US Department of Health and Human Services, Centers for Disease Control and Prevention, National Center for Chronic Disease Prevention and Health Promotion, Office on Smoking and Health.

US Department of Health and Human Services (2014). *The health consequences of smoking – 50 years of progress: A report of the surgeon general*. Atlanta: US Department of Health and Human Services, Centers for Disease Control and Prevention, National Center for Chronic Disease Prevention and Health Promotion, Office on Smoking and Health.

US Department of Health and Human Services (2016). *E-cigarette use among youth and young adults: A report of the surgeon general*. Atlanta: US Department of Health and Human Services, Centers for Disease Control and Prevention, National Center for Chronic Disease Prevention and Health Promotion, Office on Smoking and Health.

US Department of Health and Human Services (2020). *Smoking Cessation: A report of the surgeon general*. Atlanta: US Department of Health and Human Services, Centers for Disease Control and Prevention, National Center for Chronic Disease Prevention and Health Promotion, Office on Smoking and Health.

US Food and Drug Administration (2012, August 29). *Overview of the Family Smoking Prevention and Tobacco Control Act*. Retrieved from www.fda.gov/tobaccoproducts/guidancecomplianceregulatoryinformation/ucm246129.htm

US Food and Drug Administration (2016). *Deeming tobacco products to be subject to the federal food, drug, and cosmetic act, as amended by the family smoking prevention and tobacco control act; restrictions on the sale and distribution of tobacco products and required warning statements for tobacco products*. Retrieved from https://www.federalregister.gov/articles/2016/05/10/2016-10685/deeming-tobacco-products-to-be-subject-to-the-federalfood-drug-and-cosmetic-act-as-amended-by-the.

US Food and Drug Administration (2017). *Every Try Counts: Campaign overview*. Retrieved from https://fda.report/media/109497/Every-Try-Counts-Campaign-Overview.pdf

US Food and Drug Administration (2021a). *Cigarette labeling and health warning requirements*. Retrieved from https://www.fda.gov/tobacco-products/labeling-and-warning-statements-tobacco-products/cigarette-labeling-and-health-warning-requirements

US Food and Drug Administration (2021b). *Tobacco 21*. Retrieved from https://www.fda.gov/tobacco-products/retail-sales-tobacco-products/tobacco-21

US Food and Drug Administration (2022a). *Every try counts campaign*. Retrieved from https://www.fda.gov/tobacco-products/public-health-education-campaigns/every-try-counts-campaign

US Food and Drug Administration (2022b). *Smokeless Tobacco Products, Including Dip, Snuff, Snus and Chewing Tobacco.* Retrieved from https://www.fda.gov/tobacco-products/products-ingredients-components/smokeless-tobacco-products-including-dip-snuff-snus-and-chewing-tobacco

US Office of Personnel Management (2013). *Section II: Guidelines for the development of effective agency tobacco cessation programs.* Retrieved from www.opm.gov/policy-data-oversight/worklife/reference-materials/tobacco-cessation-guidance-on-establishing-programs-designed-to-help-employees-stop-using-tobacco/#Program

Vallone, D., Duke, J., Cullen, J., McCausland, K., & Allen, J. A. (2011). Evaluation of EX: A national mass media smoking cessation campaign. *American Journal of Public Health, 101*, 302–309.

Walton, K., Gentzke, A. S., Murphy-Hoefer, R., Kenemer, B., & Neff, L. J. (2020). Exposure to second-hand smoke in homes and vehicles among us youths, United States, 2011-2019. *Preventing Chronic Disease, 17*(E103), 1–5.

Wang, Y., Sung, H., Lightwood, J., Yao, T., & Max, B. W. (2022). Healthcare utilisation and expenditures attributable to current e-cigarette use among US adults. *Tobacco Control,* (May 23). doi:10.1136/tobaccocontrol-2021-057058.

Weng, S. F., Ali, S., & Leonardi-Bee, J. (2013). Smoking and absence from work: systematic review and meta-analysis of occupational studies. *Addiction, 108*(2), 307–319.

World Health Organization (2012, May). *Tobacco: Fact sheet no. 339.* Retrieved from www.who.int/mediacentre/factsheets/fs339/en/index.html

Xu, X., Shrestha, S., Trivers, K. F., Neff, L., Armour, B. S., & King, B. A. (2021). U.S. healthcare spending attributable to cigarette smoking in 2014. *Preventive Medicine, 150* https://doi.org/10.1016/j.ypmed.2021.106529.

CHAPTER 5

EATING BEHAVIORS

Food Choices, Trends, Programs, and Policies

Maya Maroto

Nutrition and food have taken center stage in many discussions related to promoting public health, and for good reason. The Global Burden of Disease study (2019) estimates that 11 million deaths per year are due to non-communicable diseases attributable to poor diet and that suboptimal diet is responsible for more deaths than any other risk globally, including tobacco smoking. The vast majority of Americans fall far short of meeting the nutrition goals set out by the **Dietary Guidelines for Americans (DGA)**, a national healthy-eating guide developed jointly by the US Departments of Health and Human Services and Agriculture.

Furthermore, estimates indicate that approximately 10% of US households are **food insecure**, meaning that they struggle to access adequate food due to lack of money and other resources (US Department of Agriculture: Economic Research Service, 2022a). Rates of food insecurity remain significantly higher among single-parent households as well as among African American and Hispanic households. More recently, the US government has advanced the broader concept of **nutrition security**, which is defined as "consistent access, availability, and affordability of foods and beverages that promote well-being, prevent disease, and if needed, treat disease, particularly among racial/ethnic minority populations, lower-income populations and rural and remote populations including, tribal communities and insular areas" (US Department of Agriculture: Food and Nutrition Service, 2022). Health promotion professionals have an excellent opportunity to successfully promote healthier dietary habits if an ecological approach is adopted to address individual and community-level drivers of food choice while also creating environments and policies that make healthier choices more accessible, available, and affordable.

LEARNING OBJECTIVES
After reading this chapter, the student will be able to:

- Define the factors that influence people's eating patterns.

- Identify the relationship between eating patterns and health.

- Identify the benefits of healthy eating.

- Discuss the history of eating patterns.

- Explain historical changes to the food environment in America.

- Restate educational programs that assist people in making healthy food choices.

- Discuss local, state, and national policies that encourage healthy eating.

- Summarize nutrition programs at the community, worksite, school, and individual levels.

Introduction to Health Promotion, Second Edition. Edited by Anastasia Snelling.
© 2024 John Wiley & Sons Inc. Published 2024 by John Wiley & Sons Inc.
Companion Website: www.wiley.com/go/snelling2e

Eating Behaviors

Why did you eat that? People make around two hundred personal decisions related to food every day and report a multitude of drivers for their eating habits, many of which lie outside of health and nutrition (International Food Information Council, 2021; Cohen & Babey 2012; Wansink, 2007). As an entrant into the field of health promotion, it is important to understand the range of potential drivers of food choices in order to approach the notion of dietary change from a realistic and informed viewpoint. Steptoe, Pollard, and Wardle (1995) reported "health is clearly not the only factor people take into account when choosing their food, and a focus on health may lead to exclusive emphasis on a set of motives that are of limited significance for many people" (p. 268).

An ecological approach is one that involves change through different spheres to influence behavior modification. This involves individual behavior, along with family, school, workplace, community, and policy change. By targeting each level, improved health changes are more likely to be practiced.

Our diet has changed more in the last 100 years than in the last 10,000, probably with the result that it is affecting our health.

—Michael Pollan, food author; journalist; and University of California,

Berkeley, professor

Dietary Guidelines for Americans (DGA) nutrition guidelines jointly issued and updated every five years by the Departments of Health and Human Services and Agriculture; provides advice on what to eat and drink to meet nutrient needs, promote health, and prevent disease. The DGA are developed and written for a professional audience, including policymakers, healthcare providers, nutrition educators, and Federal nutrition program operators.

Taste

Perhaps not surprisingly, taste is Americans' number one consideration when they make food purchasing decisions (International Food Information Council, 2021; Scheibehenne, Miesler, & Todd, 2007). The flavor of food is highly related to a person's preference. Research indicates that humans have biological preferences toward foods that are sweet, salty, and fatty. These characteristics may have been helpful for survival during early history because humans focused on foods that were calorically dense, physiologically beneficial, and safe to eat. Today's world offers an abundance of technologically created and heavily marketed ultra-processed foods that are high in refined grains, added sugar, salt, and added fat, and low in nature's healthiest elements, such as vitamins, minerals, fiber, omega 3-fatty acids, high-quality protein, and phytochemicals (plant chemicals) (Monteiro, Cannon, Lawrence, Louzada, & Machado, 2019). Foods are often processed and manufactured in ways that make them "hyperpalatable" with various combinations of fat and sodium, fat and simple sugar, or carbohydrates and sodium (Fazzino, Rohde, & Sullivan, 2019). Rising rates of ultra-processed food consumption have coincided with global increases in rates of overweight and obesity (Popkin, Adair, & Ng, 2012). Furthermore, studies suggest that for certain individuals, fat, sugar, and salt induce changes to the brain structure that are similar to those induced by addictive narcotics (Moss, 2021).

Emotions

In addition to taste, food also delivers a sense of enjoyment, often described as satisfaction, happiness, or comfort, depending on the situation. For example, a person may feel a sense of happiness in eating a healthy meal of fish, broccoli, and rice after a workout, but that same person may derive happiness from eating pizza after a night out with friends or eating "comfort" foods when stressed (Antin & Hunt, 2012). There is no denying the important role of emotions and feelings in driving food choice. Numerous studies have linked increased stress levels with craving and consuming foods high in calories, sugar, and fat (Laran & Salerno, 2013; Tryon, Carter, DeCant, & Laugero, 2013; Zellner et al., 2006). Other studies have shown that individuals residing in lower-opportunity neighborhoods and people from historically marginalized racial and ethnic groups have higher levels of chronic stress in the United States (Roubinov, Hagan, Boyce, Adler, & Bush, 2018; Williams, 2018). The links between stress, income, race, body weight, and eating habits are hot topics among nutrition and neuroscience researchers, who wish to explain the pathways between life circumstances and food choices.

Price

Cost is an important consideration for many people when selecting foods. Recent data indicate that in 2021, price was an important factor in food choices for 66% of consumers (International Food Information Council, 2021). Although there is controversy within the world of economists about which foods are least expensive, much evidence suggests that the foods delivering the most calories for the least cost include refined grains (grains largely stripped of their fiber, vitamins, and minerals) and processed foods high in added sugar, fat, and salt. These foods tend to be tasty, highly convenient, and readily available (Drewnowski & Darmon, 2005). Other researchers contend that "low energy density" diets with more servings of fruits, vegetables, and fiber and fewer added sugars and added fats did not cost more than "high energy density" diets, which tended to be higher in total fat, saturated fat, added sugars, and grains—including a higher proportion of fast food and takeout meals (Vernarelli & DiSarro, 2021). A recent analysis indicates that Americans can consume the amount of fruits and vegetables recommended by the DGA at a cost of $2.10–$2.60 per day (Stewart & Hyman, 2019). It is important to note that while obtaining healthy, whole food ingredients to prepare meals from scratch can be an affordable option, the psychological bandwidth, skills, and equipment required to carry out meal planning, food acquisition, food preparation, and kitchen cleanup are significant barriers that may be especially challenging for people struggling with aspects of poverty (Fielding-Singh, 2022).

Convenience

Americans are in a rush—to do everything. Today's economy increasingly requires adult family members to work outside of the home, leaving less time and energy for food preparation. Research indicates that even in the twenty-first century, women continue to do the vast majority of household food preparation (Anekwe & Zeballos, 2019). The amount of time Americans spend cooking varies based on employment. For example, women who do not work outside of the home spend significantly more time on food preparation than women who are employed full-time (Mancino & Newman, 2007; Sliwa, Must, Peréa, & Economos, 2015). This creates a demand for accessible, affordable, quick, and easy-to-prepare meals that include "ingredients" such as canned soups or "heat and eat" meals. Unfortunately, the less time people spend cooking, the more likely they are to be overweight or obese (Kolodinsky & Goldstein, 2011).

The convenience food market is built on a shifting culture in which everyone seems to have a shortage of time. Consumer habits have drastically changed, and many people are spending additional cash in exchange for already-prepared meals. The focus of the convenience food industry is on products that can easily be divided into helpings, are resealable, and are easily prepared in a microwave oven. Grocery stores have picked up on the convenience food trend and are now offering entrees and side dishes ready for the oven, microwave, and dinner plate. The demand for convenient foods, including ready-to-cook meals and snacks (requiring water and/or heating before consuming), ready-to-eat meals and snacks (requiring no preparation), and meals and snacks from fast food and sit-down restaurants, is on the rise and is especially in-demand among households with children (Okrent & Kumcu, 2016).

> In general, moms' decision to cook *more* entailed a choice to spend *less* recreational time with kids and on themselves. It meant feeling *more* exhausted than they already felt and even *less* connected to the kids who they hadn't seen all day.
> —Dr. Priya Fielding Singh, food author; professor, University of Utah

The rise in popularity of online grocery shopping is another important aspect of food convenience, with approximately 42% of US adults shopping for groceries online at least monthly in 2021, compared to 27% in 2019 (International Food Information Council, 2021). Interestingly, younger consumers (aged eighteen to thirty five), African American consumers, and parents were most likely to shop for groceries online. The rise in popularity of online grocery shopping was undoubtedly accelerated by changes in shopping habits experienced during the COVID-19 pandemic.

Health and Nutrition

Health and nutrition are also factors influencing food selection. Many consumers are interested in foods that will help them improve their well-being and physical health, lose weight, and manage health conditions. Although health concerns play a role in food selection for some people, personal appearance is a distinct factor reported as well. Beyond selecting foods to lose weight or avoid chronic diseases such as type 2 diabetes and heart disease, consumers also report seeking foods that provide health benefits including improved energy levels, digestive health, endurance, sleep, and immunity (International Food Information Council, 2021).

According to a large study, the top sources of information about what foods to eat or avoid include healthcare professionals, friends/family, health-focused websites, information from registered dietitians, news articles, and social media (International Food Information Council, 2021). Also, 49% of consumers reported that they look at the Nutrition Facts label "always" or "most of the time" when buying a food product for the first time. The top items that consumers look for on the Nutrition Facts label are calories, total sugar, sodium, and serving size (US Food and Drug Administration, 2021).

Food manufacturers have responded to consumers' desire for healthier products with an array of packaged foods bearing various front-of-package (FOP) claims like "all natural," "GMO-free," "sustainable," "low-carb/fat/sugar/sodium." Consumers report that they find it most helpful when packages include front-of-pack labels that identify what ingredients are included/excluded and that summarize nutrition content per serving. Consumers also perceive that products that are described as "plant-based," have a short list of familiar-sounding ingredients, are fresh (versus frozen), or are described as "all natural" as being associated with healthfulness (International Food Information Council, 2021).

Culture and Familiarity

Food selection is also influenced by culture and familiarity. Think back to a food you loved as a child and how it made you feel to consume that food. You may be flooded with powerful memories. Many people have strong connections to the foods native to their culture and upbringing. Foods are attached to a sense of identity and are a central feature of people's social lives, cultural identities, religious traditions, and holiday celebrations. Food is a powerful cultural identifier, reflecting unique values and beliefs related to food cultivation, production, preparation, and consumption (Sibal, 2018).

Environment

Foods readily available to consumers affect food selection. What types of food are near consumers' homes, schools, or workplaces? Consumers purchase food in a variety of venues, influenced by what is nearby and accessible, including grocery stores, farmer's markets, corner stores, liquor stores, fast food outlets, and coffee shops. Food availability affects food selection. The term *food desert* has historically been used to describe low-income areas that lack access to the array of foods carried in grocery stores. *Food swamp* may be a more appropriate term to describe the multitude of geographic areas with access to numerous corner stores, fast food outlets, and grocery stores. In a US Department of Agriculture report regarding food access, findings indicated that "easy access to all food, rather than lack of access to specific healthy foods, may be a more important factor in explaining increases in BMI and obesity" (Ploeg et al., 2009). The term *food apartheid* is also increasingly being used to describe areas that lack access to healthy, affordable foods, as the term "apartheid" communicates that systematic, discriminatory planning and policy decisions have precipitated pervasive race and income-based inequities in the current food system (Brones, 2018).

Marketing

Finally, food marketing influences food selection. Research has shown that individuals who are exposed to unhealthy food advertising in an experimental setting are almost 30% more likely to consume unhealthy snacks than those exposed to nonfood advertising, and that the effect becomes even more pronounced when participants are "multi-tasking" another cognitive task (Zimmerman & Shimoga, 2014). Cohen (2008) contends that the "omnipresence of food advertising is artificially stimulating people to feel hungry and overconsume. Given the increasing availability of food over time, this stimulation follows suit, potentially explaining the continuing rises in obesity" (p. S138). Advances in food marketing research have identified the most effective methods to persuade and entice consumers to consume the foods being marketed. Food marketing research enables companies to design advertisements and packaging that immediately capture and hold consumer attention. Companies have also mastered the art of "branding," which creates an automatic and powerful connection between a product and consumer emotions (Cohen, 2008). Research indicates that foods most often marketed to children are sugary breakfast cereals, soft drinks, candy, salty snacks, and fast foods, and that African American and Hispanic youth are exposed to more targeted marketing of unhealthy food than White youth, contributing to health inequities affecting youth in communities of color (Taillie, Busey, Stoltze, & Dillman Carpentier, 2019; UConn Rudd Center for Food Policy and Health, 2020a).

Nutrition, Eating Habits, and Health

Americans are eating poorly and suffering from high rates of numerous chronic diseases, including heart disease, cancer, stroke, and diabetes. Poor nutrition, along with inadequate physical activity, tobacco use, and excessive alcohol use, are linked to the nation's leading chronic diseases (Raghupathi & Raghupathi, 2018).

As identified in Table 5.1, in 2020, of the top ten leading causes of death in the United States, five were chronic diseases that were nutrition-related. The following section covers the links between various foods and nutrients and heart disease, cancer, stroke, diabetes, and kidney disease. It is notable that the nutrients that decrease the risk of these diseases

Table 5.1   Leading Causes of Death: Number of Deaths (United States, 2020)

- Heart disease: 696,962
- Cancer: 602,350
- COVID-19: 350,831
- Accidents (unintentional injuries): 200,955
- Stroke (cerebrovascular diseases): 160,264
- Chronic lower respiratory diseases: 152,657
- Alzheimer's disease: 134,242
- Diabetes: 102,188
- Influenza and pneumonia: 53,544
- Nephritis, nephrotic syndrome, and nephrosis (kidney disease): 52,547

Note: Nutrition-related causes of death are in grey background.
Source: Centers for Disease Control and Prevention (Adapted from Murphy, Kochanek, Xu, & Arias, 2020).

are usually only protective when consumed from foods—studies of nutrients from dietary supplements have generally not shown the same powerful positive effects as nutrient-rich diets.

Heart Disease

Heart disease is the leading cause of death for men, women, and people of most racial and ethnic groups in the United States (Centers for Disease Control and Prevention, 2022d). Diseases of the heart result from a buildup of plaque inside artery walls, which may ultimately lead to a heart attack. Heart disease is most prevalent among populations with unhealthy diets, individuals who smoke, individuals who consume excessive alcohol, individuals who are obese, and in those who are not physically active.

> **Heart disease** generally refers to conditions that involve narrowed or blocked blood vessels that can lead to a heart attack, chest pain (angina), or stroke

The link between nutrition and heart disease has been researched for more than one hundred years; the first studies were conducted in the early 1900s (Roberts & Barnard, 2005). Several foods and dietary patterns have been strongly linked with increased risk of heart disease, including ultra-processed foods, industrially produced trans fat, processed meats, excessive sodium (salt), sugar-sweetened beverages (SSB), sweets/desserts, refined grains, and "greater than moderate" alcohol use. Studies have shown that people consuming diets rich in fruits, vegetables, whole grains, nuts/seeds, legumes, lean meat, seafood, yogurt, and certain vegetable oils have a reduced risk of heart disease (Lichtenstein et al., 2021; Mozaffarian, 2016). Additionally, maintaining a healthy body weight is also considered an important component of heart disease prevention (Lichtenstein et al., 2021). Uncertainty exists about the benefits or harms of cheese, whole-fat dairy products, eggs, and butter with respect to heart disease risk (Mozaffarian, 2016).

Following a healthy dietary pattern can decrease the risk of multiple chronic diseases. The dietary patterns that are protective against heart disease are also protective against hypertension (high blood pressure), which is a risk factor for heart disease (Ndanuko, Tapsell, Charlton, Neale, & Batterham, 2016). Hypertension is also a leading cause of kidney disease, which means these dietary patterns will also help decrease the risk of kidney disease, another leading nutrition-related cause of death. Research shows that individuals who are obese can decrease their risk of heart disease by improving their diet and physical activity, even if weight loss is not achieved (Ndanuko, Tapsell, Charlton, Neale, & Batterham, 2016).

Cancer

Cancer is the second-leading killer in the United States and will affect one in three people in their lifetime. Numerous studies suggest that lifestyle factors including smoking, sun exposure, tanning beds, excessive alcohol use, being overweight or obese play a major role in the development of cancer (Centers for Disease Control and Prevention, 2022a). Globally, around one-third of cancers are due to factors such as tobacco use, high body mass index, alcohol consumption, low fruit and vegetable intake, and lack of physical activity (World Health Organization, 2022).

> **Cancer** term used for diseases in which abnormal cells divide without control and are able to invade other tissues

Specific nutrients have been studied for their possible relationship to cancer. Cancer is a heterogeneous disease with various etiologies due to site and tumor type, which complicates the ability of researchers to make direct causal connections between nutrients or foods and cancer risk. The American Cancer Society recommends a general healthy eating pattern high in a variety of vegetables, fruits, and whole grains and lower in red meat, processed meat, SSB, ultra-processed foods, refined grain products, and alcohol to decrease the risk of developing cancer (Rock et al., 2020).

Stroke

Stroke
occurs when the blood supply to part of the brain is interrupted or severely reduced, depriving brain tissue of oxygen and food; within minutes, brain cells begin to die

Stroke is the fifth leading cause of death in the United States and a leading cause of functional impairment in Americans, causing reduced mobility in more than half of stroke survivors aged sixty five and older (Centers for Disease Control and Prevention, 2022e). Research indicates that five factors—blood pressure, diet, physical inactivity, smoking, and abdominal obesity—account for up to 90% of strokes (Kleindorfer et al., 2021). High blood pressure is a major contributor to stroke; following dietary guidance to reduce the risk of heart disease and high blood pressure will indirectly decrease the risk of stroke as well (Medeiros, Casanova, Fraulob, & Trindade, 2012).

Several dietary patterns and foods have been associated with the risk of stroke. The Mediterranean and DASH diets (see Table 5.2 for more details) have been associated with a decreased risk of stroke. Nearly all prospective studies demonstrate that increased intake of fruits, vegetables, nuts, legumes, olive oil, and seafood is associated with decreased risk of stroke. Studies have shown that diets high in SSB, processed meats, and sodium are associated with increased risk of stroke (Larsson, 2017).

Type 2 Diabetes

Type 2 Diabetes
once known as adult-onset or noninsulin-dependent diabetes; is a chronic condition that affects the way the body metabolizes sugar (glucose), the body's main source of fuel; with type 2 diabetes, the body either resists the effects of insulin—a hormone that regulates the movement of sugar into the cells—or does not produce enough insulin to maintain a normal glucose level; untreated, can be life-threatening

Type 2 diabetes develops when a person's body becomes resistant to the effects of insulin and the body is no longer able to produce sufficient insulin to overcome this resistance. These changes lead to elevated levels of glucose (a sugar) in the blood. Type 2 diabetes is

Table 5.2   Selected Dietary Patterns, Their Characteristics, and Disease Risk Impact

Dietary Pattern	Characteristics	Disease Risk Impact
Typical American or **Westernized diet**	High in calories, added sugars, solid fats, refined grains, and sodium Low in whole grains, vegetables, fruits, and milk, dietary fiber, vitamin D, calcium, potassium, and omega-3 fatty acids (usually found in fish)	Increased risk for obesity, premature death, cardiovascular disease (CVD), type 2 diabetes, and some cancers
DASH (dietary approaches to stop hypertension)- style eating pattern	High in vegetables, fruit, and low-fat milk; includes whole grains, poultry, seafood, **olive oil**, and nuts Low in red meat, sweets, sodium, and sugar-containing beverages	Lower blood pressure, improved blood lipids, lower blood glucose, lower CVD risk, and improve control of type 2 diabetes
Mediterranean-style dietary pattern	High in plant foods, bread, vegetables, fruits, nuts, seafood, unrefined cereals, olive oil, fish, cheese, and yogurt; includes red wine with meals; ~40% of calories from monounsaturated fat Low in red meat, sweets, saturated fat, meat, and full-fat dairy products	Lower risk of coronary heart disease, lower risk of blood pressure, lower risk of stroke, lower risk of CVD, lower risk of mortality

Source: https://www.ncbi.nlm.nih.gov/books/NBK482514/ and https://www.ncbi.nlm.nih.gov/pmc/articles/PMC5902736/

increasing most rapidly in populations with unhealthy diets, among individuals living with overweight or obesity, and among those who are not physically active.

Several nutrition therapy interventions have been found to decrease the risk of developing type 2 diabetes. The strongest evidence for type 2 diabetes prevention comes from the Diabetes Prevention Program, which focuses on weight reduction via healthy eating and physical activity. DPP interventions have been shown to reduce the incidence of type 2 diabetes in adults with overweight or obesity and impaired glucose tolerance by 58% over three years. Several dietary patterns have been studied for their impact on reducing hemoglobin A1c (a long-term indicator of blood glucose levels) and have found that low and very-low-carbohydrate diets, Mediterranean-style diets, and vegetarian or vegan diets can all be helpful in normalizing HbA1C. Overall, the key factors in any of these dietary patterns are an abundance of non-starchy vegetables, minimal added sugars and refined grains, and choosing whole foods over ultra-processed foods to the extent possible (Evert et al., 2019).

Obesity

The prevalence of obesity has soared from 13% in the early 1960s to over 40% in 2018, and researchers are increasingly aware of the complex environmental, neurological, and hormonal factors behind this alarming phenomenon (Fryar, Carroll, & Afful, 2020; Hall et al., 2022). Predominant theories related to population-wide weight gain are moving beyond the "calories in-calories out" model to more advanced theories considering the impacts of hyper-palatable, ultra-processed foods on the brain, hormonal systems, epigenetics, and gut microbiota (Hall et al., 2022). Overall, a dietary pattern with higher amounts of fruits, vegetables, legumes, whole grains, low- or non-fat dairy, lean meats, poultry, seafood, nuts, and unsaturated oils and lower amounts of processed meat, sugar-sweetened foods and beverages, and refined grains is associated with lower risk of obesity (US Department of Agriculture and US Department of Health and Human Services, 2020).

Obesity can be a serious health issue because it has been linked to increased risk for premature death, type 2 diabetes, hypertension (high blood pressure), dyslipidemia (abnormalities in blood such as high low-density lipoprotein cholesterol levels), heart disease (may lead to heart attack), stroke, gall bladder disease, sleep apnea, arthritis, depression, anxiety, and several kinds of cancer (Centers for Disease Control and Prevention, 2022c) (Figure 5.1).

Selected Healthy Eating Patterns

The previous section identified the links between dietary patterns and disease and illustrated that there are several dietary patterns that either increase or decrease the risk of most common chronic diseases. Several dietary patterns, including the Mediterranean diet and the DASH diet, are widely recognized for their health promotion potential due to being studied extensively in large for many years. The typical American or **Westernized diet**, which is high in calories, processed foods, added sugars, solid fats, refined grains, and sodium, is associated with increased risk for obesity and several major chronic diseases. Human history is full of examples of healthy, nutrient-dense diets from all corners of the globe, not just the Mediterranean, and a full listing of all healthy global dietary patterns is

---

Westernized Diet
high in calories, processed foods, added sugars, solid fats, refined grains, and sodium; is associated with increased risk for obesity and several major chronic diseases

DASH (dietary approaches to stop hypertension)-style Eating Pattern
a low-sodium regimen for patients with hypertension that emphasizes fruits, vegetables, low-fat dairy foods, whole-grain products, fish, poultry, and nuts; low in saturated and total fat, cholesterol, red meat, sweets, and sugared beverages; high in magnesium, potassium, calcium, protein, and fiber

Mediterranean-style Dietary Pattern
emphasizes eating primarily plant-based foods, such as fruits and vegetables, whole grains, legumes, and nuts; replacing butter with healthy fats, such as olive oil; using herbs and spices instead of salt to flavor foods; limiting red meat to no more than a few times a month; eating fish and poultry at least twice a week; drinking red wine in moderation (optional)

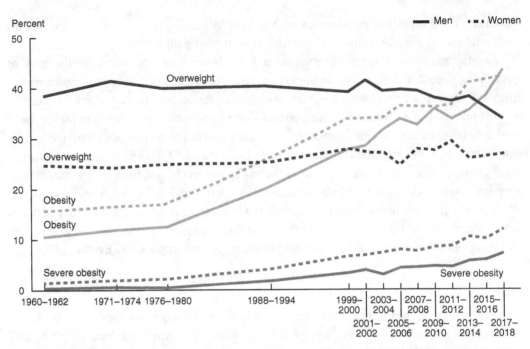

NOTES: Data are age adjusted by the direct method to U.S. Census 2000 estimates using age groups 20–39, 40–59, and 60–74. Overweight is body mass index (BMI) of 25.0–29.9 kg/m². Obesity is BMI at or above 30.0 kg/m². Severe obesity is a BMI at or above 40.0 kg/m². Pregnant women are excluded from the analysis.
SOURCES: National Center for Health Statistics, National Health Examination Survey and National Health and Nutrition Examination Surveys.

Figure 5.1 Age-Adjusted Trends in Overweight, Obesity, and Severe Obesity Among Men and Women Aged 20–74: United States, 1960–1962 Through 2017–2018
Source: https://www.cdc.gov/nchs/data/hestat/obesity-adult-17-18/Estat-adults-fig.png

beyond the scope of this chapter. The chronic disease impacts of selected eating patterns that have been the subject of intensive studies are identified in Table 5.2.

Recommended Nutrition and Dietary Intake

Starting in 1980, the United States federal government has released updated DGA every five years. The guidelines are released jointly by the Departments of Agriculture and Health and Human Services and are based on reviews of current nutrition science published in a report by scientific experts on the Dietary Guidelines Advisory Committee (DGAC). During the DGA development process, the public is encouraged to participate in nominating individuals to serve on the DGAC, to provide input on the draft nutrition science questions the committee will research, and to provide oral and written comments during the DGAC deliberation process. The DGA are intended to be used by professionals, including policymakers, nutrition educators, healthcare providers, and federal nutrition program operators, to assist with providing advice on how their patients or clients can meet nutrient needs and avoid development of nutrition-related chronic diseases (US Department of Agriculture and US Department of Health and Human Services, 2020). The guidelines are translated into a consumer resource called "MyPlate" (see Figure 5.2), which replaced the Food Guide Pyramid starting in 2011.

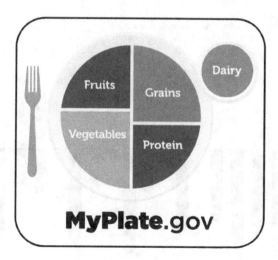

Figure 5.2   MyPlate Icon
Source: MyPlate.gov (n.d.)

The MyPlate icon and website (www.MyPlate.gov) provide consumer-oriented tools, resources, and recipes to guide consumers toward dietary choices consistent with the latest DGA.

The 2020–2025 DGA and MyPlate icon are intended to encourage Americans to increase their intake of certain foods while decreasing or limiting their intake of others. Americans are advised to choose a dietary pattern comprised of whole grains, vegetables, whole fruits, low-fat dairy products or fortified soy beverages, seafood, lean meat, lean poultry, eggs, beans, peas, and lentils, nuts, and seeds, while minimizing intake of foods and beverages high in added sugars, refined grains, sodium, and saturated fat. The advice to consume lean meat, poultry, and seafood does not apply to vegetarians. Vegetarians are encouraged to meet their protein needs with eggs, beans, peas, and lentils, nuts, seeds, and soy products (US Department of Agriculture and US Department of Health and Human Services, 2020).

Figure 5.3 compares the typical American diet to the dietary goals and limits set by the USDA and the Department of Health and Human Services in the 2020–2025 DGA.

History of Nutrition and Dietary Patterns

Historical changes in civilization have dramatically affected the dietary patterns of our species and our country. Not too long ago, Americans' food consumption and physical activity were not out of balance on a large scale. It was only in the late 1980s and 1990s that obesity levels began to rise rapidly. However, obesity is not the only indicator of a lifestyle that is out of balance; the rates of cancer, heart disease, kidney disease, and type 2 diabetes are also rising among people of all weights, particularly affecting those who are carrying excess weight. This section provides information regarding how the human diet changed over thousands of years and more recently, in the United States, with the advancement of technology and an increasing population.

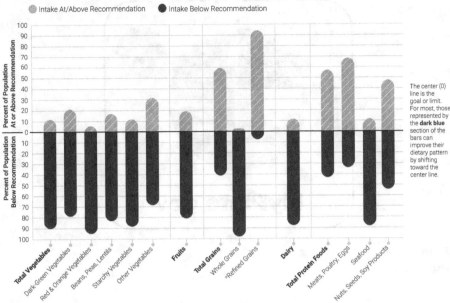

*NOTE: Recommended daily intake of whole grains is to be at least half of total grain consumption, and the limit for refined grains is to be no more than half of total grain consumption.

Data Source: Analysis of What We Eat in America, NHANES 2013-2016, ages 1 and older, 2 days dietary intake data, weighted. *Recommended Intake Ranges:* Healthy U.S.-Style Dietary Patterns (see **Appendix 3**).

Figure 5.3   Dietary Intakes Compared to Recommendations: Percent of the US Population Ages 1 and Older Who are Below, At and Above Each Dietary Goal https://www.dietaryguidelines.gov/sites/default/files/2021-11/DGA_2020-2025_CurrentIntakesSnapshot.png
Source: https://www.dietaryguidelines.gov/figures-infographics / last accessed February 06, 2023

What are the historic dietary patterns associated with the rise in chronic diseases (also called noncommunicable diseases)? Dr. Barry Popkin, a prominent nutrition researcher at the University of North Carolina at Chapel Hill, described five distinct dietary patterns that have emerged throughout human history.

Pattern 1: Paleolithic and Hunter-gatherers

Foraging, food hunting, and gathering have been the dominant forms of food acquisition sustaining the human race for the vast majority of human history. Preagricultural societies were largely omnivorous and consumed a variety of plant and animal species, including nuts, seeds, wild grasses, meat, and fish. Compared to the typical, current American diet, prehistoric diets were more than twice as rich in fiber, potassium, and calcium but contained very little sodium (Caballero & Popkin, 2002). Nutritional deficiencies were uncommon among hunter-gatherer populations (Popkin, 2006). The prehistoric diet was the dominant eating pattern for approximately the first 140,000 years of human history. Research suggests that many of our preagricultural ancestors had adult life spans of more than seventy years and were largely free of the chronic illnesses that are the leading causes of death in our culture today, including heart disease, cancer, and type 2 diabetes (Gurven & Kaplan, 2007).

Pattern 2: Advent of Agriculture

Approximately ten thousand years ago, with the advent of traditional agriculture, societies began shifting away from the hunter-gatherer diet. Human diets became heavily dominated by cereal grains (rice, wheat, and corn), supplemented with legumes (beans), tubers (such as potatoes), and oil. Dietary variety was greatly reduced from prehistoric patterns, and most diets in the early agricultural era were "highly monotonous and not very palatable" (Caballero & Popkin, 2002, p. 30). Archeological evidence suggests that average adult height during this period significantly decreased. Dependence on agriculture also subjected people to the harsh realities of famine, crop failure, and other natural disasters. However, farming enabled a tremendous increase in food calories per acre, which facilitated population growth and the formation of stratified civilizations (Caballero & Popkin, 2002). Early agriculture was based on processes such as crop rotation, cover crops, and the use of animals and human labor. All foods consumed during this era would be considered "organic" by today's standards because chemical pesticides and fertilizers had not yet been invented.

Pattern 3: Industrialization and Receding Famine

With the introduction of nonrenewable fossil fuels and electricity, farmers were able to transition to more modern farming methods. Modern farming relies on agricultural machinery for crop processing tasks and on synthetic fertilizers and pesticides to grow fruits, vegetables, and grains. Pharmaceuticals were also introduced to promote animal growth. The use of these technologies saw a marked rise in the 1960s during what was known as the "green revolution." In addition, crop varieties were developed that produced more reliable yields, and agricultural monoculture (growing of a single type of crop on a farm) began to replace agriculturally diverse farming. Modern farming methods have significantly increased crop production, providing affordable food for a much larger number of people (Popkin & Gordon-Larsen, 2004). However, one of the major drawbacks of modern agriculture is the environmental damage caused by the use of synthetic pesticides, herbicides, and fertilizers. Additionally, concentrated animal feeding operations pose a threat to animal welfare and are a source of air and water pollution (Jacobson, 2006). This dietary pattern is characterized by increased consumption of fruits, vegetables, and animal protein and decreased consumption of starchy staple foods. However, diets continued to lack variety, similar to diets in pattern 2.

Pattern 4: Noncommunicable Disease

The noncommunicable disease dietary pattern is currently most dominant in the United States and is becoming the leading pattern globally as well. Barry Popkin writes that in the last two decades of the twentieth century, "modern societies seem to be converging on a diet high in saturated fats, sugar, and refined foods but low in fiber, often termed the 'Western diet,' and on lifestyles characterized by lower levels of activity" (Popkin & Gordon-Larsen, 2004, p. S2). This dietary pattern emerged because of the convergence of many factors, including modern food processing, marketing, and distribution; consumer demand for processed food, in part because of more women entering the workforce, leaving less time for food preparation; global agricultural policies that have decreased the cost of grains and animal products; and global food advertising, among others (Popkin, 2006). In many countries, this dietary pattern is characterized by an increase in meals consumed away from home, larger portion sizes, rising consumption of animal foods, increased consumption of ultra-processed foods, and the replacement of water and milk by SSB. This dietary pattern is associated with an increase in chronic diseases (cancer, heart disease, type 2 diabetes) and obesity (Popkin, 2006).

Pattern 5: Desired Societal and Behavior Change

In the United States, this pattern would be considered optimal adherence to the US federal government's dietary guidance, the DGA and MyPlate, as described in the previous section. It is not currently the dominant pattern in the United States, but it is the pattern that many health promotion professionals encourage to reduce chronic disease risk.

Changes to the American Food Environment

In the United States, since the 1980s, significant environmental changes have affected our diets and eating habits.

Food Supply and Consumption

Today's food environment presents people with a plethora of accessible, inexpensive food options. In 1970, there were 2,054 calories available in the food supply, per day, for every person in America; by 2010, that total had increased by more than 450 calories to 2,510 calories per person (US Department of Agriculture: Economic Research Service, 2022b). In other words, there are more calories available, and, as more calories have become available in the food supply, people have tended to eat them. But what are the sources of increased calories? In the following section, food availability and food consumption trends will be described. Table 5.3 summarizes the changes to the food supply in pounds of food available per person from the early 1900s until 2009.

Table 5.3 illustrates the major food-group level shifts in consumption of grains, vegetables, protein foods, sweeteners, fats, and oils. Additional insight on each of these is included in the subsequent section.

Grains

Grains

any food made from wheat, rice, oats, cornmeal, barley, or another cereal grain, such as bread, pasta, oatmeal, breakfast cereals, tortillas, and grits

A large part of the gain in calories available in the United States is a result of the increased production of flour and cereal products. These products rose from 95 pounds per person in 1970 to 122 pounds per person in 2019. Foods produced from these flours and cereals include grain-based snack foods and bakery items (e.g., crackers, cakes, cookies), as well as breads, buns, dough, and tortillas. These foods are frequently consumed away from home (Morrison, Buzby, & Wells, 2010). Americans are overconsuming refined grains and falling far short of recommended whole-grain intakes (US Department of Agriculture and US Department of Health and Human Services, 2020; Wells & Buzby, 2008). From a public

Table 5.3   Food Availability in Pounds per Person

Food Group	Loss Adjusted Food Availability (Pounds/Person/Year)	
	1970s	2010–2019
Grains	95	122 (2019)
Vegetables*	150	171 (2018)
Fruit*	108	108 (2019)
Dairy**	231	153 (2019)
Meat, fish, eggs, and nuts	162	180 (2018)
Sweeteners***	70	73 (2019)
Fats and oils	36	57 (2010)
Total calories in food supply	2,054	2,510 (2010)

*Fresh, Canned, and Frozen
**Milk, Cream, Cheese, and Frozen Dairy Products
***Sugar, Corn Sweeteners, Honey, and Syrup
Source: https://www.ers.usda.gov/data-products/food-availability-per-capita-data-system/food-availability-per-capita-data-system/#Loss-Adjusted%20Food%20Availability

health perspective, grains are important contributors of several nutrients, including dietary fiber, B vitamins (thiamin, riboflavin, niacin, and folate), and minerals (iron, magnesium, and selenium) (MyPlate.gov, 2022a).

Fruits and Vegetables

There are currently more vegetables available in the food supply than there were in 1970. In 2018, there were 171 pounds of vegetables (fresh and processed) available per person, up from 150 pounds per person in 1970. Although this may sound like good news, it is not so simple. Potatoes and tomatoes are the top two most consumed vegetables, and the majority of intake is in the form of French fries and pizza sauce. The third most consumed vegetable is onions, followed by carrots, lettuce, and corn (US Department of Agriculture: Economic Research Service, 2022c). Americans are eating less than the recommended amounts and are also not eating the recommended pattern of vegetables, which should include ample amounts of dark green vegetables, orange/red vegetables, starchy vegetables, beans, and peas. In order to meet the most current guidelines, intakes of all categories of vegetables, including starchy vegetables, would need to increase to meet DGA recommendations (US Department of Agriculture and US Department of Health and Human Services, 2020).

Fruit intake has remained relatively stable since 1970. Orange juice and apple juice are the most common contributors of fruit in the American diet. Considering only whole fruits, bananas are the most consumed fruit, followed by apples, grapes, watermelon, strawberries, and oranges (US Department of Agriculture: Economic Research Service, 2022c).

Fruits and vegetables contribute several important nutrients to the diet, including potassium, dietary fiber, vitamin C, folate, and vitamin A (ChooseMyPlate.gov, 2022b).

Fruits and vegetables
Nutritionally similar, generally lower in calories and fat than animal products; also contain health-enhancing plant compounds, such as fiber and antioxidants, vitamins, and minerals

Dairy

Milk consumption declined from 0.9 to 0.5 cups per person per day from 1979 to 2019 (US Department of Agriculture: Economic Research Service, 2022c). The consumption of lower-fat milk began to increase in the 1990s as knowledge about cholesterol, saturated fat, and calories became more widely known by Americans (Putnam & Allshouse, 2003). Americans are currently not meeting the dietary guidelines for daily recommended milk intake, which is promoted for its contribution of nutrients (including calcium, vitamin D, potassium, protein, vitamin B12, riboflavin, niacin, phosphorus, and pantothenic acid); potential for improving bone health; and possible role in decreasing risk of type 2 diabetes and CVD (US Department of Agriculture and US Department of Health and Human Services, 2020). While milk availability has decreased, cheese availability has doubled from 1970 to 2020 and now accounts for the largest share of dairy intake in US diets.

Another contributor to the decline in cow's milk intake is the rising popularity of plant-based dairy alternatives, including soy milk, oat milk, almond milk, rice milk, and other plant-based milk alternatives. Currently, fortified soy beverages are the only beverage considered by the US government nutrition guidelines to be nutritionally comparable to cow's milk due to the contribution of high-quality soy protein as well as calcium and vitamin D (US Department of Agriculture: Economic Research Service, 2022c). A recent study compared the nutritional profile of other nondairy milk alternatives (beyond soy milk) to cow's milk and concluded that due to lower levels of protein, vitamins, and minerals, they are "not nutritionally similar to cow's milk and are not a good substitute when the goal is to provide a beverage nutritionally similar to cow's milk for growing children" (Schuster, Wang, & Hawkins 2018). Although plant-based milk is growing in popularity, its rise only explains a small portion of the decline in US fluid milk consumption, which is mainly due to generational changes in milk consumption, where newer generations are consuming less milk than preceding generations as each decade brings a wider selection of beverage choices at supermarkets, restaurants, and other food outlets (Stewart & Kuchler, 2022).

Meat and Other Protein Foods

Meat and other protein foods
all foods made from meat, poultry, seafood, beans and peas, eggs, processed soy products, nuts, and seeds

The total amount of meat, eggs, and nuts available for consumption grew from 162 pounds per person in 1970 to 180 pounds in 2018. A large portion of this increase is due to increased production of chicken, which has more than doubled from under 30 pounds per person in 1970 to over 65 pounds per person in 2018. This increase was due to technological and pharmaceutical innovations facilitating the production of very large, meaty broiler chickens, and the development of boneless chicken breasts, chicken nuggets, and ready-to-eat products, such as precooked chicken strips. Although the consumption of chicken has been on the rise, red meat and egg consumption have steadily declined since the 1970s, with increasing awareness of cholesterol and saturated fat. Seafood remains under-consumed among all age groups in the United States, and intakes have remained relatively stable since the 1970s (US Department of Agriculture and US Department of Health and Human Services, 2020; US Department of Agriculture: Economic Research Service, 2022c). Several varieties of seafood are higher in essential omega-3 fatty acids while being lower in methylmercury, including salmon, anchovies, sardines, Pacific oysters, and trout. Consumption of at least two servings of these foods per week may have beneficial effects on heart health as well as child and infant health and neurodevelopment (US Department of Agriculture and US Department of Health and Human Services, 2020).

Added Sweeteners, Fats, and Oils

SSB are the leading sources of added sugar in the American diet. Frequent consumption of SSB is associated with weight gain, obesity, type 2 diabetes, heart diseases, nonalcoholic liver disease, dental cavities, gout, and arthritis (Centers for Disease Control and Prevention, 2022b). The good news is that studies indicate that intake of SSB is declining; Between 2003–2004 and 2013–2014, the proportion of the population consuming at least one SSB per day declined from 80% to 61% among children and from 62% to 50% among adults. Between 2003–2004 and 2015–2016, heavy SSB intake (defined as >500 calories/day) declined from 11% to 3% among children and 12% to 9% among adults (Vercammen, Moran, Soto, Kennedy-Shaffer, & Bleich, 2020). Despite these improvements in SSB intake, most Americans are still consuming excessive amounts of added sugars, which are recommended to make up no more than 10% of daily calories according to the 2020–2025 DGA (US Department of Agriculture and US Department of Health and Human Services, 2020). Beginning in 2020, food manufacturers are required to list "added sugars" in grams and % Daily Value on the Nutrition Facts label in order to assist Americans with identifying the added sugar content of foods (US Food and Drug Administration, 2022a).

> **Added sweeteners, fats, and oils** found in a variety of processed foods, including soft drinks, breads, sauces, and desserts; added fats and oils found in processed foods such as French fries, baked goods, and snacks, and also used in food preparation and cooking

Added fats and oil availability have increased by almost 30 pounds per person per year between 1970 and 2010. Interestingly, the intake of animal fats, including butter, lard, beef, and tallow, has dropped while intake of vegetable oils has trended upward by 87% and salad and cooking oil has increased by 248% during this time period (Bentley, 2017). These shifts are in line with the recommendations in the 2020–2025 DGA, which recommend consuming liquid oils in place of saturated fats/animal fats (US Department of Agriculture and US Department of Health and Human Services, 2020).

Table 5.4 compares the 2020–2025 DGA with the most recent dietary consumption data with regards to grains; fruits and vegetables; milk, meats, and protein; added sweets; and fats and oils.

Where Americans Eat

Americans are increasingly consuming meals away from home, which tend to be higher in fat, sugar, and salt than home-prepared meals. From 1987 to 2010, the percentage of food dollars spent on meals away from home increased from 44% to 52.2%. Data indicate that Americans cut back on spending on restaurant meals due to the economic recession of 2007–2009 and were preparing slightly more meals at home (Kumcu & Kaufman, 2011). Home cooking spiked during the early part of the COVID-19 pandemic, and as of 2022, "cooking fatigue" has set in for many families. Retailers are responding by offering additional fresh prepared and meal kit options, as well as "shoppable recipes" that link shopping lists with TikTok videos and other social media (Crawford, 2022; Febrey & Tibbetts, 2022).

> **Beverages** include soft drinks, juices, and juice drinks, tap water and bottled water, coffee, tea, and milk (dairy and nondairy)

Table 5.4   A Comparison of the 2020–2025 Dietary Guidelines for Americans and the Average American Diet

	Dietary Guidelines Recommendations (2020–2015)*	Average American Consumption (2014)	Main Contributing Food Sources	DGA Foods to Increase
Grains	6 ounces, half of which should be whole grains	6.7 ounces	Grain-based snack foods and bakery items (such as crackers, cakes, and cookies) as well as breads, buns, dough, and tortillas	Brown rice, whole grain breads, whole wheat pastas, oatmeal, and other whole grain foods
Fruits and vegetables	2 cups of fruit 2.5 cups of vegetables	.9 cups of fruit 1.6 cups of vegetables	Orange and apple juice Potatoes, tomatoes, onions, and lettuce	Leafy green vegetables, orange vegetables, and beans, starchy vegetables
Dairy	3 cups	1.5 cups	Cheese	Fat-free and reduced-fat milk products and soy-based milk alternatives
Meats and proteins	5.5 ounces	7.1 ounces	Chicken and processed chicken products	Fish and seafood, beans, peas, nuts, and seeds
Added sugars	12.5 teaspoons (limit)	23 teaspoons	Soft drinks and high fructose corn	N/A
Fats and oils	27 grams	63 grams	Vegetable oils and fats	Vegetable oils and fats

*All recommendations are based on a two-thousand-calorie-per-day diet.
Source: https://www.ers.usda.gov/webdocs/publications/82220/eib-166.pdf?v=7719.5

The Food Industry: Friend, Foe, or Both?

The food industry spends almost $14 billion per year marketing its products to American consumers each year, and more than 80% of this advertising promotes SSB, fast food, candy, and ultra-processed snacks (UConn Rudd Center for Food Policy and Health, 2020b). Marketing is a powerful driver of increased caloric intake from high-calorie foods and beverages. High-calorie–low-nutrient foods are highly available and heavily marketed, creating a perfect combination for people to eat them (Institute of Medicine, 2012). Many of the foods marketed to consumers are the very foods people should cut back on, according to the DGA.

The food industry has adopted a number of voluntary initiatives to address public health concerns about their products. In 2006, several leading US food and beverage companies created the Children's Food and Beverage Advertising Initiative (CFBAI) to commit to uniform advertising standards for foods marketed to children under the age of thirteen. This group of twenty companies has committed to either not advertise foods or beverages to children at all or to advertise only products that meet CFBAIs uniform nutrition criteria, which include limits on calories, saturated fat, sodium, and added sugars and include minimum requirements for important food groups and key nutrients (BBBPrograms, n.d.). While there has been a small decrease in the percentage of foods high in sodium, saturated fat, and added sugar advertised to children since the inception of CFABI, analysis indicates that children aged two to eleven continue to view more than eleven food-product ads per day and that 72% of those ads are for fast foods, cereals, candy, snacks, and sugary drinks, and less than 10% of ads are for yogurt, dairy, bottled water, fruits, and vegetables. Industry has reformulated many popular products to conform with CFBAI nutrition standards by reducing the amount of sugar in cereals and adding whole grains, vitamins, and minerals. The jury is still out on whether "better for you" versions of low-nutrient density foods are truly improving the health of the nation's children (Fleming-Milici & Harris, 2020). Other companies are committing to improving their entire portfolio of products to meet certain nutrition criteria and to shift their marketing dollars toward their healthier products as part of their corporate responsibility initiatives (Partnership for a Healthier America, 2021). Food retailers are also becoming involved with point-of-sale promotions of healthier products, provision of nutrition education through in-store registered dietitians, and expansion of initiatives to bring mobile grocery units to low-access areas (Register, 2022). At this time, such initiatives are purely voluntary, as any efforts to establish mandatory national industry-wide nutrition standards for commercially available products have failed.

Farm Subsidies: The Culprit?

Farm subsidies are also a popular topic of discussion among nutrition-minded health professionals. Some argue that the billions of federal dollars paid to producers of corn and soybeans—often used in HFCS and other processed foods, oils, or cheap animal feed—are artificially lowering the price of less healthy food. However, a deeper dive into comparing the costs of highly processed foods (such as Twinkies) with fresh vegetables (such as carrots) reveals that redirecting farm subsidies could bring the price of Twinkies from $0.99 to $1.00 and could bring the cost of carrots from $2.99 to $2.97 per bunch. The reason that "junk foods" are so much cheaper than fruits and vegetables has more to do with the fact that most ultra-processed foods are made from shelf-stable ingredients (usually wheat, corn, and/or soy) compared to fresh produce, which involves substantial costs to grow and harvest as well as to keep fresh during storage and shipping. Redirecting subsidies to fresh produce may not actually make a huge dent in the price differential between carrots and Twinkies (Haspel, 2017).

Farm subsidies
paid to farmers and agribusinesses to supplement their income, manage the supply of agricultural commodities, and influence the cost and supply of such commodities; examples include wheat, feed grains (grains used as fodder, such as maize or corn, sorghum, barley, and oats), cotton, milk, rice, peanuts, sugar, tobacco, oilseeds such as soybeans, and meat products such as beef, pork, and lamb and mutton

Portion Sizes: Bigger but Not Better

The foods that Americans eat the most are generally tasty (by many people's standards), easy to get, cheap to buy, heavily marketed, and served in gigantic portions. Since the 1970s, portions have expanded at restaurants, grocery stores, and in prepackaged foods. Many studies suggest that when people are presented with larger portions of food, they tend to eat more. Restaurant meals are extremely large, often offering enough calories for an entire family in a single dish. Studies find that since the 1970s, people have eaten larger portions of salty snacks, soft drinks, hamburgers, French fries, Mexican dishes, grains and cereals, and many beverages, such as orange juice, juice drinks, soft drinks, and alcohol (beer and wine) (Division of Nutrition and Physical Activity, 2006).

Recent Efforts to Promote Healthy Eating

Despite the numerous negative trends described in this chapter, there are also many positive developments in the world of health and nutrition that may enable the country to create future progress in improving eating habits. Nutrition promotion initiatives are most likely to be successful when they work on multiple levels of the ecological model, affecting public policy (national, state, and local), communities, organizations, interpersonal relationships, and the individual. Examples of nutrition-related efforts operating on several levels of the ecological model are explained in chapter 3 under the program planning models.

National Policy Actions

Nutrition is being addressed at the national level through various government initiatives. In September 2022, the Biden–Harris administration convened the first White House Conference on Hunger, Nutrition, and Health in over 50 years and released a national strategy to address the overarching goal of "ending hunger in America and increasing healthy eating and physical activity by 2030 so that fewer Americans experience diet-related diseases—while reducing health disparities." The national strategy is divided into five pillars, including: (1) improving food access and affordability, (2) integrating nutrition and health, (3) empowering all consumers to make and have access to healthy choices, (4) supporting physical activity for all, and (5) enhancing nutrition and food security research. The national strategy calls for many actions, such as increasing access to free and nourishing school meals, expanding access to the Supplemental Nutrition Assistance Program (SNAP) and incentivizing fruits and vegetable purchases among SNAP recipients, expanding "food is medicine" meal delivery programs via Medicare and Medicaid, proposing a "front-of-package" nutrition labeling for packaged foods, lowering added sugars and sodium in packaged foods, connecting people to parks and outdoor spaces, and focusing on research to inform nutrition and food security policies. Many of these actions will require Congressional action to move forward, and ultimately, the success of the national strategy on hunger, nutrition, and health will take several years to assess.

Other recent national policy actions to address nutrition and chronic disease include mandatory disclosure of calories on chain restaurant menus (US Food and Drug Administration, 2020), the removal of industrially produced trans-fats from the food supply (US Food and Drug Administration, 2018), and updates to the Nutrition Facts label to include an easier-to-use format and disclosure of added sugars (US Food and Drug Administration, 2022b), updates to nutrition standards for childcare and school meal programs to provide additional fruits and vegetables and whole grains with less sugar and sodium (US Department of Agriculture, 2014).

The United States government operates several programs aimed at improving the nutrition of Americans. One of those programs is the **Women, Infants, and Children (WIC) program**, which provides supplemental food for low-income pregnant women and mothers with children up to the age of five. Currently, 43% of all infants in the United States are served by the WIC program, making it one of the most important federal nutrition programs (US Department of Agriculture: Economic Research Service, 2022d). In 2007, the WIC food package was updated to align with the DGA; WIC began providing increased amounts of vegetables and low-fat dairy as well as fruit, whole grains, tofu, and soy milk for the first time. The updated packages cut the amount of juice, cheese, and whole milk provided to participants (US Department of Agriculture: Food and Nutrition Service, 2009). The USDA is expected to issue a proposed rule for another update of the WIC food packages

Women, Infants, and Children (WIC) program
provides supplemental food for low-income pregnant women and mothers with children up to the age of five

in response to a 2017 report by the National Academies of Science, Engineering, and Medicine (National Academies of Sciences, Engineering, and Medicine, 2017). Some believe that SNAP (the Supplemental Nutrition Assistance Program; commonly referred to as "food stamps") should also change to align with the dietary guidelines because the program currently allows participants to purchase almost any food or beverage with this government benefit (besides hot food and alcoholic beverages). Others argue that such changes to SNAP are paternalistic and that restrictions are unnecessary. While SNAP remains a program that does not have nutritional limitations on what foods can be purchased with benefits, USDA offers a grant-based program called the Gus Schumacher Nutrition Incentive Program (GusNIP) that funds projects that provide incentives to SNAP participants at the point of purchase to boost fruit and vegetable consumption, although at the current time, this program is only available to a small fraction of SNAP recipients (John et al., 2021; US Department of Agriculture: National Institute of Food and Agriculture, 2022).

Finally, the federal government remains involved in providing dietary guidance to encourage Americans to make healthy food choices and to serve as a guide for nutrition policy. The *Dietary Guidelines for Americans*, released jointly by the Department of Health and Human Services and the USDA every five years, serves as the nation's nutrition guidance for policymakers, nutrition, and health professionals. The federal government has also released different versions of food guidance for the public over the years, including the Food Guide Pyramid, My Pyramid, and most recently MyPlate (www.myplate.gov), which can serve as an eating guide for individuals.

State Policy Actions

California provides an example of a state that has enacted a state-wide program to offer and cover medically tailored meals to members of its Medicaid health plans. Starting in 2022, people with chronic conditions such as diabetes, stroke, cancer, HIV, CVD, or behavioral health disorders, or those who have been discharged from a hospital or nursing facility with a high-risk of readmission, can receive up to three home-delivered meals per day for up to 12 weeks or longer if medically necessary. This program is based on data showing that medically tailored meals can improve health outcomes, reduce healthcare costs, and improve patient satisfaction. Similar programs covering meals are also available in New York, Massachusetts, North Carolina, and Oregon through their Medicaid-managed care plans (Sheldon, 2021).

Local Policy Actions

Many local areas are using policy in attempts to improve the nutrition and health of their populations. The New York City Department of Health required calorie listings on chain restaurant menus well before federal regulations mandated the practice and was also the first city to require chain restaurants to post a warning icon next to menu items that contain at least 2,300 mg of sodium (NYC Health, n.d.-c). The city also has a policy establishing nutrition standards for foods served in hospitals, nursing homes, homeless shelters, and all city vending machines. A city program called *Health Bucks* extends the buying power of SNAP recipients to purchase fresh fruits and vegetables at participating farmers' markets

(NYC Health, n.d.-b), and the *Get the Good Stuff* program provides extra funding for SNAP participants to purchase fruits, vegetables, and beans in participating supermarkets (NYC Health, n.d.-a). Perhaps most controversially, the New York City Health Department passed an ordinance restricting the sale of soft drinks in sizes exceeding sixteen ounces; however, the New York appeals court struck down the ruling, stating that the Department of Health exceeded its legal authority by limiting the size of a soda (Grynbaum, 2012; New York City Obesity Task Force, 2012).

Community Nutrition Efforts

Numerous communities are working together to promote healthy eating. Local and community efforts range from attracting more supermarkets to food deserts, to encouraging corner stores in urban areas to offer healthier food choices, to promoting farmers' markets, to providing nutrition education directly to consumers in grocery stores.

Many community organizations are actively engaged in nutrition outreach. The Philadelphia-based Food Trust is an organization that aims to increase healthy food access for all members of the community. Their Healthy Corner Store Initiative has increased nutritious offerings in corner stores by providing stores with training, equipment, and marketing materials to store and display healthy items (The Food Trust, n.d.). Community organizations can receive grant funding to implement programs to increase access to healthy food through the Healthy Food Financing Initiative (HFFI). HFFI has helped leverage more than $220 million in grants and $1 billion in additional financing to support nearly 1,000 grocery and healthy food retail projects in more than 35 states across the country (America's Healthy Food Initiative, 2020). Additionally, the USDA offers a Community Food Projects Competitive Grant program to provide grants to community organizations seeking to improve their local food systems to increase nutrition security among vulnerable populations (US Department of Agriculture: National Institute of Food and Agriculture, n.d.).

Worksite Wellness

Worksite environments significantly influence health behaviors and are increasingly popular as employers aim to lower health care costs and improve employee productivity. Approximate 82% of large firms and 53% of small employers in the United States offer a wellness program, making worksite wellness an $8 billion industry (Song & Baicker, 2019). Worksite wellness often includes not only nutrition workshops, modules, and challenges but also activities related to physical activity, stress reduction, and mental health support. Many programs also offer financial incentives for completing training or meeting specific goals.

In addition to formal programs and trainings, worksites can also offer healthier environments for employees. The CDC considers nutrition a key component of worksite wellness programs. CDC encourages workplace nutrition programs that encourage healthy eating among all employees and emphasize the importance of fruits, vegetables, whole grains, low-fat dairy products, lean meats, poultry fish, and legumes (Centers for Disease Control and Prevention, 2016). Millions of people consume meals and snacks at work every day; applying nutrition standards to foods offered in workplace cafeterias and vending machines can promote employee health and wellbeing. Additionally, providing nutrition education to employees while they are at work may also have a positive impact on their productivity and overall health—ultimately benefiting the employer's bottom line. The Biden–Harris National Strategy on Hunger, Nutrition, and Health proposed implementing and updating the Federal Food Service Guidelines to promote increased availability of fruits, vegetables, whole grains, low-fat dairy, low-sodium options, and plant-based options to millions of federal employees and other people who access food at government facilities.

Employers are also increasingly looking toward implementing high-tech, personalized medicine programs such as Virta Health. This program offers participants with type 2 diabetes access to an app to track blood sugars and symptoms, which are monitored by physicians and health coaches who are available to offer remote real-time support and tailored nutrition advice that can save employers an average of $5,500 per member per year and reduce diabetes prescription volume by an average of 59% (Virta Health, n.d.).

School Food Environments

Most children spend a substantial amount of time at school during their impressionable developmental years. Children who participate in the National School Lunch Program and School Breakfast Program obtain nearly half of their calories at school (Gleason & Dodd, 2009). School meals are often debated as a contributor to childhood obesity and other health issues. The **Healthy Hunger-Free Kids Act of 2010** made inroads toward ensuring that school lunches and a la carte options are aligned with current health standards. Beginning in 2012, all school meals in the United States were required to include more fruits, vegetables, whole grains, low-fat milk, and less sodium and saturated fat (US Department of Agriculture: Food and Nutrition Service, 2012). The Healthy Hunger-Free Kids Act also calls for an update of nutrition standards for "competitive foods" (foods sold in addition to the school meals, such as a la carte and vending options), which is important because improving the nutritional profile of those foods has been shown to significantly decrease children's intake of calories, total fat, and saturated fat (Snelling & Yezek, 2012).

> **Healthy Hunger-free Kids Act of 2010**
> act that requires all school meals in the United States to include more fruits, vegetables, whole grains, low-fat milk, and less sodium and saturated fat; also calls for an update of nutrition standards for "competitive foods" (foods sold in addition to the school meals, such as a la carte and vending options)

Not only can schools promote health by improving nutritious food offerings, but they can also provide nutrition education to students. The USDA has developed a variety of resources through their Team Nutrition initiative, including recipe books, curricula, posters, and best practices documents that can be ordered free of charge to all schools and child care centers that participate in the Federal Child Nutrition Programs (US Department of Agriculture: Food and Nutrition Service, n.d.).

Programs for the Individual

Recent studies affirm the effectiveness of one-on-one nutrition programs to improve food selection and promote positive health outcomes. Nutrition education programs implemented in supermarkets to assist shoppers with making healthy choices have been shown to positively affect people's purchases of fruits and vegetables (Milliron, Woolf, & Appelhans, 2012). Many people receive nutrition counseling from registered dietitians or other qualified health professionals; researchers have found that one-on-one counseling can have a lasting effect on weight loss, lowering the risk of type 2 diabetes, hypertension (high blood pressure), and high cholesterol (Dansinger, Tatsioni, Wong, Chung, & Balk, 2007).

Summary

The importance of nutrition for maintaining good health is without question. Many of the leading causes of death and disability worldwide can be traced, at least in part, to poor dietary quality. Changes in dietary habits have occurred very recently in human history, with dramatic effects on the health of our species and our planet. The US food supply provides ample opportunities for individuals to consume foods that are low in nutrients and high in calories, in the form of inexpensive processed foods and large restaurant meals and portions. Health promotion professionals must be able to make changes to the food environment as well as encourage individual behavior change through education and coaching in order to create successful and lasting dietary change.

KEY TERMS

1. **Dietary Guidelines for Americans:** nutrition guidelines jointly issued and updated every five years by the Departments of Health and Human Services and Agriculture; provide authoritative advice for Americans ages two and older about consuming fewer calories, making informed food choices, and being physically active to attain and maintain a healthy weight, reduce risk of chronic disease, and promote overall health

2. **Heart disease:** generally refers to conditions that involve narrowed or blocked blood vessels that can lead to a heart attack, chest pain (angina), or stroke

3. **Cancer:** term used for diseases in which abnormal cells divide without control and are able to invade other tissues

4. **Stroke:** occurs when the blood supply to part of the brain is interrupted or severely reduced, depriving brain tissue of oxygen and food; within minutes, brain cells begin to die

5. **Type 2 diabetes:** once known as adult-onset or noninsulin-dependent diabetes; is a chronic condition that affects the way the body metabolizes sugar (glucose), the body's main source of fuel; with type 2 diabetes, the body either resists the effects of insulin—a hormone that regulates the movement of sugar into the cells—or does not produce enough insulin to maintain a normal glucose level; untreated, can be life-threatening

6. **Westernized diet:** high in calories, processed foods, added sugars, solid fats, refined grains, and sodium; is associated with increased risk for obesity and several major chronic diseases

7. **DASH (dietary approaches to stop hypertension)-style eating pattern:** a low-sodium regimen for patients with hypertension that emphasizes fruits, vegetables, low-fat dairy foods, whole-grain products, fish, poultry, and nuts; low in saturated and total

fat, cholesterol, red meat, sweets, and sugared beverages; high in magnesium, potassium, calcium, protein, and fiber

8. **Mediterranean-style dietary pattern:** emphasizes eating primarily plant-based foods, such as fruits and vegetables, whole grains, legumes, and nuts; replacing butter with healthy fats, such as olive oil; using herbs and spices instead of salt to flavor foods; limiting red meat to no more than a few times a month; eating fish and poultry at least twice a week; drinking red wine in moderation (optional)

9. **Grains:** any food made from wheat, rice, oats, cornmeal, barley, or another cereal grain, such as bread, pasta, oatmeal, breakfast cereals, tortillas, and grits

10. **Fruits and vegetables:** nutritionally speaking, similar to each other; generally lower in calories and fat than animal products; also contain health-enhancing plant compounds, such as fiber and antioxidants; loaded with vitamins and minerals

11. **Beverages:** include soft drinks, juices, juice drinks, tap water and bottled water, coffee, tea, and milk (dairy and nondairy)

12. **Meat and other protein foods:** all foods made from meat, poultry, seafood, beans and peas, eggs, processed soy products, nuts, and seeds

13. **Added sweeteners, fats, and oils:** found in a variety of processed foods, including soft drinks, breads, sauces, and desserts; added fats and oils found in processed foods such as French fries, baked goods, and snacks, and also used in food preparation and cooking

14. **Farm subsidies:** paid to farmers and agribusinesses to supplement their income, manage the supply of agricultural commodities, and influence the cost and supply of such commodities; examples include wheat, feed grains (grains used as fodder, such as maize or corn, sorghum, barley, and oats), cotton, milk, rice, peanuts, sugar, tobacco, oilseeds such as soybeans, and meat products such as beef, pork, and lamb and mutton

15. **Women, Infants, and Children (WIC) program:** provides supplemental food for low-income pregnant women and mothers with children up to the age of five

16. **Healthy Hunger-Free Kids Act of 2010:** act that requires all school meals in the United States to include more fruits, vegetables, whole grains, low-fat milk, and less sodium and saturated fat; also calls for an update of nutrition standards for "competitive foods" (foods sold in addition to the school meals, such as a la carte and vending options)

17. **Ultra-processed foods:** the NOVA food classification system groups foods into four groups, including: (1) **unprocessed and minimally processed** foods, including plants, animals, fungi, algae, and water; (2) **processed culinary ingredients**, including oils, butter, lard, sugar, and salt; (3) **processed foods** made by combining group 1 and 2 foods, which could include canned foods, preserved animal foods, breads, and cheeses, and which retain the basic identity of the original group 1 food; and (4) **ultra-processed foods**, which are formulations of industrially created ingredients, where group 1 foods are either missing or are present in small amounts.

REVIEW QUESTIONS

1. What are the factors that influence people's eating patterns?

2. How have these factors changed over the decades?

3. What are the trends of overweight and obesity for children and adults in the United States?

4. What are the benefits of healthy eating?

5. What educational tools are available to guide healthy eating?

6. What are the five historic dietary patterns of eating?

7. What has been the availability of food over the past one hundred years?

8. How does the food industry influence eating patterns?

9. What are some national and state policies to promote healthy eating?

10. What is the school food environment doing to promote healthy eating?

GENERAL

STUDENT ACTIVITIES

1. Review the following quote from Cohen (2008, p. S141):

    A more accurate conceptualization of the obesity epidemic is that people are responding to the forces in their environment, rather than lacking in will power and self-control. A metaphor that more truly captures the phenomenon is the tsunami. The environmental tsunami of cues and stimuli artificially make people hungry and lead them to unintentionally overconsume and to remain excessively sedentary. The societal response to the tsunami has been to provide swimming lessons and cheerleaders. The response has clearly not been proportional to the threat. People cannot change their responses to cues they do not perceive. Unless we focus on a more appropriate response, the obesity epidemic will continue. The real solution would be to control and reduce those forces that are causing the tsunami, change the cues we are exposed to on a daily basis or make explicit the cues we cannot change. Only then will people be able to make good use of the swimming lessons they receive, and bring themselves into energy balance according to their individual preferences.

    a. What do you think this quote means when it refers to "swimming lessons and cheerleaders"?

b. Do you believe the forces identified in the first question are substantial enough to change the public's eating habits and begin to reduce obesity? If so, why? If not, why not?

c. What do you think Cohen means when referring to the "forces that are causing the tsunami"? How do you think those forces play into nutrition choices?

d. Do you agree with Cohen's quote? Please explain why or why not.

2. Several examples of nutrition programs on various levels of the ecological model were provided in the chapter. Find three additional examples of nutrition programs operating on various levels of the ecological model. Write a brief description of the program and outline your opinions on the strengths and weaknesses of each program.

3. Draw a schematic of leading causes of death and the nutrition factors.

References

Afshin, A., Sur P., Fay K., Cornabay, L., Ferrara, G., Salama, J. S., . . .Murray, C. J. (2019). Health effects of dietary risks in 195 countries, 1990–2017: A systematic analysis for the global burden of disease study 2017. *The Lancet, 393*(10184), 1958–1972. doi: https://doi.org/10.1016/S0140-6736(19)30041-8

America's Healthy Food Finance Initiative. (2020). *About America's healthy food finance initiative.* Retrieved from https://www.investinginfood.com/about-hffi

Anekwe, T. D., & Zeballos, E. (2019). *Food-related time use: Changes and demographic differences.* United States Department of Agriculture, Economic Research Service.

Antin, T.M.J. and Hunt, G. (2012). Food choice as a multidimensional experience. A qualitative study with young African American women. *Appetite 58*(3): 856–863.

BBBPrograms. (n.d.). *Children's food & beverage advertising initiative.* Retrieved from https://bbbprograms.org/programs/all-programs/cfbai

Bentley, J. (2017). *U.S. trends in food availability and a dietary assessment of loss-adjusted food availability, 1970–2014.* United States Department of Agriculture, Economic Research Service.

Brones, A. (2018). Karen Washington: It's not a food desert, it's food apartheid. *Guernica Magazine* (7 May).

Caballero, B. and Popkin, B.M. (2002). *The nutrition transition: Diet and disease in the developing world.* Amsterdam: Academic Press.

Centers for Disease Control and Prevention. (2016). *Workplace health strategies: Nutrition.* Retrieved from https://www.cdc.gov/workplacehealthpromotion/health-strategies/nutrition/index.html

Centers for Disease Control and Prevention. (2022a). *Cancer.* Retrieved from https://www.cdc.gov/chronicdisease/resources/publications/factsheets/cancer.htm

Centers for Disease Control and Prevention. (2022b). *Get the facts: Sugar-sweetened beverages and consumption.* Retrieved from https://www.cdc.gov/nutrition/data-statistics/sugar-sweetened-beverages-intake.html

Centers for Disease Control and Prevention. (2022c). *Health effects of overweight and obesity.* Retrieved from https://www.cdc.gov/healthyweight/effects/index.html

Centers for Disease Control and Prevention. (2022d). *Heart disease facts*. Retrieved from https://www.cdc.gov/healthyweight/effects/index.html

Centers for Disease Control and Prevention. (2022e). *Stroke*. Retrieved from https://www.cdc.gov/stroke/facts.htm

ChooseMyPlate.gov. (2022a). *Grains*. Retrieved from https://www.myplate.gov/eat-healthy/grains

ChooseMyPlate.gov. (2022b). *MyPlate*. Retrieved from https://www.myplate.gov/

ChooseMyPlate.gov. (n.d.). *MyPlate graphic resources*. Retrieved from https://www.myplate.gov/resources/graphics/myplate-graphics

Cohen, D.A. (2008). Obesity and the built environment: Changes in environmental cues cause energy imbalances. *International Journal of Obesity 32* (Suppl. 7): S137–S142.

Cohen, D. A. & Babey, S. H. (2012). Contextual influences on eating behaviours: Heuristic processing and dietary choices. *Obesity Reviews, 13*(9), 766–779. doi: https://doi.org/10.1111/j.1467-789X.2012.01001.x

Crawford, E. (2022). *Waning interest in cooking at home creates opportunities, challenges for retailers, brands.* Retrieved from https://www.foodnavigator-usa.com/Article/2022/07/05/waning-interest-in-cooking-at-home-creates-opportunities-challenges-for-retailers-brands

Dansinger, M.L., Tatsioni, A., Wong, J.B. et al. (2007). Meta-analysis: The effect of dietary counseling for weight loss. *Annals of Internal Medicine 147*(1): 41–50.

Division of Nutrition and Physical Activity (2006). *Research to practice series no. 2: Portion size.* Atlanta: Centers for Disease Control and Prevention.

Drewnowski, A. and Darmon, N. (2005). The economics of obesity: Dietary energy density and energy cost. *American Journal of Clinical Nutrition 82* (Suppl. 1): 265S–273S.

Evert, A., Dennison, M., Gardner, C., W. T. Garvey, K. H. K. Lau, J. MacLeod, J. Mitri, R. F. Pereira, K. Rawlings, S. Robinson, L. Saslow, S. Uelmen, P. B. Urbanski, W. S. Yancy, Jr. (2019). Nutrition therapy for adults with diabetes or prediabetes: A consensus report. *Diabetes Care, 42*(5), 731–754. doi: https://doi.org/10.2337/dci19-0014

Fazzino, T., Rohde, K., & Sullivan D. (2019). Hyper-palatable foods: Development of a quantitative definition and application to the US food system database. *Obesity, 27*(11), 1761–1768. doi: https://doi.org/10.1002/oby.22639

Febrey, A., & Tibbetts, R. (2022). *From sourdough-mania to cooking fatigue: Food preparation habits in a post-lockdown world*. Retrieved from https://www.fmi.org/blog/view/fmi-blog/2022/07/14/from-sourdough-mania-to-cooking-fatigue-food-preparation-habits-in-a-post-lockdown-world

Fielding-Singh, P. (2022). *How the other half eats: The untold story of food and inequality in America.* New York: Little, Brown Spark.

Fleming-Milici, F., & Harris, J. L. (2020). Food marketing to children in the United States: Can industry voluntarily do the right thing for children's health? *Physiology & Behavior, 227*, 113139–113139. doi: https://doi.org/10.1016/j.physbeh.2020.113139

Fryar, C. D., Carroll, M. D., & Afful, J. (2020). Prevalence of overweight, obesity, and severe obesity among adults aged 20 and over: United States, 1960–1962 through 2017–2018. *NCHS health e-stats*, 1–7.

Gleason, P. M., & Dodd, A. H. (2009). School breakfast program but not school lunch program participation is associated with lower body mass index. *Journal of the American Dietetic Association, 109*(Suppl. 2) S118–S128. doi: https://doi.org/10.1016/j.jada.2008.10.058

Grynbaum, M. (2012). Health panel approves restriction on sale of large sugary drinks. *New York Times.* Retrieved from www.nytimes.com/2012/09/14/nyregion/health-board-approves-bloombergs-soda-ban.html

Gurven, M. and Kaplan, H. (2007). Longevity among hunter-gatherers: A cross-cultural examination. *Population and Development Review 33*(2): 321–365.

Hall, K., Farooqi, S., Friedman, J., S. Klein, R. J. F. Loos, D. J. Mangelsdorf, S. O'Rahilly, E. Ravussin, L. M. Redman, D. H. Ryan, J. R. Speakman, D. K. Tobias (2022). The energy balance model of obesity: Beyond calories in, calories out. *The American Journal of Clinical Nutrition, 115*(5), 1243–1254. doi: https://doi.org/10.1093/ajcn/nqac031

Haspel, T. (2017). *Junk food is cheap and healthful food is expensive, but don't blame the farm bill.* Retrieved from https://www.washingtonpost.com/lifestyle/food/im-a-fan-of-michael-pollan-but-on-one-food-policy-argument-hes-wrong/2017/12/04/c71881ca-d6cd-11e7-b62d-d9345ced896d_story.html

Institute of Medicine (2012). *Accelerating progress in obesity prevention: Solving the weight of the nation.* Washington, DC: National Academies Press.

International Food Information Council. (2021). *2021 Food & health survey.* Retrieved from https://foodinsight.org/2021-food-health-survey/

Jacobson, M. (2006). *Six arguments for a greener diet.* Washington, DC: Center for Science in the Public Interest.

John, S., Lyerly, R., Wilde, P., Cohen, E. D., Lawson, E., & Nunn, A. 2021). The case for a national SNAP fruit and vegetable incentive program. *American Journal of Public Health, (1971), 111*(1), 27–29. doi: https://doi.org/10.2105/AJPH.2020.305987

Kleindorfer, D., Amytis T., Seemant, C., K. M. Cockroft, J. Gutierrez, D. Lombardi-Hill, H. Kamel, W. N. Kernan, S. J. Kittner, E. C. Leira, O. Lennon, J. F. Meschia, T. N. Nguyen, P. M. Pollak, P. Santangeli, A. Z. Sharrief, S. C. Smith Jr, T. N. Turan, L. S. Williams (2021). 2021 Guideline for the prevention of stroke in patients with stroke and transient ischemic attack: A guideline from the American Heart Association/American Stroke Association. *Stroke, 52*(7), e364–e467. doi: https://doi.org/10.1161/STR.0000000000000375

Kolodinsky, J. M. & Goldstein, A. B. (2011). Time use and food pattern influences on obesity. *Obesity, 19*(12), 2327–2335. doi: https://doi.org/10.1038/oby.2011.130

Kumcu, A., & Kaufman, P. (2011). Food spending adjustments during recessionary times. *Amber Waves.* Retrieved from www.ers.usda.gov/amber-waves/2011-september/food-spending.aspx#.UvAMCbRn1Ns

Laran, J. and Salerno, A. (2013). Life-history strategy, food choice, and caloric consumption. *Psychological Science 24* (2): 167–173.

Larsson, S.C. (2017). Dietary approaches for stroke prevention. *Stroke, 48*(10), 2905–2911. doi: https://doi.org/10.1161/STROKEAHA.117.017383

Lichtenstein, A., Appel, L., Vadeiveloo, M., F. B. Hu, P. M. Kris-Etherton, C. M. Rebholz, F. M. Sacks, A. N. Thorndike, L. Van Horn, J. Wylie-Rosett (2021). Dietary guidance to improve cardiovascular health: A scientific statement from the American Heart Association. *Circulation, 144*(23), e472–e487. doi: https://doi.org/10.1161/CIR.0000000000001031

Mancino, L., & Newman, C. (2007). *Who has time to cook? How family resources influence food preparation* (No. 55961). Washington, DC: US Department of Agriculture, Economic Research Service.

Medeiros, F., Casanova, M., Fraulob, J. C., & Trindade, M. (2012). How can diet influence the risk of stroke? *International Journal of Hypertension*, 763507. doi: https://doi.org/10.1155/2012/763507

Milliron, B.-J., Woolf, K., and Appelhans, B.M. (2012). A point-of-purchase intervention featuring in-person supermarket education affects healthful food purchases. *Journal of Nutrition Education and Behavior 44*(3): 225–232.

Monteiro, C. A., Cannon, G., Lawrence, M., Louzada, M. D. C., & Machado, P. P. (2019). *Ultra-processed foods, diet quality, and health using the NOVA classification system.* Food and Agricultural Association of the United Nations.

Morrison, R. M., Buzby, J. C., & Wells, H. F. (2010). Guess who's turning 100? Tracking a century of American eating. *Amber Waves.* Retrieved from www.purl.umn.edu/122141

Moss, M. (2021). *Hooked: Food, free will, and how the food giants exploit our addictions.* New York: Random House.

Mozaffarian, D. (2016). Dietary and policy priorities for cardiovascular disease, diabetes, and obesity. *Circulation, 133*(2),187–225. doi: https://doi.org/10.1161/CIRCULATIONAHA.115.018585

Murphy S., Kochanek K., Xu J. Q., & Arias, E. (2020). Mortality in the United States. *NCHS data brief,* no 427. Hyattsville, MD: National Center for Health Statistics. doi: https://dx.doi.org/10.15620/cdc:112079

National Academies of Sciences, Engineering, and Medicine. (2017). *Review of WIC food packages: Improving balance and choice: Final report.* Washington, DC: The National Academies Press. doi: https://doi.org/10.17226/23655.

Ndanuko, R. N., Tapsell, L. C., Charlton, K. E., Neale, E. P., & Batterham, M. J. (2016). Dietary patterns and blood pressure in adults: A systematic review and meta-analysis of randomized controlled trials. *Advances in Nutrition, 7*(1), 76–89. doi: https://doi.org/10.3945/an.115.009753

New York City Obesity Task Force. (2012). *Reversing the epidemic: The New York City Obesity Task force plan to prevent and control obesity.* Retrieved from www.nyc.gov/html/om/pdf/2012/otf_report.pdf

NYC Health. (n.d.-a). *Get the good stuff.* Retrieved from https://www.nyc.gov/site/doh/health/health-topics/free-produce-snap.page

NYC Health. (n.d.-b). *Health bucks.* Retrieved from https://www.nyc.gov/site/doh/health/health-topics/health-bucks.page

NYC Health. (n.d.-c). *Sodium initiatives.* Retrieved from https://www.nyc.gov/site/doh/health/health-topics/national-salt-reduction-initiative.page#:~:text=Sodium%20Warning%20Rule%20in%20NYC,at%20least%202300mg%20of%20sodium

Okrent, A.M. and Kumcu, A. (2016). *U.S. households' demand for convenience food.* Washington, DC: United States Department of Agriculture, Economic Research Service.

Partnership for a Healthier America. (2021). Keurig Dr Pepper advances corporate responsibility agenda through commitment with partnership for a healthier America. Press release (30 June).

Ploeg, M. V., Breneman, V., Farrigan, T., Hamrick, K., Hopkins, D., Kaufman, P. . . . Kim, S. (2009). Access to affordable and nutritious food measuring and understanding food deserts and their consequences. *Administrative Publication, 160* (AP-036).

Popkin, B.M. (2006). Global nutrition dynamics: The world is shifting rapidly toward a diet linked with noncommunicable diseases. *American Journal of Clinical Nutrition 84*(2): 289–298.

Popkin, B., & Gordon-Larsen, P. (2004). The nutrition transition: Worldwide obesity dynamics and their determinants. *International Journal of Obesity, 28*, S2–S9. doi: https://doi.org/10.1038/sj.ijo.0802804

Popkin, B. M., Adair, L. S., & Ng, S. W. (2012). Global nutrition transition and the pandemic of obesity in developing countries. *Nutrition Reviews, 70*(1), 3–21. doi: https://doi.org/10.1111/j.1753-4887.2011.00456.x

Putnam, J., & Allshouse, J. (2003). Trends in U.S. per capita consumption of dairy products, 1909 to 2001. *Amber Waves: The Economics of Food, Farming, Natural Resources, and Rural America.*

Raghupathi, W., & Raghupathi, V. (2018). An empirical study of chronic diseases in the United States: A visual analytics approach to public health. *International Journal of Environmental Research and Public Health, 15*(3), 431. doi: https://doi.org/10.3390/ijerph15030431

Register, K. (2022). *The food industry is working to improve nutrition security*. Retrieved from https://www.fmi.org/blog/view/fmi-blog/2022/08/15/the-food-industry-is-working-to-improve-nutrition-security

Roberts, C. K., & Barnard, R. J. (2005). Effects of exercise and diet on chronic disease. *Journal of Applied Physiology, 98*(1), 3–30. doi: https://doi.org/10.1152/japplphysiol.00852.2004

Rock, C., Thomson, C., T. Gansler, Gapstur, S. M., McCullough, M. L., Patel, A. V., . . . & Doyle, C. (2020). American Cancer Society guideline for diet and physical activity for cancer prevention. *CA: A Cancer Journal for Clinicians, 70*(4), 245–271. doi: https://doi.org/10.3322/caac.21591

Roubinov, D. S., Hagan, M. J., Boyce, W. T., Adler, N. E., & Bush, N. R. (2018). Family socioeconomic status, cortisol, and physical health in early childhood: The role of advantageous neighborhood characteristics. *Psychosomatic Medicine, 80*(5), 492–501. doi: https://doi.org/10.1097/PSY.0000000000000585

Scheibehenne, B., Miesler, L., & Todd, P. M. (2007). Fast and frugal food choices: Uncovering individual decision heuristics. *Appetite, 49*(3), 578–589. doi: https://doi.org/10.1016/j.appet.2007.03.224

Schuster, M., Wang, X., & Hawkins, T. (2018). Comparison of the nutrient content of cow's milk and nondairy milk alternatives: What's the difference? *Nutrition Today, 53*(4), 153–159. doi: https://doi.org/10.1097/NT.0000000000000284

Sheldon, M. (2021). *Medically tailored meals become a covered service option in California*. Retrieved from https://www.nycfoodpolicy.org/food-policy-snapshot-medically-tailored-meals-california-medicaid/

Sibal, V. (2018). Food: Identity of culture and religion. *Scholarly Research Journal for Interdisciplinary Studies, 6*(46): 10908–10915.

Sliwa, S. A., Must, A., Peréa, F., & Economos, C. D. (2015). Maternal employment, acculturation, and time spent in food-related behaviors among Hispanic mothers in the United States. Evidence from the American Time Use Survey. *Appetite,* 8710–19. doi: https://doi.org/10.1016/j.appet.2014.10.015

Snelling, A. M., & Yezek, J. (2012). The effect of nutrient-based standards on competitive foods in 3 schools: Potential savings in kilocalories and grams of fat. *Journal of School Health, 82*(2), 91–96. doi: https://doi.org/10.1111/j.1746–1561.2011.00671.x

Song, Z., & Baicker, K. (2019). Effect of a workplace wellness program on employee health and economic outcomes: A randomized clinical trial. *Journal of the American Medical Association, 321*(15), 1491–1501. doi: https://doi.org/10.1001/jama.2019.3307

Steptoe, A., Pollard, T. M., & Wardle, J. (1995). Development of a measure of the motives underlying the selection of food: The food choice questionnaire. *Appetite, 25*(3), 267–284. doi: https://doi.org/10.1006/appe.1995.0061

Stewart, H. and Hyman, J. (2019). Americans still can meet fruit and vegetable dietary guidelines for $2.10–$2.60 per day. *Amber Waves,* 1–6.

Stewart, H. and Kuchler, F. (2022). Fluid milk consumption continues downward trend, proving difficult to reverse. *Amber Waves,* 1–9.

Taillie, L. S., Busey, E., Stoltze, F. M., & Dillman Carpentier, F. R., (2019). Governmental policies to reduce unhealthy food marketing to children. *Nutrition Reviews, 77*(11), 787–816. doi: https://doi.org/10.1093/nutrit/nuz021

The Food Trust. (n.d.). *Health in the heart of the community*. Retrieved from https://thefoodtrust.org/what-we-do/corner-stores/

Tryon, M.S., Carter, C.S., DeCant, R., and Laugero, K.D. (2013). Chronic stress exposure may affect the brain's response to high calorie food cues and predispose to obesogenic eating habit. *Physiology & Behavior 120*: 233–242.

UConn Rudd Center for Food Policy and Health. (2020a). *Targeted marketing*. Retrieved from https://uconnruddcenter.org/research/food-marketing/targetedmarketing/#

UConn Rudd Center for Food Policy and Health. (2020b). *Food marketing*. Retrieved from https://uconnruddcenter.org/research/food-marketing/#a1

US Department of Agriculture. (2014). Fact sheet: Healthy, hunger-free kids act school meals implementation. Press release (20 May).

US Department of Agriculture and US Department of Health and Human Services. (2020). *Dietary guidelines for Americans, 2020–2025*. Retrieved from https://www.dietaryguidelines.gov/sites/default/files/2021-03/Dietary_Guidelines_for_Americans-2020-2025.pdf

US Department of Agriculture: Economic Research Service. (2022a). *Food security and nutrition assistance*. Retrieved from https://www.ers.usda.gov/data-products/ag-and-food-statistics-charting-the-essentials/food-security-and-nutrition-assistance/#:~:text=The%20prevalence%20of%20food%20insecurity,had%20very%20low%20food%20security

US Department of Agriculture: Economic Research Service. (2022b). *Food availability (per capita) data system*. Retrieved from https://www.ers.usda.gov/data-products/food-availability-per-capita-data-system/food-availability-per-capita-data-system/#Loss-Adjusted%20Food%20Availability

US Department of Agriculture: Economic Research Service. (2022c). *Food availability and consumption*. Retrieved from https://www.ers.usda.gov/data-products/ag-and-food-statistics-charting-the-essentials/food-availability-and-consumption/?topicId=080e8d1d-e61e-4bd8-beac-51f0f1d1f0fe

US Department of Agriculture: Economic Research Service. (2022d). *WIC program*. Retrieved from https://www.ers.usda.gov/topics/food-nutrition-assistance/wic-program/

US Department of Agriculture: Food and Nutrition Service. (2009). *Special supplemental nutrition program for women, infants and children (WIC): Revisions in the WIC food packages—Interim rule*. Retrieved from www.fns.usda.gov/wic/interim-rule-revisions-wic-food-packages

US Department of Agriculture: Food and Nutrition Service. (2012). *Nutrition standards for school meals*. Retrieved from www.fns.usda.gov/cnd/governance/legislation/nutritionstandards.htm

US Department of Agriculture: Food and Nutrition Service. (2022). *USDA actions on nutrition security*. Retrieved from https://www.usda.gov/sites/default/files/documents/usda-actions-nutrition-security.pdf

US Department of Agriculture: Food and Nutrition Service. (n.d.). *Team nutrition*. Retrieved from https://www.fns.usda.gov/team-nutrition

US Department of Agriculture: National Institute of Food and Agriculture. (2022). *Gus Schumacher nutrition incentive program*. Retrieved from https://www.nifa.usda.gov/grants/programs/hunger-food-security-programs/gus-schumacher-nutrition-incentive-program

US Department of Agriculture: National Institute of Food and Agriculture. (n.d.). *Community food projects competitive grants program*. Retrieved from https://www.nifa.usda.gov/grants/funding-opportunities/community-food-projects-competitive-grants-program

US Food and Drug Administration. (2018). *Trans fat*. Retrieved from https://www.fda.gov/food/food-additives-petitions/trans-fats

US Food and Drug Administration. (2020). *Menu labeling requirements*. Retrieved from https://www.fda.gov/food/food-labeling-nutrition/menu-labeling-requirements

US Food and Drug Administration. (2021). *2019 Food safety and nutrition survey report.* Retrieved from https://www.fda.gov/food/science-research-food/2019-food-safety-and-nutrition-survey-report

US Food and Drug Administration. (2022a). *Added sugars on the new nutrition facts label.* Retrieved from https://www.fda.gov/food/new-nutrition-facts-label/added-sugars-new-nutrition-facts-label

US Food and Drug Administration. (2022b). *Changes to the nutrition facts label.* Retrieved from https://www.fda.gov/food/food-labeling-nutrition/changes-nutrition-facts-label

Vercammen, K. A., Moran, A. J., Soto, M. J., Kennedy-Shaffer, L., & Bleich, S. N. (2020). Decreasing trends in heavy sugar-sweetened beverage consumption in the United States, 2003 to 2016. *Journal of the Academy of Nutrition and Dietetics, 120*(12), 1974–1985.e5. doi: https://doi.org/10.1016/j.jand.2020.07.012

Vernarelli, J. A., & DiSarro, R. (2021). Debunking the high cost of healthy diets: Consumer behavior predicts dietary energy density in a nationally representative sample of US adults. *American Journal of Health Promotion, 35*(4), 543–550. doi: https://doi.org/10.1177/0890117120970123

Virta Health. (n.d.). *Employers: Virta health.* Retrieved from https://www.virtahealth.com/employers

Wansink, B. (2007). *Mindless eating: Why we eat more than we think.* New York: Bantam-Dell.

Wells, H. F., & Buzby, J. C. (2008). *Dietary assessment of major trends in U.S. food consumption, 1970–2005* (EIB-33). Washington, DC: US Department of Agriculture Economic Research Service. Retrieved from www.ers.usda.gov/publications/eib-economic-information-bulletin/eib33.aspx#.UzrtG4VgHl8

Williams, D. R. (2018). Stress and the mental health of populations of color: Advancing our understanding of race-related stressors. *Journal of Health and Social Behavior, 59*(4), 466–485. doi: https://doi.org/10.1177/0022146518814251

World Health Organization. (2022). *Cancer.* Retrieved from https://www.who.int/news-room/fact-sheets/detail/cancer

Zellner, D.A., Loaiza, S., Gonzalez, Z. et al. (2006). Food selection changes under stress. *Physiology & Behavior 87*(4): 789–793.

Zimmerman, F. J., & Shimoga, S. V. (2014). The effects of food advertising and cognitive load on food choices. *BMC Public Health, 14*(1), 342–342. doi: https://doi.org/10.1186/1471-2458-14-342

PHYSICAL ACTIVITY BEHAVIORS

Benefits, Trends, Programs, and Policies

Jennifer Childress

People do not stop moving because they grow old; they grow old because they stop moving. We are designed to be physically active. Yet, with an increasing number of barriers, including personal, social, physical, and environmental factors such as lack of time, limited access to safe walking paths and sidewalks, longer commutes, sedentary jobs, weather, and lower levels of health, people move less on a daily basis.

More than 75% of adults in the United States do not meet government-recommended physical activity guidelines for aerobic and muscle-strengthening activities. Similarly, more than 75% of U.S. adolescents do not participate in enough aerobic physical activity to meet the guidelines (US Department of Health and Human Services, 2022a). To combat physical inactivity, the Centers for Disease Control and Prevention (CDC) created the "Active People, Healthy Nation® Initiative, with the goal to help 27 million Americans become more physically active by 2027. If the goal is met, the risks associated with at least 20 chronic diseases will be reduced (US Department of Health and Human Services, 2022b).

As a nation, we have many opportunities to engage and encourage people to be more physically active where they work, live, play, and pray, through enhancing and supporting access to places and raising awareness on opportunities to move more and sit less. As health promotion professionals, increasing physical activity among the population is a simple yet complex issue to address. As health promoters, we can learn from efforts that have been proven effective and strive to build on and innovate them.

Lead by example! While reading this chapter, get up and move for two minutes every half hour.

LEARNING OBJECTIVES

After reading this chapter, the student will be able to:

- Define five different types of physical activity.

- Explain the benefits of being physically active.

- Identify the amount of physical activity recommended for individuals.

- Explain societal trends that have influenced physical activity patterns.

- Discuss the barriers to regular physical activity.

- Identify recent educational efforts to promote physical activity behaviors.

- Summarize local, state, and national policies that are designed to promote physical activity.

Introduction to Health Promotion, Second Edition. Edited by Anastasia Snelling.
© 2024 John Wiley & Sons Inc. Published 2024 by John Wiley & Sons Inc.
Companion Website: www.wiley.com/go/snelling2e

Physical Activity

Physical activity and exercise are often used interchangeably. However, there is a difference between the two terms. **Physical activity** is defined as any bodily movement produced by skeletal muscles that requires energy expenditure (World Health Organization, 2022a). Any movement during the day is physical activity, including walking, climbing stairs, and doing housework. **Exercise** is a subset of physical activity that is planned, structured, and repetitive and has as a final or an intermediate objective to improve or maintain physical fitness level (Caspersen, Powell, & Christenson, 1985). In aiming to reduce sedentary behavior, the U.S. government's health-related organizations typically focus on "lifestyle activity," the incorporation of physical activity into everyday life, such as taking the stairs, doing yard work or housework, brisk walking, and participating in recreational activities.

There are three primary types of physical activity: aerobic, muscle-strengthening, and bone-strengthening. Balance and flexibility activities are also beneficial (National Heart, Lung, and Blood Institute, 2022).

physical activity
any bodily movement produced by skeletal muscles that requires energy expenditure

exercise
a subset of physical activity that is planned, structured, and repetitive and has a final or an intermediate objective to improve or maintain physical fitness level

---

aerobic (endurance) activity moves large muscle groups in the body (arms and legs), and results in increased heart rate and breath, which over time make your heart and lungs stronger. Examples include gardening, walking, pushing a grocery cart around a store, hiking, swimming, bicycling, dancing, and playing sports. Aerobic activities can be done with varying levels of intensity, including: light (doesn't require much effort); moderate (produces noticeable increases in breathing and heart rate); and vigorous (heart, lungs, and muscles work hard). Moderate- and vigorous-intensity aerobic activities are more beneficial for your heart compared to light-intensity activities. However, light-intensity activities are better than no activity at all.

muscle-strengthening activities improve muscular strength, power, and endurance. Examples include doing pushups, lifting weights, climbing stairs, and digging in the garden.

bone-strengthening activities improve bone density by causing impact on the musculo-skeletal system. Examples include jumping rope, running, walking, and lifting weights.

balance activities improve your ability to resist forces that can make you fall. Examples include walking backward, standing on one leg, walking heel-to-toe, and practicing standing from a sitting position.

flexibility activities improve flexibility and joint mobility. Examples include touching your toes, reaching over your head, and yoga exercises.

Muscle- and bone-strengthening activities can be aerobic if heart rate increases (e.g., running, jumping jacks, speed walking).

Recommended Physical Activity Levels

Of 117 million Americans, about half have one or more preventable chronic diseases. Regular physical activity favorably influences seven of the ten most common chronic diseases. However, less than 25% of adults are meeting recommended amounts of physical

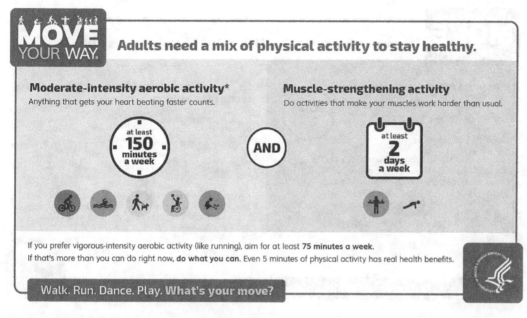

Figure 6.1 Physical Activity Recommendations for Adults (Office of Disease Prevention and Health Promotion, Office of the Assistant Secretary for Health, Office of the Secretary, U.S. Department of Health and Human Services, 2022)

activity. This is linked to approximately $117 billion in annual health care costs, and approximately 10% of premature mortality. In 2018, the US Department of Health and Human Services released the second edition of the Physical Activity Guidelines for Americans. The guidelines are an essential resource for health professionals and policymakers as they design and implement physical activity programs, policies, and promotion initiatives. The guidelines have been translated into actionable plain language messages and resources for individuals, families, and communities through the Move Your Way campaign (US Department of Health and Human Services, 2018).

Move Your Way tools help people understand the importance of being physically active, and provide safe, and fun ways to move for adults, parents, and women during and after pregnancy. Figures 6.1–6.3 show the recommendations by age/life stage.

Benefits of Physical Activity

There are many benefits of physical activity, which include lowered risk of chronic diseases including, heart disease, stroke, high blood pressure, and type 2 diabetes. Additional benefits include reduced risk of developing osteoporosis, enhanced mental health, and improved quality of life. Through physical activity, people increase their energy expenditure, helping to maintain energy balance and maintaining a desirable body weight. Being physically active helps improve self-esteem, mental activity, and energy levels. In addition, it improves learning, memory, and mood (Figure 6.4).

Evidence for the benefits of physical activity has continued to grow since the 2008 Guidelines were published. Here are just a few of the recently identified benefits:

- Improved bone health and weight status for children ages three through five years.

- Improved cognitive function for youth ages six to thirteen years.

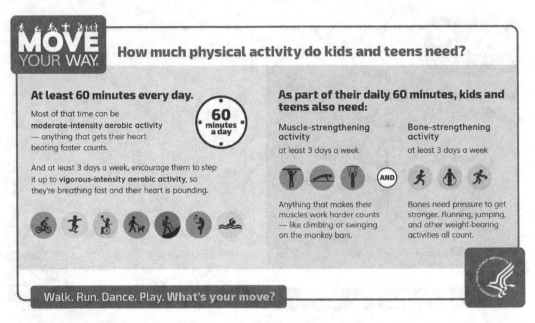

Figure 6.2   Physical Activity Recommendations for Kids and Teens (Office of Disease Prevention and Health Promotion, Office of the Assistant Secretary for Health, Office of the Secretary, U.S. Department of Health and Human Services, 2022)

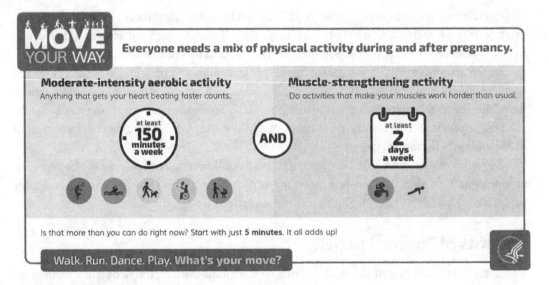

Figure 6.3   Physical Activity Recommendations for During and After Pregnancy
Source: Office of Disease Prevention and Health Promotion, Office of the Assistant Secretary for Health, Office of the Secretary, U.S. Department of Health and Human Services (2022).

- Reduced risk of cancer at a greater number of sites.

- Brain health benefits include possible improved cognitive function, reduced anxiety and depression risk, and improved sleep and quality of life.

- For pregnant women, reduced risk of excessive weight gain, gestational diabetes, and postpartum depression.

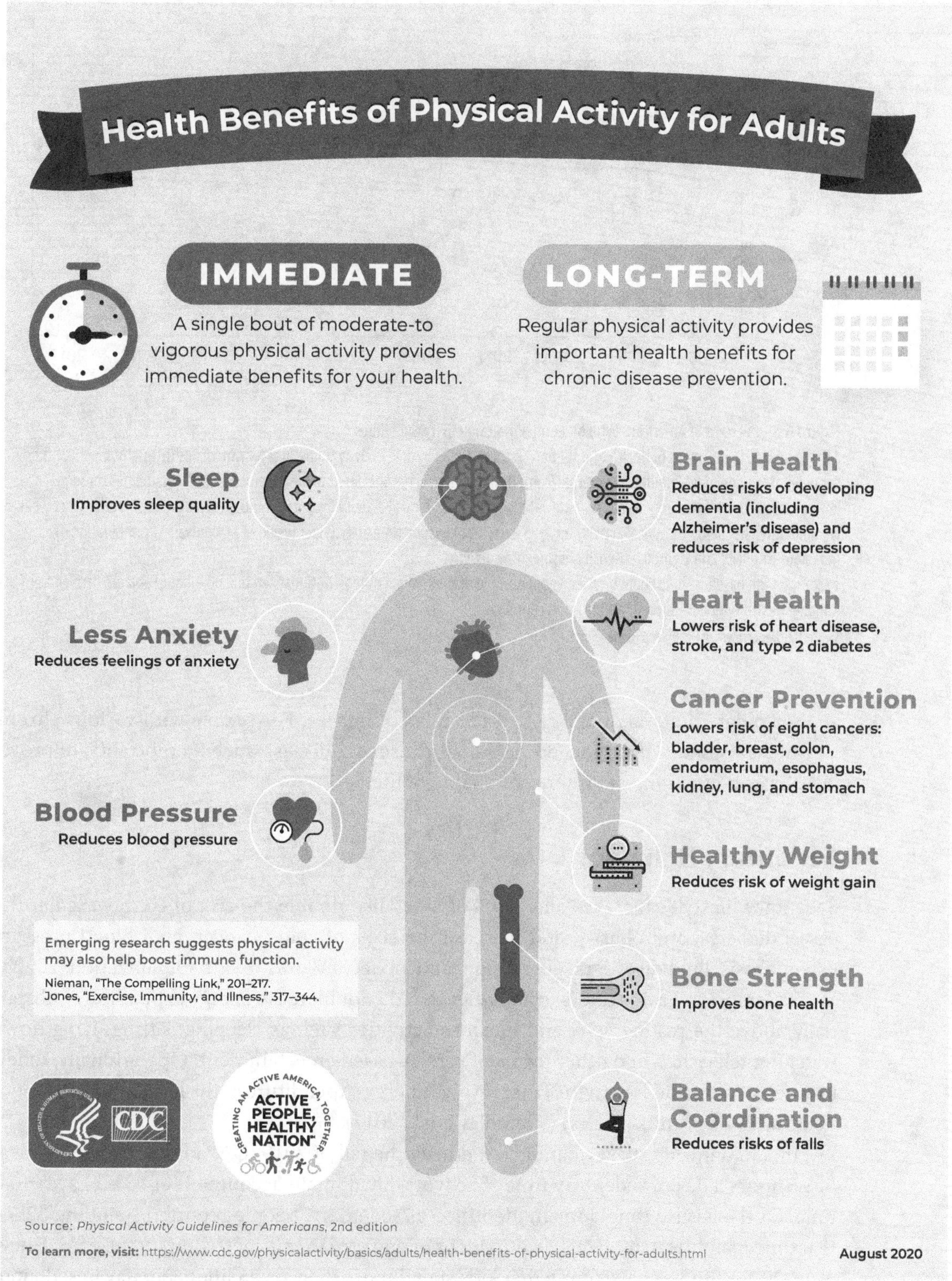

Figure 6.4   Health Benefits of Physical Activity for Adults

Source: U.S. Department of Health and Human Services.

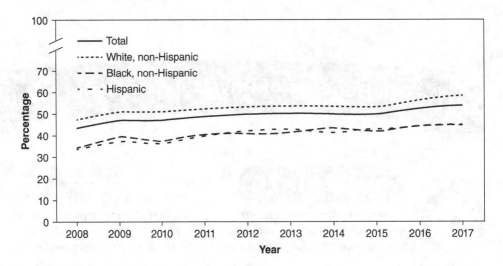

Figure 6.5   Percent of Americans Who Meet the Physical Activity Guidelines
* Based on U.S. Department of Health and Human Services 2008 Physical Activity Guidelines for Americans (https://www.health.gov/
paguidelines/guidelines/default.aspxexternal icon). Respondents were considered to meet aerobic activity guidelines through
leisure-time activity if they reported moderate-intensity aerobic physical activity for ≥150 minutes of leisure-time activity per week,
vigorous-intensity aerobic physical activity for ≥75 minutes of leisure-time activity per week, or an equivalent combination of
moderate-intensity and vigorous-intensity leisure-time activity.
† Estimates are based on household interviews of a sample of the civilian, noninstitutionalized U.S. population and are derived from the
National Health Interview Survey Sample Adult component.
Source: U.S. Department of Health and Human Services

- For older adults, reduced risk of fall-related injuries. For people with various chronic medical conditions, reduced risk of all-cause and disease-specific mortality, improved physical function, and improved quality of life

Sedentary Behavior

Sedentary lifestyles increase all causes of mortality, double the risk of cardiovascular diseases, diabetes, and obesity, and increase the risks of colon cancer, high blood pressure, osteoporosis, lipid disorders, depression, and anxiety (World Health Organization, 2022b).

Sedentary behavior refers to activities that do not increase energy expenditure substantially above the resting level and includes activities such as sleeping, sitting, lying down, watching television, and other forms of screen-based entertainment. Operationally, sedentary behavior includes activities that involve energy expenditure at the level of 1.0–1.5 metabolic equivalent units (METs) (Tremblay et al., 2017).

In a nationwide survey conducted during the fall of 2019, U.S. adults reported a mean of 9.5 hours a day of sedentary time. The work-life domain accounted for 53% of sedentary time. Of the leisure time domain identified as sedentary, people reported spending 82% of that time mainly watching television/videos or engaged in Internet/computer use (Matthews et al., 2021). Studies have found that kids spend more than seven hours per day in sedentary activities—that equates to about 50% of their waking hours. And only about half of kids stick

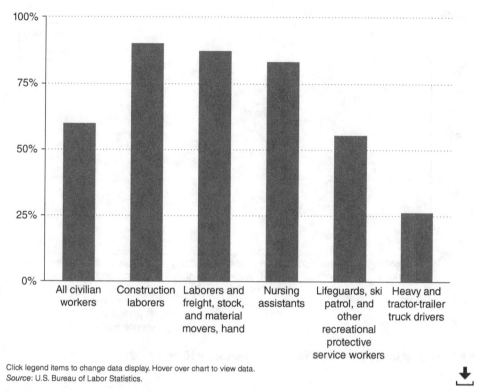

Figure 6.6 Percent of Workday Standing or Walking is Required in Selected Occupations 2017

to keeping their entertainment screen time (not school-related) to the recommended limit of one or two hours per day (New Balance Foundation Obesity Prevention Center, 2022).

Even people who are physically active can be sedentary. For example, a person can meet the physical activity guideline recommendations, yet, still spend most of their day sitting in their cars on a commute, or in front of their screens at work and home. Research shows that cardiovascular risk increases when people sit for more than ten hours (Pandey et al., 2016).

To address sedentary behaviors, the 2018 Physical Activity Guidelines for Americans first key guideline is to move more and sit less. And, emphasizes that any amount of physical activity has some health benefits.

What is Your Level of Activity?

- **Inactive** is not getting any moderate- or vigorous-intensity physical activity beyond basic movement from daily life activities.

- **Insufficiently active** is doing some moderate- or vigorous-intensity physical activity but less than 150 minutes of moderate-intensity physical activity a week, 75 minutes of vigorous-intensity physical activity a week, or the equivalent combination of the two. This level is less than the target range for meeting the key guidelines for adults.

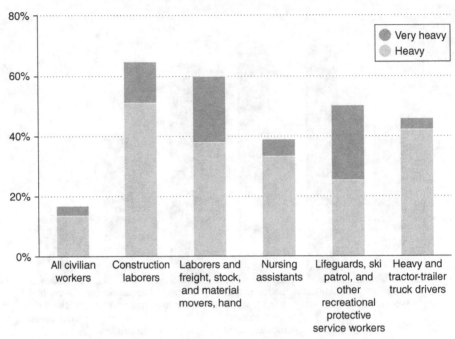

Figure 6.7   Percent of Jobs Requiring Heavy or Very Heavy Strengths, Selected Occupations, 2017

- **Active** is doing the equivalent of 150 –300 minutes of moderate-intensity physical activity a week. This level meets the key guideline target range for adults.

- **Highly active** is doing the equivalent of more than 300 minutes of moderate-intensity physical activity a week. This level exceeds the key guideline target range for adults.

Physical Activity Patterns

This section examines the trends in physical activity levels in the United States, with information provided for adolescents, adults, and older adults.

Historical Patterns

Changes in occupational patterns, advances in transportation and technology, and suburban growth have affected our nation's levels of physical activity over the past century. An examination of occupational trends since the 1960s (Church et al., 2011) suggests that almost half the jobs in private industry in the United States fifty years ago required at least moderate intensity physical activity, compared to now, where less than 20% demand that intensity. Since 1969, with the popularity of the automobile and the growth of the suburbs, there has been a steady decline in the proportion of trips to work by public transportation or walking. According to 2021 survey, the national average of people who would drive rather than walk a five-minute walk away is 32% (Blechman, 2021). A combination of changes to the built environment and more people engaging in sedentary behavior has resulted in a decrease in the amount of physical activity.

Looking back even further, when comparing the metabolic rates of Americans today with those from the early nineteenth century, researchers found that the number of total calories burned when our bodies are completely at rest has fallen about 6% since 1820. This translates into twenty seven minutes less of daily exercise (World Economic Forum, 2021).

Physical Activity Behaviors and Barriers

There are multiple variables affecting a person's decision to be physically active, such as individual factors (e.g., physical capacity, attitudes, preferences, and time demands), the built environment (e.g., land use patterns), and the social context (e.g., social norms or public policies) (Committee on Physical Activity, Health, Transportation, and Land Use, 2005).

Individual

Physical activity behavior is influenced by individual characteristics such as demographics (gender, age, ethnic background), and socioeconomic characteristics (e.g., education and income levels). And, at least three other factors play a role (Institute of Medicine, 2005):

1. Attitudes, preferences, motivations, and skills related to the behavior

2. Opportunities or constraints that make the behavior easier or more difficult to perform

3. Incentives or disincentives that encourage or discourage the desired behavior relative to competing activities.

For example, if the norm within the home is to spend all free time on phones and social media instead of playing or being active, family members are more likely to be sedentary.

Another example includes that of a single parent working multiple jobs to support their household, who has to commute to work as well as take care of children. In this instance, the person has time and financial constraints that make being physically active challenging.

A person's attitude toward physical activity is also relevant. If people do not feel they have the time or that physical activity is not important or fun, they will be less likely to be physically active. Therefore, increasing people's physical activity level also hinges on finding internal significance or reasons why the person would be more likely to engage in physical activity and continue to be physically active.

Recreation

According to the Bureau of Labor Statistics, 19.3% of the U.S. population was engaged in sports and exercise each day in 2019. Male participation was higher (20.7%) than the participation rate of women (18%). This included participation in sports, exercise, and other active leisure activities. On average, Americans spent half an hour per day doing sport, exercise, and on recreation in 2019 (Statista, 2022a).

During 2008–2017, the percentage of adults eighteen years and older who met federal guidelines for aerobic physical activity through leisure-time activity increased from 43.5% in 2008 to 54.1% in 2017. This pattern was seen in each race/ethnicity group shown, with an increase from 33.4% to 45.0% for Hispanic, 34.1% to 44.3% for non-Hispanic black, and 46.0% to 58.6% for non-Hispanic white adults. Throughout the period, non-Hispanic white adults were more likely to meet the guidelines through leisure-time activity than were non-Hispanic black and Hispanic adults (National Health Interview Survey, 2008–2017, 2019) (Figure 6.5).

Built Environment

built environment
human-made surroundings that provide the setting for human activity; the human-made space in which people live, work, and recreate on a day-to-day basis

The **built environment** touches all aspects of our lives, encompassing the buildings we live in, the distribution systems that provide us with water and electricity, and the roads, bridges, and transportation systems we use to get from place to place. It can generally be described as human-made or modified structures that provide people with living, working, and recreational spaces (Environmental Protection Agency, 2022). The role of the built environment as it relates to physical activity is an important area of research and focus. Urban sprawl, suburbs, and the "freeway era" have affected the way people travel. City engineering and design are critical components in developing areas that are conducive to promoting physical activity in the spaces where people live and work. The decline of physically active occupations, increases in labor-saving devices, housing choices, and increases in automobile use have broadly affected physical activity levels.

Occupation

Some occupations require more physical activity than others. For example, some jobs require workers to stand and walk more compared to sitting. Among all civilian jobs in 2017, workers spent an average of 60.4% of their workday standing or walking and 39.6% of their workdays sitting. Construction laborers spent more than 90% of their workday standing or walking (Bureau of Labor Statistics, 2017) (Figure 6.6).

Strength requirements are another measure of physically strenuous jobs. Strength is measured in five levels, from sedentary to very heavy. The strength required for a job depends on how much weight a worker must lift or carry, how often they lift this weight, and the amount they stand or walk in some special cases.

Nearly half (45%) of jobs in 2017 required medium strength. In some occupations, however, most jobs are classified as heavy or very heavy work. Among construction laborers, for example, 65% of jobs required heavy or very heavy work. For these occupations that require heavy or very heavy work, truck drivers were the only ones that did not also require workers to stand or walk more than half the workday (Figure 6.7).

It is also of note that while technology and machines have made work easier for most, more than 25% of older white workers and over 40% of Black and Hispanic workers have physically demanding jobs (Schwartz Center for Economic Policy Analysis The New School, 2022).

Commuting and Transportation Choices

According to the New American Driving Survey (AAA Foundation for Traffic Safety, 2021), about nine in ten U.S. residents drove at least occasionally and made an average of 2.5 driving trips daily during 2019–2020. On average, people drove nearly 30 miles daily and drove fifty nine minutes. It was estimated that 246.3 million drivers made nearly 225 billion trips and spent 89 billion hours driving nearly 3 trillion miles. While the survey results cannot be compared with previous results due to changes in methodologies and the impact of the COVID pandemic starting in early 2020, which had an impact on driving, these numbers provide a snapshot of the vast number of miles and hours driven.

Seventy-six percent of Americans largely rely on their personal cars to travel between home and work or school, according to Statista's Global Consumer Survey. Meanwhile, only 11% use public transportation, and 10% their bikes. Other forms of transportation comprising fewer than 10% response rates included ride-hailing, taxis, car sharing, motorcycles, and bike sharing (Richter, 2022).

Neighborhoods

Where people live has an impact on physical activity levels. Neighborhoods that include visually engaging, eye-catching objects and locations increase the frequency, duration, and vigorousness of residents' and visitors' exercise. Three key takeaways from the research find that:

1. If neighborhoods include features directly relevant to exercise, such as dense mixed-use developments, greenspaces, parks, sidewalks, and connected streets, people are more active and maintain better health.

2. When there are visually interesting contents that are indirectly relevant to exercise, people believe exercise is more feasible, which predicts increased physical activity.

3. As people become more physically active, they are less tempted by unhealthy food, which may counteract the detrimental effects on healthy eating posed by nearby fast-food restaurants.

Race and socioeconomic disparities coexist with the contents of neighborhoods (Balcetis, Cole, & Duncan, 2020).

Social Environment

According to the **social learning theory**, "people learn by watching other people. We can learn from anyone—teachers, parents, siblings, peers, co-workers, YouTube influencers, athletes, and even celebrities. We observe their behavior, and we mimic that behavior. In short, we do what they do. This theory is also known as social cognitive theory." (Psychology Today, 2022). Formal and informal policies and cultures affect the way people behave. For example, in an office where the expectation is that people work through their lunch breaks

social learning theory
a theory of behavior that posits personal, environmental, and behavioral factors continuously interact to influence a person's behavior, along with past experiences and actions of others

at their desks, employees might participate in less physical activity than in an office where the expectation is that people leave the building or their desks during the lunch hour. Or, if there's a corporate policy requiring that participation in health promotion activities (including being physically active) occur off the clock, employees might be less inclined to participate. A school policy preventing students from walking or riding their bikes to school would likely discourage physical activity. These types of situations create a culture or environment that does not promote physical activity.

In contrast, if a workplace has groups of people who informally get together to walk or has a policy for allowing fifteen minutes in between meetings that make standing or walking breaks possible, if teachers incorporate physical activity into learning activities, or if families play or go out for walks together, then these activities help build social environments that support being physically active.

Efforts and Initiatives to Increase Physical Activity

As the nation's working and living landscapes continue to evolve, there has been a cultural change in how people are physically active. The fitness and recreation industries recognize that people will be physically active if there are opportunities that are convenient, appealing, and social. The benefits of physical activity and its links to reducing chronic disease continue to be formally promoted by both the public and private sectors through a variety of methods.

Technology

Social support is a critical element in successful behavior change. As society becomes increasingly reliant on technology, people are using smartphones, the Internet, and online apps to manage their health and fitness, locate and participate in group physical activities, and join virtual health or fitness-focused groups to stay accountable. The private sector continually explores ways to tap into this market and find out what interests these individuals and what keeps them motivated. New and yet-to-be-developed technological tools will likely continue to support increased physical activity for adults and children.

Tracking Activity

Many people build accountability into their physical activity through virtual or online tracking, whether using their phones, smart watches, fitness apps, or subscriptions to workout platforms. These tools (such as Strava and Run Keeper) enable people to monitor, track, and share their physical activities, and, if they choose, be part of an online community. Many of these services include some type of encouragement or motivation for users, such as reminders to stand up and be active through texts or prompts.

Virtual Social Support

In addition to being able to track activities, many sites offer members the opportunity to network with one another, access information and resources, ask questions, and post comments and questions in online forums. Bodi and Peloton are some examples of companies that offer websites that provide members with a virtual social community and support in reaching physical activity or health goals. Including support and resources, such as healthy recipes and articles on health and well-being. The CDC has developed and promoted social media tools to support people in being physically active, including e-cards, badges, podcasts, and online videos, all of which are free.

Education Programs in Worksites, Schools, and Communities

There are many opportunities to connect people with opportunities for physical activity where they live, work, and play. The key is to minimize barriers and provide a variety of activities while promoting what is available. Because adults spend most of their waking hours at their jobs, and children at school, worksites and school settings provide opportunities for captive audiences. Additional community sites, such as faith-based organizations, also provide opportunities for physical activity engagement.

Workplace Health

On average, Americans working full-time spend more than one-third of their day, five days per week, at the workplace. The use of effective workplace programs and policies can reduce health risks and improve the quality of life for American workers (Centers for Disease Control and Prevention, 2019). To help promote and encourage physical activity, workplaces may offer informal opportunities, such as walking groups, or formalize their commitment to physical activity through programs and policies. Policies such as allowing employees to participate in physical activity while on the job, offering flexible work hours, and providing physical activity incentives (gym membership subsidies, gift cards, recognition, etc.) can significantly affect employee levels of physical activity (Partnership for Prevention, 2007). Increasingly, employers are modifying work environments to support physical activity, implementing walking workstations (treadmills with desks) and standing workstations, and encouraging walking meetings or huddles when team members do not require technology during a meeting. Larger employers may provide on-site fitness centers or walking and biking paths. Even smaller organizations can implement stretch breaks, post signs to encourage the use of the stairs, sponsor teams to participate in charity races (Sherwin, 2014), or provide "lunch 'n' learns" on health and fitness topics.

According to the 2017 Workplace Health in America survey, a nationally representative survey of U.S. employers (Centers for Disease Control and Prevention, 2018) physical activity programs were the most common type of health promotion program offered by worksites of all sizes and industry groups (Figures 6.8 and 6.9). Nationally, 28.5% of worksites reported offering some type of program to address physical activity, fitness, and/or sedentary behavior.

Most worksites (57.9%) offered a combination of informational and skill-building programs (Figure 6.10). Compared to most other health topics, a lower percentage of worksites offered physical activity programs that were informational only.

Respondents indicated that employee participation in physical activity programs was relatively low, with 84.3% estimating that less than 50% of employees took advantage of

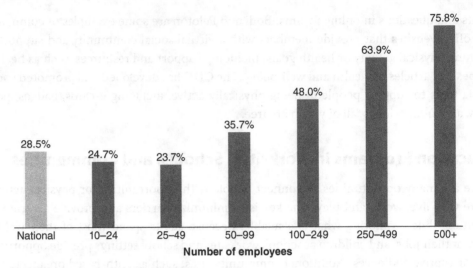

Figure 6.8   Percentage of US Worksites That Offered a Physical Activity Program by Worksite Size

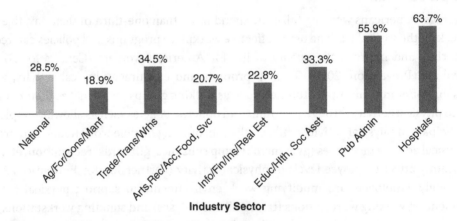

Note: Ag/For/Const/Manf = Agriculture, Forestry, Fishing; Mining; Utilities; Construction: Manufacturing

Trade/Trans/Wrhs = Wholesale/Retail Trade; Transportation; Warehousing

Arts,Rec/Acc,Food, Svc = Arts, Entertainment, Recreation; Accommodations and Food Service; Other Services

Info/Fin/Ins/Real Est = Information; Finance; Insurance; Real Estate and Leasing; Professional, Scientific, Technical Services; Management: Administration Support; Waste Management

Educ/Hlth, Soc Asst = Education Services, Health Care & Social Assistance

Pub Admin = Local, State, and Federal Public Administration.

Percentages based on weighted estimates.

Figure 6.9   Percentage of US Worksites That Offered a Physical Activity Program by Industry Group

these programs (Figure 6.11). Only 8.2% of worksites offered paid time to be physically active, and less than 20% had any evidence-based strategies in place, which may help to explain low participation.

Among all the strategies the survey asked about, the most common was subsidizing or discounting the cost of onsite or offsite exercise facilities (17.6% of worksites). This ranged

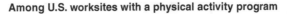

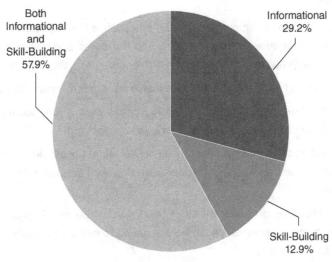

Figure 6.10   Type of Worksite Physical Activity Programs Offered to Employee

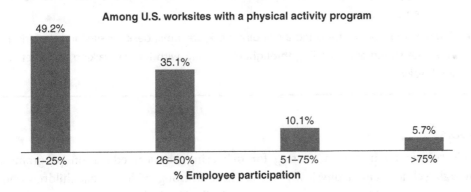

Figure 6.11   Level of Employee Participation in Worksite Physical Activity Program

from just 11.6% of the worksites with 24–49 employees to 55.3% of the worksites with at least 500 employees. Similarly, 17.2% of the worksites provided organized individual or group physical activity programs, such as walking programs or group exercise classes. These organized programs were reported by 12.6% of worksites with 24–49 employees and 51.0% of worksites with at least 500 employees. Only 8.2% of all worksites offered employees paid time to be physically active during work hours, for fitness breaks, walking meetings, or other options. This policy, which could be more expensive than some of the other strategies, was relatively uncommon even among the largest worksites. It was offered by 19.5% of worksites with more than 500 employees.

GET ACTIVE!

The American Heart Association (AHA) (2022) emphasizes the importance of being physically active to help reduce stress and anxiety and has developed resources for employers and employees with tips on how to be more active throughout the workday, including:

- When you take a break, move to a different area and stretch versus sitting in place

- If you sit at a desk, make it a habit to stand up or move every time you make or answer a phone call. March in place or pace in a circle to keep moving.

- Stuck on a long call or need an energizing break? Stand up and do some basic strength and balance exercises, like squats, desk push-ups, wall sits, calf raises, tree pose, and chair pose.

- Keep small hand weights or a resistance band at your desk for bicep curls, lateral raises, rows, and overhead presses. Watch demos online to make sure you're doing exercises correctly to avoid injury.

- Form a virtual walking club at work

- Try walking or moving for informal discussions and brainstorming meetings. Use a voice memo app on your phone to capture notes. You may find you're more creative on your feet!

- Explore your options for using a standing desk, treadmill desk, or sit-stand desk riser. Alternate sitting and standing throughout the day, with lots of walking and stretching breaks.

Schools

Schools remain an important setting for delivering physical education programs and encouraging children to be physically active. There is strong evidence that children who are physically active tend to perform better academically. Physical activity improves the brain's functioning, and different kinds of physical activity impact cognitive performance. There is a strong correlation between physical activity and the development of overall wellness and academic confidence. In addition to academic benefits, research also shows behavioral improvements in students with learning and cognitive disabilities (Rubis, 2020).

SHAPE America establishes national standards and guidelines for physical education in grades K–12 (SHAPE America, 2015). Table 6.1 displays the essential components of physical education program. Sadly, although evidence indicates that children who are physically active perform better academically, budget cuts and an increased focus on standardized testing have resulted in an astonishingly low, e.g., only 4% of elementary schools, 7% of middle schools, and 2% of high schools offering daily P.E. the entire school year. Twenty-two percent of schools have no P.E. at all (Mathews, 2022).

Table 6.1   Essential Components of Physical Education

Policy and environment	• Every student is required to take daily physical education in grades K–12, with instruction periods totaling 150 minutes/week in elementary and 225 minutes/week in middle and high school.
	• School districts and schools require full inclusion of all students in physical education.
	• School districts and schools do not allow waivers from physical education class time or credit requirements.
	• School districts and schools do not allow student exemptions from physical education class time or credit requirements.
	• School districts and schools prohibit students from substituting other activities (e.g., JROTC, interscholastic sports) for physical education class time or credit requirements.
	• Physical education class size is consistent with that of other subject areas and aligns with school district and school teacher/student ratio policy.
	• Physical activity is not assigned or withheld as punishment.
	• Physical education is taught by a state-licensed or state-certified teacher who is endorsed to teach physical education.
Curriculum	• School districts and schools should have a written physical education curriculum for grades K–12 that is sequential and comprehensive.
	• The physical education curriculum is based on national and/or state standards and grade-level outcomes for physical education.
	• The physical education curriculum mirrors other school districts and school curricula in its design and schedule for periodic review/update.
Appropriate instruction	• The physical education teacher uses instructional practices and deliberate-practice tasks that support the goals and objectives defined in the school district's/school's physical education curriculum (e.g., differentiated instruction, active engagement, modified activities, self-assessment, and self-monitoring).
	• The physical education teacher evaluates student learning continually to document teacher effectiveness.
	• The physical education teacher employs instructional practices that engage students in moderate to vigorous physical activity for at least 50% of class time.
	• The physical education teacher ensures the inclusion of all students and makes the necessary adaptations for students with special needs or disabilities.
Student assessment	• Student assessment is aligned with national and/or state physical education standards and established grade-level outcomes and is included in the written physical education curriculum along with administration protocols.
	• Student assessment includes evidence-based practices that measure student achievement in all areas of instruction, including physical fitness.
	• Grading is related directly to the student learning objectives identified in the written physical education curriculum.
	• The physical education teacher follows school and school district protocols for reporting and communicating student progress to students and parents.

Faith-based Organizations

Religion and belief in a higher purpose are linked to a person's overall well-being. According to a 2021 survey, 22% of Americans attend church or synagogue every week (Statista 2022b). Faith-based settings, therefore, are another important and effective environment for providing opportunities for and inspiring and engaging members in physical activity.

faith-placed interventions
interventions that occur within the faith-based setting but do not have a spiritual or religious component; typically delivered by health promotion professionals

faith-based interventions
interventions offering some degree of spiritual or religious involvement, referencing the Bible or other religious text, institutionalized into the faith-based organization, and delivered by trained faith-based organization volunteers

Faith-based interventions are defined as those offering some degree of spiritual or religious involvement, referencing the Bible or other religious texts, institutionalized into the faith-based organization, and delivered by trained faith-based organization volunteers. **Faith-placed interventions** do not have a spiritual or religious component but are located on the site of a faith-based organization. Among faith-based interventions, those that ranged from six to eight months showed a significant increase in physical activity among participants immediately following the program and in the one-year follow-up.

There is further need to conduct research regarding physical activity interventions within faith-based organizations to help identify evidence-based best practices that can serve as models. The Faith, Activity, and Nutrition (FAN) program was implemented in rural South Carolina, where community health advisors trained church committees and delivered telephone-based technical assistance to improve opportunities, guidelines, messages, and pastor support for physical activity and healthy eating. FAN resulted in churchgoers reporting seeing more opportunities for physical activity as well as more messages and pastor support for physical activity and healthy eating (Rural Health Information Hub, 2022).

Other Settings

Exercise is Medicine (EIM), an initiative of the American College of Sports Medicine (ACSM), encourages primary care physicians and other health care providers to include exercise in their patients treatment plans and to refer patients to evidence-based exercise programs and qualified exercise professionals. EIM is committed to the belief that physical activity promotes optimal health and is integral in the prevention and treatment of many medical conditions (www.exerciseismedicine.org). In addition to providing training and resources for medical students and doctors, ACSM also provides information, resources, and credentialing for health and fitness professionals in establishing partnerships with health care providers to promote and implement EIM.

Innovative interventions in a variety of community-based settings can be effective in planning, improving, and evaluating health promotion efforts. There are several studies that have been conducted and that are currently examining beauty salons and barber shops as settings for reaching and promoting health among African Americans. In these studies, cosmetologists and barbers are trained to deliver health messages regarding daily physical activity, blood pressure, weight management, and nutrition as part of an overall prevention message. The research has found that customers who spoke with their cosmetologists, hairstylists, and barbers about health also reported higher percentages of increased readiness for and actual behavior changes after the seven-week study and twelve months postintervention (Linnan et al., 2005; University of Maryland, 2022).

Policies That Promote Increasing Physical Activity

Policies at the national, state, and local levels have been implemented to support increasing opportunities for physical activity. These range from focusing on changing the built environment to organizing schools for successful and active kids to promoting financial and benefit polices within the workplace. The federal government has provided physical activity guidelines and funding to stimulate the design of programs to promote active lifestyles and measure their impact.

National Policy

The federal government has the capability to affect levels of physical activity for adults and children across the country through legislation, resources, funding, research, and technical assistance.

The CDC (Division of Nutrition, Physical Activity, and Obesity, National Center for Chronic Disease Prevention and Health Promotion, 2021) promotes scientifically proven strategies to increase physical activity through state and community-based programs, including:

- State Physical Activity and Nutrition Program—CDC provides funding to states to implement evidence-based strategies at state and local levels to improve nutrition and physical activity.

- High Obesity Program—CDC provides funding to land-grant universities to work with community extension services to increase access to healthier foods and safe and accessible places for physical activity in counties that have more than 40% of adults with obesity.

- Racial and Ethnic Approaches to Community Health Program (REACH)—CDC administers REACH, whose aim is to reduce racial and ethnic health disparities. Through REACH, recipients plan and carry out local, culturally appropriate programs to address a wide range of health issues among Black or African American, Hispanic or Latino, Asian, American Indian, Native Hawaiian, Pacific Islander, and Alaska Native persons.

CDC provides guidance on what others can do to implement policies that work to increase physical activity, including (Division of Nutrition, Physical Activity, and Obesity, National Center for Chronic Disease Prevention and Health Promotion, 2021b):

- Adopt combined built-environment approaches to enhance opportunities for active transportation and/or leisure-time physical activity.

- Adopt zoning code reforms that promote physical activity.

- Develop shared-use agreements that allow community members to use existing community facilities such as playgrounds, gyms, or pools.

- Promote social support interventions, such as walking or cycling groups, that create or strengthen social networks and help people increase their physical activity.

- Create bicycle or pedestrian master plans to make bicycling, walking, wheelchair rolling, and riding transit safer, more convenient, and more realistic travel options.

- Adopt Complete Streets policies for safe and convenient access to community destinations.

- Participate in Safe Routes to School programs to create safe, convenient, and fun opportunities for children to bicycle and walk to and from school.

"Complete Streets are streets for everyone. Complete Streets is an approach to planning, designing, building, operating, and maintaining streets that enables safe access for all people who need to use them, including pedestrians, bicyclists, motorists and transit riders of all ages and abilities." (Smart Growth America, 2022)

Nonprofit organizations, such as the AHA and Physical Activity Alliance, among others, advocate for and help implement policies to increase and enhance physical activity efforts.

The American Heart Association (AHA) (2022) supports various policies that support making physical activity safe and accessible for all. Ensuring access to bike and pedestrian trails and evidence-based physical education can help create more livable and active environments, which are critical to improving public health.

AHA advocates for an increase to Title IV, Part A funding, a grant program created by the Every Student Succeeds Act. They also advocate for using this funding to improve, enhance, and create physical education programs in schools. Additionally, AHA supports the Every Kid Outdoors program (www.everykidoutdoors.gov), which gives free passes to fourth graders to get outside and enjoy our national parks and lands. As strong supporters of increasing funding for walking and biking, including Safe Routes to School, AHA is currently exploring ways to improve the built environment in the upcoming transportation reauthorization.

Safe Routes to School (SRTS) is an approach that promotes walking and bicycling to school through infrastructure improvements, enforcement, tools, safety education, and incentives to encourage walking and bicycling to school. Nationally, 10–14% of car trips during morning rush hour are for school travel. SRTS initiatives improve safety and levels of physical activity for students. (U.S. Department of Transportation, 2015).

The Physical Activity Alliance engages in advocacy efforts, including facilitating the Congressional Physical Activity Caucus, which serves as a bipartisan organization committed to efforts to promote, educate, inform, and encourage others to engage in physical activity. The Caucus' mission is to educate decision-makers about the importance of physical activity for physical health, mental health, growth and development, disease prevention, reducing health care costs, the economy, disease prevention, national security, and military readiness and retention (Physical Activity Alliance, 2022).

State Policy

As mentioned above, through the State Physical Activity and Nutrition Program, states receive funding from CDC to implement evidence-based strategies at state and local levels to improve nutrition and physical activity.

Below are a few examples of what states are doing (Division of Nutrition, Physical Activity, and Obesity, National Center for Chronic Disease Prevention and Health Promotion, 2021).

Alaska—is implementing statewide and local-level interventions that support healthy nutrition, breastfeeding, and safe and accessible physical activity. They are promoting healthy foods and beverages in worksites with point-of-decision prompts and menu labeling, supporting mothers who breastfeed at the clinical and community level as well as in the workplace, and helping Alaskan children and adults be physically active through increased access to a safe and walkable transportation system with Vision Zero planning and Complete Streets policies.

Ohio—is implementing five strategies and outcomes: (1) providing training and technical assistance to local counties and their government jurisdictions on the food service guidelines; (2) providing training and technical assistance to worksites on adopting breastfeeding policies and adhering to the federal law; (3) expanding the Ohio Healthy Program; (4) providing training and technical assistance to local counties on adopting complete street policies and/or active transportation master plans; and (5) implementing and integrating physical activity standards into statewide early care and education systems.

Pennsylvania—The Pennsylvania Department of Health is implementing comprehensive strategies to increase: (1) hospitals and community settings that implement food service guidelines; (2) settings that implement supportive breastfeeding interventions; (3) places that implement community planning and transportation interventions that support safe and accessible physical activity; and (4) implementation of nutrition and physical activity standards in early care and education systems.

North Carolina's Eat Smart, Move More Initiative

North Carolina's Eat Smart, Move More initiative is a good example of the types of state actions that can influence physical activity. This initiative began with a policy strategy platform, which is a list of policy recommendations aimed at helping North Carolina meet the goals in its obesity prevention plan by influencing the environment to support healthy behavior change (Dunn & Kolasa, 2013). Eat Smart, Move More identified eight community settings and a menu of strategies to help meet the state's healthy weight goals. Below is a sampling of settings and strategies related to increasing physical activity and reducing screen time:

Setting	Strategy	Physical Activity	Screen Time
Health Care Strategies			
	Implement a practice policy to require measurement of weight and length or height in a standardized way and plotting of information on World Health Organization or CDC growth charts as part of every well-child doctor visit	X	X
	Counsel caregivers about risk factors for obesity, such as children's weight-for-length, body mass index (BMI), rate of weight gain, and parental weight status	X	X
	Practice healthy lifestyle behaviors, be role models for patients, and participate in community coalitions	X	X
	For treatment of people with severe mental illness who are at risk for overweight or obesity, consider medications that are more weight neutral, and emphasize behaviors to minimize weight gain.	X	X
	Establish policies and practices to offer counseling and behavioral interventions for adults identified as obese	X	X
	Promote physical activity for all patients, record patients' physical activity levels, and stress the importance of consistent exercise and daily physical activity	X	X
	Provide point-of-decision prompts to encourage use of stairs in clinical setting	X	X
	Advise caregivers of children ages two to five years to limit screen time to less than two hours per day, including discouraging the placement of televisions, computers, or other digital media devices in children's bedrooms or other sleeping areas		X
State level policies	Enact policies and regulations to support insurance coverage at no cost-sharing for counseling and behavioral interventions for those identified as obese.	X	
Child Care Strategies			
	Implement policies and practices to give infants, toddlers, and preschool children opportunities to be physically active throughout the day	X	
	Implement policies that ensure that the amount of time toddlers and preschoolers spend sitting or standing still is minimized by limiting the use of equipment that restricts movement.	X	
	Implement the Move More North Carolina: Recommended Standards for After-School Physical Activity in all after-school program	X	
	Implement policies that reduce screen time.		X
State level policies	Direct the North Carolina Division of Child Development to examine the current levels of physical activity that children receive in child care facilities, and review model physical activity guidelines with the goal of promoting statewide model guidelines.	X	
School Building Strategies			
	Coordinate healthy eating and physical activity policies and practices through a school health council and school health coordinator.	X	
	Use a systematic approach to assess, develop, implement, and monitor school healthy eating and physical activity policies	X	

Setting	Strategy	Physical Activity	Screen Time
	Establish policies and practices to create a school environment that encourages a healthy body image, shape, and size among all students and staff members, accepts diverse abilities, and does not tolerate weight-based teasing or stigmatizes healthy eating and physical activity	X	X
	Teach educators and other school personnel how to increase children's physical activity, decrease their sedentary behavior, and advise parents or caregivers about their children's physical activity	X	X
	Increase the amount of physical activity in physical education programs	X	
	Fully implement and monitor the North Carolina State Board of Education Healthy Active Children Policy requiring thirty minutes of physical activity per day for all K–8 students.	X	X
School District Strategies			
	Require high-quality physical education that meets North Carolina Department of Public Instruction standards in all district schools	X	
	Implement policies and practices that provide opportunities for extracurricular physical activity	X	
	Implement policies to enhance infrastructure that supports bicycling and walking.	X	
	Implement policies and practices to promote joint use and community use of facilities	X	
State level policies	Budget funding to support (1) provision of school-based and school-linked health services and (2) staffing of school nurses to improve access to needed health care for all students.	X	X
	Establish a full-time healthy living coordinator in each school district.	X	X
	Require schools to implement evidence-based healthy living curricula in schools.	X	
	Increase the number of jurisdictions with policies to locate schools within easy walking distance of residential areas	X	
College and University Strategies			
	Provide opportunities for students, faculty, and staff to volunteer with community coalitions or partnerships that address obesity	X	X
	Within student health services, include routine BMI screening, counseling, and behavioral interventions to improve physical activity and dietary choices	X	X
	Through the divisions of student life, residence life, and university recreation, increase the number of campus organizations with policies and practices that provide opportunities for physical activity	X	
	Enhance the university's infrastructure to support all students, staff, and visitors in bicycling, walking, and wheeling on campus.	X	
	Implement policies and practices to encourage joint use of fitness facilities by faculty, staff, and community members.	X	
	Implement policies and practices that enhance personal safety in university settings where people are or could be physically active.	X	
	Implement policies and practices that enhance traffic safety in areas on campus where people are or could be physically active	X	

Setting	Strategy	Physical Activity	Screen Time
	Develop and implement a campuswide comprehensive plan for land use and transportation that creates opportunities for physical activity and that aligns with comprehensive plans for the city and county.	X	
State level policies	Enact policies that enable the University of North Carolina system institutions to implement recommended strategies	X	
	Adopt a budget that supports the University of North Carolina system institutions' implementation of recommended strategies	X	

For more information, see www.eatsmartmovemorenc.com.

Local Policy

Government officials at the local level play a primary role within the community in enacting policies supporting healthy community design. Elected and appointed members of city councils and county commissions, zoning boards, and school boards, as well as government officials within transportation and planning departments, health departments, human services departments, parks and recreation departments, and school divisions, can develop and implement local policies and programs that directly affect the physical activity levels of residents. Systemic change takes time; goals for the short and long term should be set and continually measured to assess the community's performance and adjust goals as necessary (Khan et al., 2009).

Community Policy

Communities may be smaller areas within a local government jurisdiction or may bridge multiple local government jurisdictions. The Task Force on Community Preventive Services has identified fifteen interventions across three broad approaches (Behavioral and Social; Campaigns and Informational; and Environmental and Policy) where there is sufficient evidence for increasing physical activity (Guide to Community Preventive Services, 2022). Embedded within the task force recommendations are research-tested intervention programs, which provide useful information on the practical application of the task force's recommendations. These programs are designed to help health promotion professionals identify how interventions could be incorporated into their communities (see Table 6.2).

Community Partner Initiatives and Multisectoral Strategies

multisectoral approaches
partnerships among multiple sectors to leverage resources and address community member needs

Multisectoral approaches are helpful for bringing together communities to leverage resources and address community member needs. Through partnerships, communities create environments that support active living. Using the multisectoral approach broadens access to opportunities for physical activity. Cost and location are barriers to some participating in physical activity. For other communities, safety, sidewalks, and neighborhoods

Table 6.2   Community Preventive Services Task Force (CPSTF) Findings for Physical Activity—Interventions to Increase Physical Activity

Intervention	CPSTF Finding
Behavioral and Social Approaches	
Classroom-based physical activity break interventions	Recommended (sufficient evidence) March 2021
Classroom-based physically active lesson interventions	Recommended (sufficient evidence) March 2021
Digital health interventions for adults fifty five years and older	Recommended (sufficient evidence) April 2019
Enhanced school-based physical education	Recommended (strong evidence) December 2013
Family-based interventions	Recommended (sufficient evidence) October 2016
Home-based exercise interventions for adults aged sixty five years and older	Recommended (sufficient evidence) July 2022
Individually-adapted health behavior change programs	Recommended (strong evidence) February 2001
Interventions, including activity monitors, for adults with overweight or obesity	Recommended (sufficient evidence) August 2017
Social support interventions in community settings	Recommended (strong evidence) February 2001
Campaigns and Informational Approaches	
Community-wide campaigns	Recommended (strong evidence) February 2001
Stand-alone mass media campaigns	Insufficient evidence March 2010
Environmental and Policy Approaches	
Built environment approaches combining transportation system interventions with land use and environmental design	Recommended (sufficient evidence) December 2016
Creating or improving places for physical activity	Recommended (strong evidence) May 2001
Interventions to increase active travel to school	Recommended (sufficient evidence) August 2018
Park, trail, and greenway infrastructure interventions when combined with additional interventions	Recommended (sufficient evidence) July 2021
Park, trail, and greenway interventions when implemented alone	Insufficient evidence July 2021
Point-of-decision prompts to encourage use of stairs	Recommended (strong evidence) June 2005

inadvertently cause access limitations. Therefore, public–private partnerships and community collaboration are essential in successfully implementing programming.

Recognizing that there are countless venues and collaborative opportunities available, the national government, in partnership with public and private entities, developed efforts aimed at increasing physical activity from a cross-sectorial approach.

Walk Friendly Communities

Walk Friendly Communities (www.walkfriendly.org) is a national recognition program developed to encourage towns and cities across the United States to establish or recommit to a high priority for supporting safer walking environments. The WFC program recognizes communities that are working to improve a wide range of conditions related to walking, including safety, mobility, access, and comfort.

Arlington County, Virginia was recently recognized as a Walk Friendly Community for its success in transit-oriented planning, remarkable promotion and outreach, and educational offerings for staff and residents.

- Arlington's longstanding goal of emphasizing growth around transit lines and embracing multi-modal transportation is guided by the Master Transportation Plan (MTP). The Pedestrian Element of the MTP includes clear sidewalk project ranking criteria and exemption policy for sidewalks. The county does an outstanding job tracking and reporting progress with performance measures with an annual report and an online dashboard.

- In 2019, Arlington County launched a comprehensive Vision Zero effort to eliminate transportation-related deaths and severe injuries. Building upon their transportation plan, their five-year Vision Zero Action Plan represents a strong commitment to improving safety across the county. The county is working hard to implement safety improvements and measure its progress toward these goals.

- Pedestrian and walkability initiatives in Arlington are supported by a committed team of professionals who devote a large portion of their time to improving conditions for people on foot. This includes a pedestrian and bicycle planner, a WalkArlington program manager, an active transportation director, and an outreach and events coordinator.

- Arlington has a model Complete Streets program that separately addresses concerns on both arterial and neighborhood streets through context-sensitive approaches. Complete streets projects include sidewalk expansion, pedestrian lighting improvements, curb ramps, crosswalk and signal enhancements, and other improvements that support pedestrian travel.

- Arlington County has extensive pedestrian (and bicycle) data collection activities. The data is used for planning, engineering, and operations, as well as education, outreach, marketing, and research. The Bicycle and Pedestrian program in the Transportation Planning Bureau manages an in-house network of permanent and portable automatic continuous pedestrian and bicycle counters. There are thirty seven automated counters and six portable counters that detect and separately record bicycle and pedestrian trips. These counts are shared publicly with an online, map-based display.

- One of their flagship resources is the Walkabout. They offer detailed route maps for twenty five different neighborhoods that include the distance, type of terrain you'll find, and a description of the neighborhood.

- The county has demonstrated a superb understanding of market-based parking management. Parking costs are unbundled from housing, and public on-street spaces are provided at minimal cost to car-sharing programs like Zipcar, which reduce the need for private automobiles. For commercial developments, below-grade parking is the norm, and Arlington also encourages shared parking between uses. The community also provides cash-out incentives, providing employees who do not require a parking space with monetary compensation.

- The county has a comprehensive Safe Routes to School program that engages young people on topics related to walking and safety. SRTS programming takes place at every elementary and middle school in the county, and the work is led and supported by a full-time coordinator.

Rails-to-Trails

The mission of Rails-to-Trails (www.railstotrails.org/index.html) is to create a nationwide network of trails from former rail lines and connecting corridors to build places for people to become healthier. To date, Rails-to-Trails has supported the development of more than 1,600 preserved pathways that form the foundation of a growing trail system spanning communities, regions, states, and the entire country. In addition to providing places for people to walk and bike, the trails can also be used for other physical activities including in-line skating and horseback riding. Other benefits include wildlife conservation, historical preservation, stimulation of local economies by increasing tourism and promoting local businesses, and providing safe and accessible routes for commuting.

Bike Shares

In the United States, just over half of car trips are less than three miles, which translates into an approximately 20-minute bike ride. Bikeshares are examples of **micromobility**, and provide communities with to reduce air pollution and advance the country's goal of becoming carbon-neutral by 2050. Additionally, bike share programs can increase access to neighborhoods at a lower cost than cars. Bike share can be owned by municipalities, privately, or in a partnership between local organizations (nonprofits, governments, and businesses).

Micromobility transportation using lightweight vehicles, such as bicycles or scooters, that may be borrowed as part of a self-service rental program in which people rent vehicles for short-term use within a town or city.

YMCA Initiatives

The YMCA is the leading nonprofit committed to strengthening individuals and communities across the country. At the Y, we are here to help you find your "why"—your greater sense of purpose—by connecting you with opportunities to improve your health, support young people, make new friends, and contribute to a stronger, more cohesive community for all.

The Y's Healthier Communities Initiatives are built on the concept that local communities can work together to give all community members healthy choices and support the pursuit of healthy lifestyles. More than one hundred and sixty Ys are working in collaboration with community leaders to make changes in policies and the physical surroundings in those communities so that healthy living is within reach for individuals of all ages and backgrounds.

The Y has ten Active Living Strategies:

1. Increase Mixed Land Use—When people's jobs, homes, and retail activities are located close together, they are more likely to be physically active. Mixed land use policy interventions can be effective in promoting physical activity.

2. Improve Built Environment to Support Walking—When their environment provides safe, convenient places to walk, people are likely to walk more. Constructing walking trails and improving street paths has been shown to be effective in getting people physically active.

3. Improve Built Environment to Support Biking—Bicycling is an accessible, convenient form of physical activity that people will choose more often when their environment provides safe, convenient places to bike. The use of bicycling has greatly increased in countries that have policies to make bicycling safer, faster, and more convenient.

4. Locate Schools Within Easy Walking Distance of Residential Areas—Neighborhood schools have many benefits to children, families, and the environment. Schools that are located in neighborhoods near residential areas are more walkable and help children stay active by walking and biking to school.

5. Increase Active Commuting to School—Active commuting promotes higher levels of overall physical activity and fitness as well as enhanced long-term health. Policies to create a safe route to school increase students' walking or biking to school.

6. Improve Traffic Safety Through Traffic Calming Measures—In areas where safety measures have been implemented, children are more likely to play outside and walk or bike to school. Safety from traffic and related injury is an important element of getting people to be physically active.

7. Provide Opportunities for Physical Activity at the Worksite—Motivating employees to participate in physical activity can effect positive behavior change and potentially improve overall workforce health. Worksite interventions targeting physical activity have been shown to be the most effective.

8. Use Point-of-Decision Prompts to Promote Stair Use—Promoting physical activity through signs that highlight its benefits and art and music that make active environments more attractive can stimulate more physical activity in multiple settings. Simple environmental changes to encourage people to take the stairs have increased stair use in various public places.

9. Reduce Screen Time—Studies show limiting screen time in various settings can increase physical activity and lead to improved overall health. Interventions aimed at reducing television viewing were effective in reducing sedentary behaviors.

10. Implement Campaigns on Physical Activity Across Many Venues of the Community—Media advertising, websites, and public relations events support the importance of physical activity and the availability of physical activity opportunities. Community-wide campaigns to promote physical activity can be effective in increasing physical activity.

Blue Zones Project

The Blue Zones Project (www.bluezonesproject.com) is a community well-being improvement initiative designed to change the way people experience the world around them. Because healthier environments naturally nudge people toward healthier choices, Blue

Zones Project focuses on influencing the Life Radius®—the area close to home in which people spend 90% of their lives. Blue Zones Project's best practices use people, places, and policies as levers to transform those surroundings. Blue Zones communities have populations with greater well-being, improved health outcomes, reduced costs, and increased civic pride, all of which support healthy economic development.

The Blue Zones Project uses the Sharecare Community Well-Being Index (based on over three million surveys and more than six hundred elements of social determinants of health data) to measure community well-being across and within populations. The data and insights on well-being inform Blue Zones on more effective strategies that encourage the sustained lifestyle changes necessary for people to thrive and perform to their highest potential.

Summary

There are many opportunities to increase physical activity levels among the entire US population. People's decisions to be physically active are influenced not only by personal factors but also by social and environmental factors. The most successful efforts are those that are multifaceted, addressing personal, social, and environmental factors. The more variety, access, and points of confluence that exist, the more likely it is to build and sustain environments that are conducive to active living. The important thing is to just move! Be more active, and encourage others around you to be as active as they can be. Even small increases make a difference.

Additionally, health promotion professionals can advocate for health and well-being legislation by contacting local health departments, city councils, and representatives and voicing support for initiatives that promote health and physical activity.

KEY TERMS

1. **Physical activity:** any bodily movement produced by skeletal muscles that requires energy expenditure

2. **Exercise:** a subset of physical activity that is planned, structured, and repetitive and has a final or an intermediate objective to improve or maintain physical fitness level

3. **Aerobic (endurance) activity:** any activity that uses the large muscle groups in the body to increase heart rate and benefit the strength of the cardiovascular system

4. **Muscle-strengthening activities:** any activity that improves muscular strength, power, and endurance

5. **Bone-strengthening activities:** any activity that improves bone density by causing impact on the musculoskeletal system

6. **Stretching activities:** any activity in which a specific muscle or tendon is lengthened in an effort to improve flexibility and joint mobility

7. **2018 Physical Activity Guidelines for Americans (PAG):** a resource for health professionals and policymakers as they design and implement physical activity programs, policies, and promotion initiatives. Translated into actionable plain language and resources for individuals, families, and communities through the Move Your Way Campaign.

8. **Built environment:** human-made surroundings that provide the setting for human activity; the human-made space in which people live, work, and recreate on a day-to-day basis

9. **Social learning theory:** a theory of behavior that posits personal, environmental, and behavioral factors continuously interact to influence a person's behavior, along with past experiences and actions of others

10. **Faith-based interventions:** interventions offering some degree of spiritual or religious involvement, referencing the Bible or other religious texts, institutionalized into the faith-based organization, and delivered by trained faith-based organization volunteers

11. **Faith-placed interventions:** interventions that occur within the faith-based setting but do not have a spiritual or religious component; typically delivered by health promotion professionals

12. **Multisectoral approaches:** partnerships among multiple sectors to leverage resources and address
community member's needs

REVIEW QUESTIONS

1. What are the benefits of physical activity?

2. What are the health risks associated with a sedentary lifestyle?

3. What percentage of adolescents, adults, and older adults are meeting physical activity recommendations?

4. What are the individual and social barriers to achieving physical activity?

5. How do you define the variables of social environment, built environment, and individual factors as they relate to physical activity?

6. What is a multisectoral approach to physical activity?

7. Why is a policy approach important to increasing physical activity?

8. How do you describe policy approaches at the national, state, and local levels?

STUDENT ACTIVITIES

1. Identify your current level of physical activity based on the levels outlined in this chapter. Using an app of your choice, track your physical activity for two weeks. What patterns do you notice?

2. Explore your college/university's strategies to increase physical activity. What are some highlights? What are some opportunities for improvement?

3. Review the differences between the Community Preventive Services Task Force findings for the park and greenway interventions when implemented alone and when combined with additional interventions. Why is one recommended and other not? What are examples of additional interventions provided and why are they important?

References

AAA Foundation for Traffic Safety. (2021). New American Driving Survey: Updated Methodology and Results from July 2019 to June 2020 (Technical Report). Washington, DC. Retrieved from https://aaafoundation.org/new-american-driving-survey-updated-methodology-and-results-from-july-2019-to-june-2020/

American Heart Association. (2022). *How to Be More Active During the Work Day*. Retrieved from https://www.heart.org/en/healthy-living/fitness/getting-active/how-to-be-more-active-at-work

Balcetis, E., Cole, S., and Duncan, D.T. (2020). How walkable neighborhoods promote physical activity: Policy implications for development and renewal. *Policy Insights from the Behavioral and Brain Sciences* 7 (2): 173–180. https://doi.org/10.1177/2372732220939135.

Blechman, P. (2021) *Walking vs driving—New survey suggests 1/3 of Americans would rather drive than walk 5 minutes*. Retrieved from https://barbend.com/new-survey-americans-walking-vs-driving/

Bureau of Labor Statistics, U.S. Department of Labor. (2017). *The Economics Daily, Physically strenuous jobs in 2017*. Retrieved from https://www.bls.gov/opub/ted/2018/physically-strenuous-jobs-in-2017.htm

Caspersen, C.J., Powell, K.E., and Christenson, G.M. (1985). Physical activity, exercise, and physical fitness: Definitions and distinctions for health-related research. *Public Health Reports 100* (2): 126–131.

Centers for Disease Control and Prevention. (2018). *Workplace Health in America 2017. Atlanta, GA: Centers for Disease Control and Prevention, U.S. Department of Health and Human Services, 2018*. Retrieved from https://www.cdc.gov/workplacehealthpromotion/data-surveillance/summary-report.html

Centers for Disease Control and Prevention. (2019). *Workplace Health Promotion*. Retrieved from https://www.cdc.gov/workplacehealthpromotion/index.html

Church, T.S., Thomas, D.M., Tudor-Locke, C. et al. (2011). Trends over 5 decades in U.S. occupation-related physical activity and their associations with obesity. *PLoS One 6* (5): e19657. https://doi.org/10.1371/journal.pone.0019657.

Committee on Physical Activity, Health, Transportation, and Land Use (2005). Does the built environment influence physical activity? Examining the evidence. *Transportation Research Board* Special Report 282. Retrieved from http://onlinepubs.trb.org/onlinepubs/sr/sr282.pdf.

Division of Nutrition, Physical Activity, and Obesity, National Center for Chronic Disease Prevention and Health Promotion. (2021a). *Strategies to increase physical activity.* Retrieved from https://www.cdc.gov/physicalactivity/activepeoplehealthynation/creating-an-active-america.html

Division of Nutrition, Physical Activity, and Obesity, National Center for Chronic Disease Prevention and Health Promotion. (2021b). *Strategies to increase physical activity.* Retrieved from https://www.cdc.gov/nccdphp/dnpao/state-local-programs/span-1807/span-1807-recipients.html

Dunn, C. and Kolasa, K.M. (2013). Development of a movement and state plan for obesity prevention, Eat Smart, Move More North Carolina. *Journal of Nutrition Education and Behavior* 45 (6): 690–695. https://doi.org/10.1016/j.jneb.2013.07.010.

Eat Smart, Move More North Carolina (2020). *North Carolina's plan to address overweight and obesity.* Raleigh, NC: Eat Smart, Move More North Carolina. Retrieved from www.eatsmart movemorenc.com.

Environmental Protection Agency (2022). *Basic information about the built environment.* Retrieved from https://www.epa.gov/smm/basic-information-about-built-environment

Guide to Community Preventive Services. (2022). *CPSTF findings for physical activity.* Retrieved from https://www.thecommunityguide.org/pages/task-force-findings-physical-activity.html

Institute of Medicine. (2005). *Does the built environment influence physical activity?: Examining the evidence – Special Report 282.* Washington, DC: The National Academies Press. Retrieved from https://doi.org/10.17226/11203.

Khan, L.K., Sobush, K., Keener, D. et al. (2009, July 24). Recommended community strategies and measurements to prevent obesity in the United States. *MMWR* 55 (7): 1–26. Retrieved from www.cdc.gov/mmwr/preview/mmwrhtml/rr5807a1.htm.

Linnan, L.A., Ferguson, Y.A., Wasilewski, Y. et al. (2005). Using community-based participatory research methods to reach women with health messages results from the North Carolina BEAUTY and Health Pilot Project. *Health Promotion Practice* 6 (2): 164–173.

Mathews, J. (2022). What happened to P.E.? It's losing ground in our push for academic improvement. *Washington Post* (June 25). https://www.washingtonpost.com/education/2022/06/05/physical-education-classes-schools/

Matthews, C.E., Carlson, S.A., Saint-Maurice, P.F. et al. (2021). Sedentary behavior in U.S. adults: Fall 2019. *Medicine and Science in Sports and Exercise* 53 (12): 2512–2519. https://doi.org/10.1249/MSS.0000000000002751.

National Health Interview Survey, 2008–2017 (2019). QuickStats: Percentage of adults who met federal guidelines for aerobic physical activity through leisure-time activity, by race/ethnicity. *Morbidity and Mortality Weekly Report* 68: 292. https://doi.org/10.15585/mmwr.mm6812a6external icon.

National Heart, Lung, and Blood Institute. (2022). *Physical activity and your heart: Types.* Retrieved from https://www.nhlbi.nih.gov/health/heart/physical-activity/types and http://www.nhlbi.nih.gov/health/health-topics/topics/phys/types.html

New Balance Foundation Obesity Prevention Center. (2022). *Boston Children's fit kit: Sedentary time.* Retrieved from https://www.childrenshospital.org/programs/new-balance-foundation-obesity-prevention-center/boston-childrens-fit-kit/sedentary-time#:~:text=Studies%20have%20found%20that%20kids,50%20percent%20of%20waking%20hours

Office of Disease Prevention and Health Promotion, Office of the Assistant Secretary for Health, Office of the Secretary, U.S. Department of Health and Human Services. (2022). https://health

.gov/our-work/nutrition-physical-activity/move-your-way-community-resources/partner-promotion-toolkit

Pandey, A., Salahuddin, U., Garg, S. et al. (2016). Continuous dose-response association between sedentary time and risk for cardiovascular disease: A meta-analysis. *JAMA Cardiology 1* (5): 575–583. https://doi.org/10.1001/jamacardio.2016.1567.

Partnership for Prevention. (2007). *Leading by example feature sheets.* Retrieved from www.prevent.org/data/files/initiatives/lbe_profile_sheets.pdf

Physical Activity Alliance. (2022). Congressional Physical Activity Caucus. Retrieved from https://paamovewithus.org/congressional-physical-activity-caucus/

Psychology Today. (2022). *Social learning theory.* Retrieved from https://www.psychologytoday.com/us/basics/social-learning-theory

Richter, F. (2022). Public Transportation. Commuting. *Cars Still Dominate the American Commute.* Retrieved from https://www.statista.com/chart/18208/means-of-transportation-used-by-us-commuters/

Rubis, D. (2020). *Physical activity to help students perform better in the classroom.* Retrieved from https://nwcommons.nwciowa.edu/cgi/viewcontent.cgi?article=1245&context=education_masters

Rural Health Information Hub. (2022). *Faith, activity, and nutrition.* Rural Health Information Hub. Available at https://www.ruralhealthinfo.org/project-examples/1011

Schwartz Center for Economic Policy Analysis The New School. (2022). *Physically demanding jobs and involuntary retirement worsen retirement insecurity.* Retrieved from https://www.economicpolicyresearch.org/jobs-report/physically-demanding-jobs-and-involuntary-retirement-worsen-retirement-insecurity

SHAPE America. (2015). *The essential components of physical education.* Guidance document. Retrieved from https://www.shapeamerica.org/upload/TheEssentialComponentsOfPhysicalEducation.pdf

Sherwin, J. (2014, January 29). *A look into MD Anderson Cancer Center's wellness program—An employer case.* Retrieved from www.corporatewellnessmagazine.com/article/a-look-into-md-anderson-cancer-center-s-wellness-program-an-employer-case-.html

Smart Growth America (2022). Complete Streets. https://smartgrowthamerica.org/what-are-complete-streets/

Statista. (2022a). *Physical activity – Statistics & facts.* Retrieved from https://www.statista.com/topics/1749/physical-activity/#dossierKeyfigures.

Statista. (2022b). *Church attendance of Americans 2021.* Retrieved from https://www.statista.com/statistics/245491/church-attendance-of-americans/#:~:text=According%20to%20a%202021%20survey,Americans%20who%20attend%20every%20week.

Tremblay, M.S., Aubert, S., Barnes, J.D. et al. (2017). Sedentary behavior research network (SBRN) – Terminology consensus project process and outcome. *International Journal of Behavioral Nutrition and Physical Activity 14*: 75. https://doi.org/10.1186/s12966-017-0525-8.

University of Maryland. (2022). *The Health Advocates In-Reach and Research Campaign (HAIR): Maryland Center for Health Equity.* Retrieved from https://sph.umd.edu/hair

US Department of Health and Human Services. (2018). *Physical activity guidelines for Americans (2nd Ed).* Retrieved from https://health.gov/sites/default/files/2019-09/Physical_Activity_Guidelines_2nd_edition.pdf

US Department of Health and Human Services. (2022a, September 6). *Exercise/Physical Activity.* Retrieved from https://www.cdc.gov/nchs/fastats/exercise.htm

US Department of Health and Human Services. (2022b, March 24). *About Active People, Healthy Nation*. cdc.gov/ Retrieved from https://www.cdc.gov/physicalactivity/activepeoplehealthynation/about-active-people-healthy-nation.html

US Department of Transportation. (2015) *Safe routes to school programs*. Retrieved from https://www.transportation.gov/mission/health/Safe-Routes-to-School-Programs

World Economic Forum. (2021). *Are we more or less active than two centuries ago? A new study looks at the United States*. Retrieved from https://www.weforum.org/agenda/2021/11/physical-activity-health-technology-united-states/

World Health Organization. (2022a). *Physical activity*. Retrieved from https://www.who.int/news-room/fact-sheets/detail/physical-activity

World Health Organization. (2022b). *Physical inactivity a leading cause of disease and disability, warns WHO*. Retrieved from https://www.who.int/news/item/04-04-2002-physical-inactivity-a-leading-cause-of-disease-and-disability-warns-who

CHAPTER 7

STRESS, EMOTIONAL WELL-BEING, AND MENTAL HEALTH

Marty Loy

Sound mental and **emotional health** is linked to a wide range of positive outcomes, including better health status, educational achievement, productivity, higher earnings, improved interpersonal relationships, better parenting, closer social connections, greater resilience, and an overall improved quality of life (World Health Organization, 2022b).

Conversely, poor mental health can impede our capacity to realize our full potential, work productively, and make contributions to our families, work, and community. Consider the following statistics, according to the National Alliance on Mental Illness (2022b):

- One in five adults will experience a mental health disorder in any given year; one in twenty lives with a serious mental illness (SMI) such as schizophrenia, major depression, or bipolar disorder; and 1 in 6 children ages 6–17 suffer from a mental or emotional disorder.

- Major depressive disorder affects 8% of adults, or about 21 million Americans, and it is the leading cause of disability worldwide.

- Anxiety disorders, including panic disorder, generalized anxiety disorder, and phobias, affect about 19% of adults, an estimated forty million. Obsessive-compulsive disorder (OCD) affects about 3 million Americans, and post-traumatic stress disorder (PTSD) affects approximately 9 million.

- Suicide is the twelfth leading cause of death in the United States and the third leading cause of death for people ages fifteen to twenty-four years.

- Less than one-half of adults and children with a diagnosable mental disorder receive mental health services in a given year, and those rates are even lower among racial and ethnic minority groups.

LEARNING OBJECTIVES
After reading this chapter, the student will be able to:

- Define the elements of mental and emotional health.

- Describe the stress response or the fight-or-flight response.

- Identify statistics that support the rising levels of stress in our country.

- Describe how stress is linked to chronic disease and stress physiology.

- Explain the opportunities for managing stress.

- Identify strategies for managing individual and organizational stress.

- Describe mental health disparities.

- Summarize how stress affects children.

Introduction to Health Promotion, Second Edition. Edited by Anastasia Snelling.
© 2024 John Wiley & Sons Inc. Published 2024 by John Wiley & Sons Inc.
Companion Website: www.wiley.com/go/snelling2e

emotional health
our ability to attend to our own emotional needs and the skill with which we are able to deal with everyday life

- Youth ages 6–17 with a mental, behavioral, or emotional condition are three times more likely to have to repeat a grade, and high school students with depression are two times more likely to drop out compared to their same-aged peers.

- About 32% of U.S. adults (17 million) with a mental illness also experienced a substance use disorder in 2020.

The Origins of the Term *Stress*

Physician Hans Selye first introduced the term *stress* to the biologic science community in 1936. That does not mean that stress did not exist until then; it certainly did. Early humans probably struggled to find food and protect their young. Depression-era families certainly struggled to survive. Even so, recent research indicates that stress may be at an all-time high. Consider the following statistics, according to the American Psychological Association (2009):

- More than 70% of Americans experience regular physical and psychological stress symptoms; over half rate their stress levels as moderate to high and a third of those report living with extreme stress. The American Academy of Family Physicians estimates that two-thirds of all office visits to family physicians are because of stress-related symptoms.

- At work, eight out of 10 employees report job-related stress, and nearly half say they need help managing stress.

- Chronic stress is associated with a greater risk for many illnesses, such as depression, cardiovascular disease, diabetes, autoimmune diseases, upper respiratory infections, and poorer wound healing.

Consider the following statistics, according to the American Psychological Association (2018), regarding GenZ (GenZ is generally considered to be anyone born between the late 1990s and 2010):

- Over 50% of the GenZ population in the U.S. reports feeling stressed about issues in the news such as mass shootings, global warming, and widespread sexual harassment and assault reports.

- 91% of people aged 18–21 experienced at least one physical or emotional symptom due to stress in the past month, compared to 74% of adults.

- Only half of the GenZ population feels they do enough to manage their stress.

Mental health and emotional well-being depend on our ability to deal with stress and maintain control our emotions and behaviors. The first step is to understand how the body handles stress.

The Fight-or-flight Response

"Fight or flight" was a phrase first introduced to the literature by Walter Cannon in 1914. Cannon, a Harvard physiologist, used the term to describe our body's physiologic response that produces the energy to either "fight" or "flee" when we are confronted with a stressor.

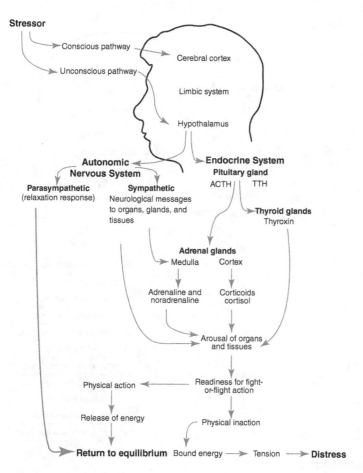

Figure 7.1   Stress Response
Source: Adapted from Seaward (2004 p. 38).

The **fight-or-flight response**, also known as the *stress response,* begins with the interpretation of an event (conscious or unconscious). Once recognized as a threat, a physiologic reaction occurs activating the nervous and endocrine systems, leading to the arousal of protective bodily functions. When the stressor is gone, the body returns to homeostasis (see figure 7.1).

The fight-or-flight response is often characterized by describing the two options cavemen had when confronted by a lion and their instinctive response to either stay and fight the animal or run away from it. Fight or flight is easily recognized when the stressor is physical in nature; however, the urge to fight or flee is also a reaction brought on by nonphysical stressors, such as pressure of an upcoming exam or a big project at work, a verbal encounter with someone. In some cases, even our imagination can elicit the stress response; consider the effects of a scary dream or the thought that a loved one who has not returned home on time may be lost.

Cannon identified physiologic reactions that occur to prepare for fighting or fleeing that have clear protective functions. For example, when under stress, our heart rate increases, carrying more oxygen to our muscles, arteries dilate in order to redirect blood flow to

fight-or-flight response
a human body's physiological response to stress; the response produces the energy needed to either fight back against a stressor or flee from it

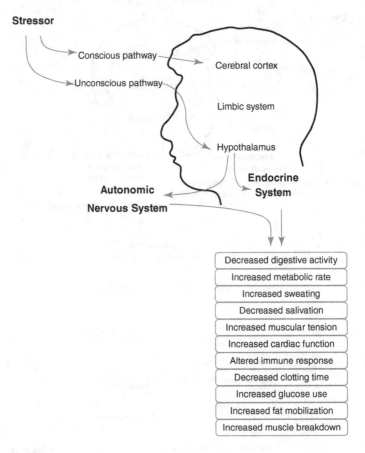

Figure 7.2   Protective Adaptations
Source: Adapted from Blonna (2005, p. 117).

muscles and organs that need it, and we perspire more, using our body's innate cooling system (see figure 7.2).

Stress Physiology

The autonomic nervous system, endocrine system, and immune system are three physiologic pathways involved in the stress response and the stress-illness relationship (see figure 7.3).

The **autonomic nervous system (ANS)**, is part of the peripheral nervous system (brain, spinal cord, and nerves) that regulates involuntary body functions. Autonomic functions are automatic or reflexive, regulating many of our vital body functions, such as heart rate and respiration. This system has two parts: (1) the sympathetic nervous system, recognized as the stress system because it excites and speeds you up, and (2) the parasympathetic nervous system, known for stimulating the relaxation response and helping the body return to a relaxed, normal state. Inciting the sympathetic system releases chemicals and hormones that initiate the stress response, increasing capabilities of essential organs of the body and constraining organs that are not essential.

autonomic nervous system (ANS)
the part of the peripheral nervous system that regulates involuntary bodily functions such as heart rate and respiration

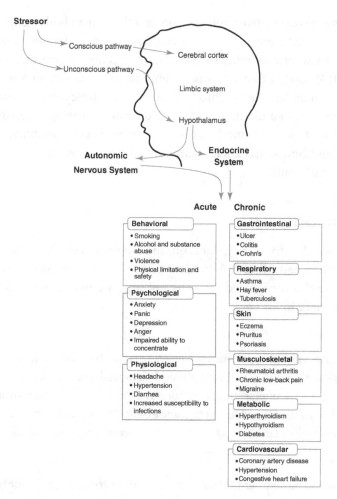

Figure 7.3   Effects of Stress on Health
Source: Adapted from Hesson (2010, p. 34).

The **endocrine system** is made up of glands that secrete hormones into the bloodstream. Three major glands involved in the stress response are the pituitary, the thyroid, and the adrenal glands. The pituitary, a pea-sized gland located at the base of the skull, is often called the master gland because it controls all other glands. Pituitary hormones trigger hormone release in other organs. The thyroid gland, located in the front of the neck below the larynx, regulates metabolism, and in reaction to stress, its hormones increase the rate at which the body can use energy. Adrenal glands, located on the top of each kidney, have two distinct parts: an outer part called the cortex, which produces steroid hormones such as cortisol, aldosterone, and testosterone, and an inner part called the medulla, which produces adrenaline and noradrenaline. The adrenal cortex produces a glucocorticoid called cortisol, which increases blood sugar and assists in metabolizing fat, protein, and carbohydrates. In recent years, there has been growing interest in using cortisol as an objective marker of stress because it is easy to trace in urine, saliva, and plasma. Cortisol has also been shown to affect immune function.

endocrine system
a system of glands responsible for secreting hormones into the blood-stream

immune system
a system of biological structures responsible for protecting the human body from infectious external agents such as bacteria and viruses and against the body's own disease-causing agents

The **immune system** primary role is to protect the human body against infections such as bacteria, viruses, and cancerous cells. Stress has long been known to suppress immune function and increase susceptibility to infections and cancer; however, recent observations by Dhabhar (2014) suggest that stress may suppress immune function under some conditions and enhance it under others. Chronic or long-term stress seems to suppress immunity by decreasing immune cell numbers and function and increasing regulatory T cells; however, during acute stress, immune function can be enhanced (Dhabhar, 2014). The more that we learn about how stress affects immunity, the more we can see how our emotions influence illness and health.

Eustress and Distress

eustress
"good" stress; stress that can be beneficial to the experiencer

distress
"bad" stress; stress that can be harmful to the experiencer, especially in excess amounts

Not all stress is bad. The frequency, duration, and intensity each play a role in whether stress is good (**eustress**) or bad (**distress**). In his 1956 book titled *The Stress of Life*, noted endocrinologist Hans Selye recognized stress as not only a demand but also commonly quite helpful. In the preface to his book, he wrote,

> No one can live without experiencing some degree of stress all the time. You may think that only serious diseases or intensive physical or mental injuries can cause stress. This is false. Crossing a busy intersection, exposure to a draft, or even sheer joy are enough to activate the body's stress mechanism to some extent. Stress is not even necessarily bad for you; it is also the spice of life, for any emotion or any activity causes stress. (Selye, 1956, p. vii)

It is important to remember that stress is most often good; after all, our body's physiologic response to a stressor is designed to help us achieve success and protect us from physical and psychological demands. Indeed, humans need stress to be healthy, happy, and productive. The Yerkes–Dodson law (Yerkes & Dodson, 1908) was conceptualized by two psychologists to show the interaction between arousal and performance. Applied more broadly, it demonstrates that having either too little or too much stress can create distress and harmful effects. People perform at peak levels when they are in the zone of optimal stress (see figure 7.4).

general adaptation syndrome (GAS)
the physical response to a stressor involves three stages: alarm, resistance, and exhaustion

Hans Selye's research demonstrated that our bodies respond to stress in remarkably similar ways and that the physical response to a stressor goes through three predictable stages known as the **general adaptation syndrome (GAS)**: alarm, resistance, and exhaustion. The alarm stage, previously described as the fight-or-flight response, prepares our body for action. During the resistance stage, our body reduces arousal levels to more appropriate and manageable levels, which are necessary to continue to protect us for a longer duration. Our body's defenses against stress cannot go on forever, and once our protective resources are depleted, we reach a state of exhaustion in which our body can no longer meet the demands placed on it and it fails to function properly. This is when chronic and serious illnesses can develop. For example, the chronic immune activation associated with prolonged exposure to stress can lead to health issues that resemble chronic inflammatory diseases like rheumatoid arthritis and other autoimmune diseases (Morey, Boggero, Scott, & Segerstrom, 2015). Even when our

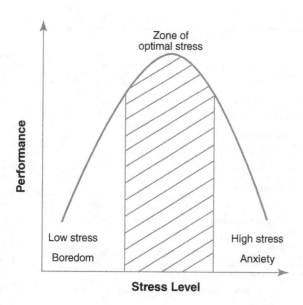

Figure 7.4   Optimal Stress Zone
Source: Adapted from Seaward (2004, p. 8).

stress is not particularly intense, if prolonged, it can still lead to poor performance, poor mental health, depression, and illness (Cohen, Janicki-Deverts, & Miller, 2007).

Life Stress and Illness

Two early researchers, Thomas Holmes and Richard Rahe (1967), studied the link between stress and illness. Holmes and Rahe found significant correlations between the severity of the life events (positive and negative) and medical histories of their study participants. Based on what they learned, they designed a Social Readjustment Rating Scale. Their scale assigned "life-change units" (LCUs) to each of forty-three stressful, yet common life events. According to Holmes and Rahe, a score of 150 LCUs or above indicated the potential for major health-related problems (see figure 7.5).

Trauma and high levels of stress exposure in childhood are linked to similar outcomes. The CDC defines adverse childhood experiences (ACEs) as potentially traumatic events that occur before the age of 18. ACEs can include things like physical abuse or exposure to substance use disorders, among others. Childhood exposure to toxic stress can affect brain development and impact the body's physical response to stress. ACEs can be linked to mental health problems and chronic health issues. Consider the statistics from the Centers for Disease Control and Prevention (2019):

- 1 in 6 adults experienced more than 4 ACEs. Females and racial/ethnic minorities are at a higher risk for experiencing 4 or more ACEs.

- 5 of the 10 leading causes of death are associated with ACEs.

- Prevention of ACEs could lower the number of adults with depression by 44%.

INSTRUCTIONS: Mark down the point value of each of these life events that has happened to you during the previous year. Total these associated points.

Life Event	Mean Value
1. Death of spouse	100
2. Divorce	73
3. Marital Separation from mate	65
4. Detention in jail or other institution	63
5. Death of a close family member	63
6. Major personal injury or illness	53
7. Marriage	50
8. Being fired at work	47
9. Marital reconciliation with mate	45
10. Retirement from work	45
11. Major change in the health or behavior of a family member	44
12. Pregnancy	40
13. Sexual difficulties	39
14. Gaining a new family member (i.e. birth, adoption, older adult moving in, etc.)	39
15. Major business readjustment	39
16. Major change in financial state (i.e. a lot worse or better off than usual)	38
17. Death of a close friend	37
18. Changing to a different line of work	36
19. Major change in the number of arguments w/ spouse (i.e. either a lot more or a lot less than usual)	35
20. Taking on a mortgage (for home, business, etc.)	31
21. Foreclosure on a mortgage or loan	30
22. Major change in responsibilities at work (i.e. promotion, demotion, etc.)	29
23. Son or daughter leaving home (marriage, attending college, joined mil.)	29
24. In-law troubles	29
25. Outstanding personal achievement	28
26. Spouse beginning or ceasing work outside the home	26
27. Beginning or ceasing formal schooling	26
28. Major change in living condition (new home, remodeling, deterioration of neighborhood or home etc.)	25
29. Revision of personal habits (dress manners, associations, quitting smoking)	24
30. Troubles with the boss	23
31. Major changes in working hours or conditions	20
32. Changes in residence	20
33. Changing to a new school	20
34. Major change in usual type and/or amount of recreation	19
35. Major change in church activity (i.e. a lot more or less than usual)	19
36. Major change in social activities (clubs, movies, visiting, etc.)	18
37. Taking on a loan (car, tv, freezer, etc.)	17
38. Major change in sleeping habits (a lot or a lot less than usual)	16
39. Major change in number of family get-togethers	15
40. Major change in eating habits (a lot more or less food intake, or very different meal hours or surroundings)	15
41. Vacation	13
42. Major holidays	12
43. Minor violations of the law (traffic tickets, jaywalking, disturbing the peace, etc.)	11
150pts or less means a relatively low amount of life change and a low susceptibility to stress-induced health breakdown	
150 to 300pts implies about a 50% chance of major health breakdown in the next 2 years	
300pts or more raises the odds to about 80%, according to the Holmes- Rahe statistical predication model	

Figure 7.5   Holmes and Rahe Stress Scale

Source: Adapted from Holmes and Rahe (1967).

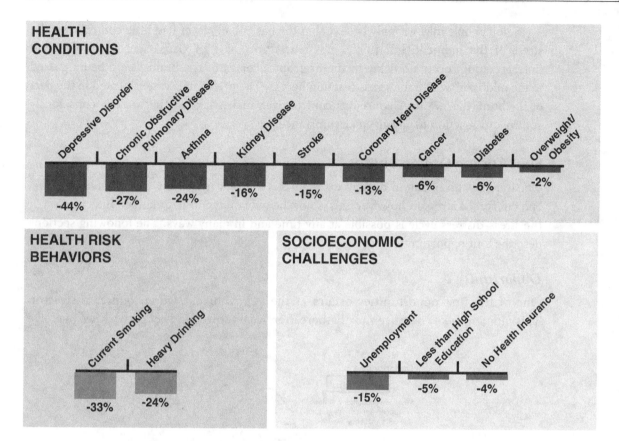

Figure 7.6   Lifetime Health Benefits of Reduced Exposures to Adverse Childhood Experiences

Source: Adapted from CDC Vital Signs (2019).

Prevention of ACEs can lower a person's risk for an array of health-related conditions and help them to thrive later in life (see figure 7.6).

Coping: Stress Management Techniques

Most scholars agree that it is not the circumstance that is stressful, but the perception and interpretation of the circumstance (Seaward, 2011). How we interpret a situation or event will have a great deal to do with the stress that results and the outcome of the situation.

A basketball player is standing at the free throw line getting ready to take a shot that will determine the outcome of a championship game. The game is on the line. If she makes the shot her team wins; if she misses they will lose. It is the same shot she has easily made many times in practice: the rim is at the same height, she is standing the exact same distance from the hoop, and every ball is the same size and weight. The only difference is her perception. If she interprets the situation accurately she will maintain perspective and find herself in a state of eustress. Effectively having coped with the situation, she will in all likelihood make the shot to win the game.

Some people may wrongly believe that the basketball player had little control over the stress of the moment, but this is not true. Processing of visual sensory information (interpretation) occurs quickly in the prefrontal cortex of the brain *before* being passed to the midbrain, where the stress reaction begins. The prefrontal cortex, located in the part of the brain that we have conscious control over, makes it clear that we *can* consciously control our reaction to any given circumstance.

Four Coping Opportunities

One important moment in dealing with stress is the very moment we encounter, perceive, and interpret a stressor; however, this is not the only moment that matters. Intervention in the stress-distress cycle is possible at any time and in many ways. The following sections describe four opportunities (see figure 7.7).

Opportunity 1

One of the first opportunities occurs at the very moment we encounter a stressor. This moment is key because shortly thereafter, we interpret and act on what we perceive

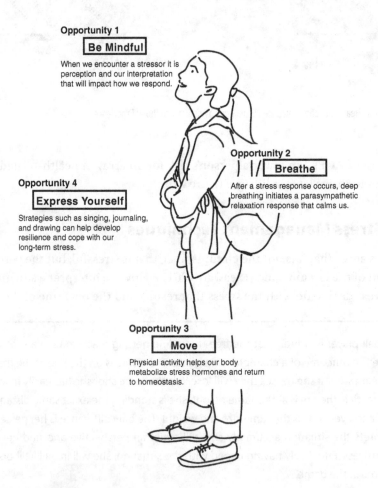

Opportunity 1
Be Mindful
When we encounter a stressor it is perception and our interpretation that will impact how we respond.

Opportunity 2
Breathe
After a stress response occurs, deep breathing initiates a parasympathetic relaxation response that calms us.

Opportunity 4
Express Yourself
Strategies such as singing, journaling, and drawing can help develop resilience and cope with our long-term stress.

Opportunity 3
Move
Physical activity helps our body metabolize stress hormones and return to homeostasis.

Figure 7.7   Four Coping Opportunities

as a threat. This interpretation is what sets the physiologic stress response in motion. If we view a threat as being more or less than it really is, we risk being ineffective at dealing with it, and we will be harmed either by the stressor itself or by the stress hormones being produced. A few other stress management approaches that can help manage perceptions are mindfulness, spirituality, finding purpose and meaning, visualization and self-talk, gratitude, and managing our environment. Let us consider mindfulness as an example.

Mindfulness, at its core, is a way of paying attention, perceiving things as they truly are, and living in the moment. Being mindful enables us to recognize habitual, often unconscious, emotional, and physiological reactions to everyday events. Considering the role of perception in stress, it is easy to see how mindfulness can help accurately interpret and initiate an appropriate stress response.

mindfulness
a way of paying attention, perceiving things as they truly are, and living in the moment

Although mindfulness stems from Buddhist tradition, it is neither a religious concept nor is it affiliated with any religious, cultural, or belief system. It is secular in nature; however, mindfulness practice has been shown to foster a sense of purpose and meaning and feelings of being grounded and connected with one's own spirituality. It is not uncommon for companies, hospitals, and community centers to provide mindfulness instruction to their employees, patients, or residents as a way of helping them succeed, reduce stress, cope with mental illness, or deal with chronic pain.

Mindfulness is a way of thinking and a skill that takes time and practice to learn. It can be practiced in a number of ways, but is most often taught through meditation. One of the most frequently cited contemporary authorities on mindfulness is Jon Kabat-Zinn, professor of medicine at the University of Massachusetts Medical School. Kabat-Zinn developed an eight-week meditation-based training called Mindfulness-Based Stress Reduction (MBSR). MBSR has demonstrated benefits for a wide range of emotional and physical issues, including stress, anxiety, depression, and psychological distress in people with chronic pain (Creswell, 2017). Mindfulness is a useful strategy to help react to stress appropriately, cope in the short and long term, and develop resiliency.

Opportunity 2

Shortly after the stress response occurs, we have a second opportunity to cope. The act of breathing is a simple yet powerful way to bring about a parasympathetic relaxation response that stops the flow of stress hormones, calms us, and returns our body to equilibrium. Deep breathing is a common technique used, but just about any type of breathing will work. All relaxation techniques, as well as meditation, have breathing as a core component. Imagery, progressive muscle relaxation, meditation, touch and massage, and anchoring are also effective ways to produce calm when under stress.

People who first try meditation or other stress management techniques often leave with the attitude that the relaxation exercise was quieting, but they have a limited sense of its benefits. That is because starting a formal relaxation routine in many ways is similar to starting a formal exercise routine, and similar to exercise, it takes time for the benefits to become apparent. If you were asked to describe what it felt like after your first day of strength training, you would probably say "sore"; if asked again after six weeks, you would probably say that your muscles feel tighter and stronger; and if asked after six months, you would probably notice other people admiring your new look and say that strength training is a routine that you cannot live without. The same is true with any formal relaxation routine; at first, it may seem only vaguely helpful, but as you progress, you will begin to experience its benefits, and at some point, you will begin to rely on your routine, and it will become an activity that you cannot live without.

There are many relaxation activities to choose from, and all include or are enhanced by breathing; however, all relaxation techniques also have characteristics that are unique. Visualization and anchoring are two examples that illustrate how different techniques can be used to manage stress.

Visualization serves three purposes: (1) to bring calm to a stressful situation, (2) to support behavior change by enabling opportunities to experience the benefits of the desired change through imagining their benefits, and (3) to provide an opportunity to mentally rehearse and prepare for a potentially stressful situation. Visualization has been used extensively among athletes to help them practice desired standards of performance and think through potential stressful situations before they happen. In this way, visualization enables athletes to think through and rehearse their game plan and plan ahead of time for any stressful situation that might occur, so they will be able to maintain perspective and keep stress at optimal levels when under the pressure of a big game. Considering its purposes, it is easy to see the many uses of visualization in day-to-day life.

Anchoring, which is different from visualization, is a tactic that helps prepare in advance for stress. An anchor is a physical or mental cue (e.g., touching our thumb and forefinger together, imagining our favorite beach) that stimulates a desirable conditioned response. For example, if we use a physical cue such as touching our thumb and forefinger whenever we are in a relaxed state, this conditions our body to associate the touching of our finger to our thumb with the state of relaxation. Practice this enough and it becomes a conditioned response that can be used to trigger relaxation whenever a stressful situation arises.

Opportunity 3

Exercise is one of *the* most helpful stress management techniques. To understand why, recall the stress physiology section of this chapter, and in particular the bottom of figure 7.1. Physical action, such as exercise, is one way of following through on the fight-or-flight response. By using major muscle groups during exercise, our body metabolizes excess blood sugar, fats, and stress hormones (adrenalin and cortisol), and with the hormones gone, our body can return to homeostasis. Not only does exercise help with the stress of the moment, but it is believed that regular exercise over time reduces the amount of adrenalin and cortisol released during other stressful times (Olpin & Hesson, 2016) and may weaken neural mechanisms involved in the stress response, resulting in lower sympathetic nervous system activity in response to perceived stress (Kelley, 2009).

There is much evidence of the positive and lasting relationship between exercise and emotional health for the mentally healthy as well as psychiatric populations. For example, a number of studies have demonstrated a positive relationship between exercise and mental health in people with emotional and mental health issues that range from hostility and drug and alcohol abuse to clinical depression and schizophrenia (Daley, 2002). Studies have shown that physically active people, even if that physical activity is limited to walking for a period of time each day, are less prone to depression than people who live a more sedentary lifestyle (Dasgupta, 2018).

Exercise has long been known to improve mood and reduce anxiety. It increases daily energy levels, boosts self-confidence, and creates a sense of accomplishment. Brain chemicals such as endorphins and serotonin are released during exercise and produce a feeling of euphoria sometimes called a "runners' high." These uplifting feelings can last for hours after the exercise is completed. All types of exercise can contribute to emotional and mental health, and activities such as yoga, tai chi, and qi gong can bring additional coping benefits, such as breathing work, being grounded, and maintaining perspective.

Opportunity 4

Music, art, and writing are each considered expressive coping strategies that are available to help manage stress and build resilience over time. Other examples of expressive therapies are drama, photography, dance, drumming, and play. These activities cater to a greater variety of communication styles, for example, verbal, visual, tactile, and so on, and provide supportive ways to communicate effectively and authentically. Expressive strategies help individuals quickly communicate relevant issues in ways that talk cannot accomplish. Expressive strategies can be particularly helpful for people with limited language skills, such as children, trauma victims, or older persons who may have suffered a stroke or are dealing with dementia. Each expressive strategy has its own unique properties and can play a variety of roles in sustaining emotional health and building resilience.

Music as a coping strategy can be as simple as a change in your emotional state by listening to uplifting music when feeling depressed. Music is routinely used by companies to achieve desired emotional effects or to sell products. Consider the use of "elevator music" as a way to calm clients who are waiting to be seen by a physician, rock and roll to excite players and fans at a professional sporting event, or jazz at a nightclub to portend romance. According to the American Music Therapy Association (2005), music can also effect positive changes in psychological, physical, cognitive, and social functioning, and it has the ability to break down strong emotional defenses and enable the expression of feelings. Not only is listening to music helpful, but also creating, singing, and moving to music can be therapeutic. Participating in music creates positive relationships, enhances social and community engagement, and creates joyful experiences (Damsgaard & Jensen, 2021); all of which could have a positive impact on mental health.

Art therapy, according to the American Art Therapy Association (2022), is the use of art media, the creative process, and the resulting artwork to help people explore and express feelings, deal with emotions, gain self-awareness, improve self-esteem, and reduce stress, fear, and anxiety. In some cases, such as with children, difficult emotions and information about stressful or traumatic events can be more easily expressed through drawings than through conversation. Art can also inspire a sense of freedom and personal well-being.

Writing is another expressive therapy that helps us understand and communicate perceptions, make reasoned interpretations, and consider appropriate responses. It can take many forms, such as journaling, poetry, letter writing, and blogging. Expressive writing provides opportunities to express and release emotions, make sense of stressful events, and process their meanings. If shared, writing can facilitate social support and enable opportunities to receive feedback and advice.

Only a few of the many available healthy coping strategies have been touched on here. Unfortunately, poor coping is all too common in response to stress. Overeating, using tobacco products, or consuming alcohol are unhealthy and counterproductive and can lead to a cycle of unresolved stress and a wide range of lifestyle illnesses. Thus, it is important to make healthy lifestyle choices and maintain a variety of healthy coping strategies.

Stress at Work

Stress is bad for business, and it places workers at alarming levels of risk. The American Institute of Stress reports that 25% of people consider their job to be their number one stressor (2022). A review of the literature completed by the American Psychological Association (2022) suggests that employees exposed to high levels of stress in the workplace are more likely to miss work and show less engagement and commitment to their work. The estimated cost of job stress in the United States could be as much as $187 billion. Research shows that health care expenditures for employees with high stress are 47% higher than for those with low stress (Goetzel et al., 1998). Conversely, as organizations reduce stress, they also reduce the associated costs, and, as data suggests, their companies will also outperform their competitors (Brown, 2006), their workers will suffer fewer sick days, and they will become more productive and more engaged. Putting policies in place to support the well-being of workers costs companies money, time, and energy, however, evidence from the APA (2022) shows that neglecting to support employees' mental, emotional, and psychological health could be far higher.

Demand and Control

The work of Karasek (1979) and later Karasek and Theorell (1990) have led to a deeper understanding of what factors play the greatest role in job stress. Their work looked specifically at the relationships between psychological demands of any given job and the amount of control one has in his or her position. When looking at the demand-control relationship, it is somewhat surprising to learn that control is a greater predictor of job stress than demand is. As one might expect, the combination of high job demands coupled with low decision-making authority can place any job among the most stressful; however, because control is the variable that is most predictive of stress, the least stressful and often most satisfying jobs can be those that are among the most demanding (see figure 7.8).

When people have ownership over their work, they gain a sense of meaning, purpose, and control. Meaning and purpose will not only make a worker more productive and

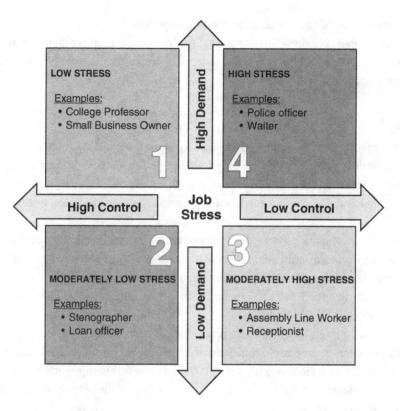

Figure 7.8   Demand-Control Support Model
Source: Adapted from de Lange, Taris, Kompier, Houtman, and Bongers (2003, p. 282).

creative (Whyte, 1994), but also it will lower stress and provide greater personal satisfaction. Finding meaning in your work will increase control and confidence and lead to a more creative, productive, and fulfilling work life (Loy, 2001).

This concept is described in a story that is common among corporate culture experts.

A STORY ABOUT VISION, MEANING, AND LOW STRESS

A manager came upon three of his workers who were each busy breaking large pieces of granite, so he stopped to ask them, "What are you doing?" The first one sarcastically replied, "What does it look like I'm doing? I'm trying to break this granite." The second worker said, "I'm breaking granite so it can be chiseled to be sold as a corner stone." The third worker enthusiastically responded, "I'm part of a team of people who are building a beautiful cathedral."

This story illustrates the importance that having clear vision and purpose has on worker satisfaction and stress. Taking into account the importance of perceived control on stress, one could predict that stress levels became lower as the vision of their work became more meaningful.

Understanding the demand-control relationship provides insights that health promotion professionals can rely on when designing strategies that help workers see purpose and meaning in their jobs and when providing more decision-making authority, greater flexibility, and greater control at the worksite.

Worksite Stress Management

worksite stress management
a worksite program designed to (1) create a healthier workplace and (2) build the capacity of employees to cope with stress through targeted stress management programs

The primary objectives of **worksite stress management** are to (1) create a healthier workplace and (2) build the capacity of employees to cope with stress through targeted stress management programs (Girdano, Everly, & Dusek, 2009). Workplace stressors can come from the physical and social work environment, organizational policies, and from workers themselves.

The most obvious work environment stressors are noise, lighting, ergonomics (equipment design factors), temperature, and repetitive tasks. Other stressors found within particular work environments might include those caused by the psychosocial work environment or those found within specific job functions, such as the demands of shift work or excessive travel requirements.

There is broad recognition that the psychosocial environment at work can have profound emotional impact on people, individually and collectively. The National Institutes of Occupational Safety and Health (Howard, 2007) lists the following work environment factors that affect physical and mental health as well as organizational outcomes such as work performance and effectiveness:

• Racism and racial and ethnic prejudice

• Sexism and sexual harassment

• Gender and racial discrimination

• Work-family integration and balance

• Support for diversity in the workplace and workforce

Organizational policies can also contribute to a stressful workplace (Greenberg, 2009). Wages, advancement opportunities, and career guidance will each play a role in job satisfaction and employee self-image and confidence levels. For example, employees who are in positions in which they are appropriately challenged and have opportunities to develop new skills and advance within their companies are far less stressed than those in companies with few advancement opportunities. Conversely, work that exceeds individual capacities through overspecialization, excessive time pressures, and job or decision-making complexity will cause stress. It is important to note that it is not only work that is too difficult that can be stressful. Low-demand or meaningless work can also lead to boredom, low job satisfaction, and stress.

Job satisfaction among employees is closely related to quality of performance (Sypniewska, 2014), demonstrating that investing in employee satisfaction benefits companies as a whole. Employees who are better informed are more satisfied, feel more involved in the company, and ultimately contribute more to its success. In particular, communication that reveals shared values and reflects common commitments to organizational goals enables coworkers to forge and sustain productive relationships in organizations (Herriot, 2002).

Companies in which internal communication is a priority are more likely to have motivated employees who are focused on company goals, resolve conflicts, and improve employee productivity. The best workplace communication is open and honest and values ethics, transparency, and accountability (Proctor & Doukakis 2003). Among many functions of corporate communication are listening, information sharing, decision-making, influencing, coordinating, and motivating (Cheney, Christensen, Zorn, & Ganesh, 2011). Job satisfaction is higher when supervisors are open and honest with their employees, share information, convey both good and bad news, evaluate job performance regularly, create a supportive climate, solicit input, and make appropriate disclosures.

Having clear policies, procedures, work objectives, job descriptions, and expectations are also essential characteristics of worksite communication that affect employee stress. Too much bureaucracy, commonly called "red tape" because of its complex and seemingly arbitrary rules, can stifle employee creativity and lead to frustration, dissatisfaction, and stress.

Newer-generation employees tend to value schedule flexibility more than past generations because their priority is work-life balance (Andrade, Westover, & Kupka, 2019). Furthermore, they tend to value relationships in the workplace, which can also be influenced by corporate and personal communication (Jablin & Krone, 1994). As self-managed work teams become commonplace in organizations, communication among and between employees becomes more important than ever before. New communication technologies (e.g., social networks, Twitter, blogs, photo sharing, and writing communities) show great promise for helping employers manage changing work environments and enhance internal communication.

Mental Health in Communities

Health statistics clearly show that mental health is one of our most pressing community health issues. For many healthy Americans, exposure to stressful lifestyles represents an increased risk of mental illness (McKenzie, Pinger, & Kotecki, 2008). Mental disorders are common throughout the United States. According to the National Institute of Mental Health (NIMH), approximately 1 in 5 U.S. adults lives with a mental illness; this totaled nearly 53 million people in the year 2020 (NIMH 2022a). What is most notable about NIMH data is that only a fraction of those affected by mental illness receive treatment.

The social costs of mental illness are staggering. The latest data available from the Centers for Disease Control and Prevention (2022) indicates a steady rise in US suicide deaths each year since 2000, with 45,979 suicide deaths reported in 2020. According to the CDC, there is a death by suicide every 11 minutes in the United States and suicide is one of the top 10 leading causes of death among Americans ages 10–64. In 2020, suicide was the second-leading cause of death for ages 10–14 and 25–34, and an estimated 12.2 million adults had serious thoughts about suicide. A look at the most prescribed medications by drug class is another indicator of mental health in the United States. Antidepressants are the third most prescribed class of drugs in the United States (Masiero, Mazzonna, & Steinbach, 2020), and an estimated 12% of Americans over the age of 12 report taking antidepressants at any given time (Masiero, Mazzonna, & Steinbach, 2020). Perhaps the most disappointing observation that can be made about community mental health is that the United States still does not have an adequate mental health program.

Stress, as a contributor to mental health problems, is likely to remain important as life becomes increasingly complex. Even Americans who believe they have good mental health carry out their everyday activities under considerable stress (McKenzie, Pinger, & Kotecki, 2008). Although there will be opportunities for community health promotion professionals to directly affect stress and mental health in community populations through programming, much of the work will be directed toward referral and mental health policy change.

Meeting Community Mental Health Needs

Health promotion professionals play an important role in creating and advocating for community health policies at local, state, and national levels. When thoughtfully conceived, mental health policy improves the coordination of essential prevention and treatment services to ensure care is delivered to people in need while improving continuity and eliminating redundancies in the health system. Any community mental health plan must start with predetermined goals, objectives, and outcome measures and be designed using evidence-based strategies. It should clarify the roles of multiple stakeholders in implementing the activities of the plan.

The World Health Organization's (2010) section on mental health policy planning and service development suggests an optimal mix of mental health services and that most mental health care can be self-managed or managed informally through community mental health services; in doing so, health care costs could be greatly reduced (see figure 7.9).

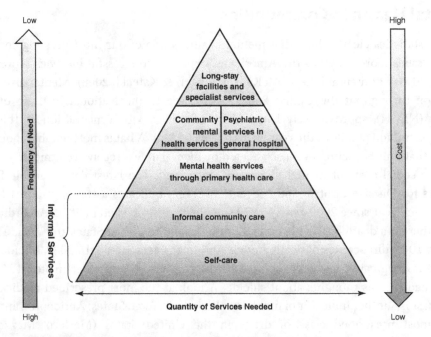

Figure 7.9   World Health Organization's Optimal Mix of Mental Health Services
Source: Department of Mental Health and Substance Abuse (2007).

Prevention is more cost-effective and humane than treatment; thus, it must be the first goal of any community mental health promotion strategy. There are many examples of preventive mental health programming in community settings (e.g., grief support groups, suicide prevention training, depression education) that is designed to address mental health issues before they manifest as mental health problems. For example, grief support groups are generally designed to normalize the grief experience, provide support, and teach coping strategies that will protect participants from mental health issues, such as depression or prolonged grief disorder. Prevention programs for children that teach resilience are particularly beneficial, for example, art, music, poetry, martial arts, or dance focused on the expression of emotions, coping, healing, and community building (Mental Health Services Oversight and Accountability Commission, 2011).

Mental health treatment refers to the provision of systematic mental health intervention, support, and assistance for those already affected by a mental health issue. Treatment services provide appropriate medical, psychiatric, psychopharmacologic, and emotional support to those affected. Psychotherapy, cognitive behavioral therapy, assertive community treatment, supportive housing, self-help groups, support groups, and peer support services are all examples of treatment options for mental health issues. Assertive community treatment, for example, is an intense, integrated approach to community mental health services in which severely mentally ill recipients receive multidisciplinary round-the-clock staffing from a psychiatric team (e.g., psychiatry, social work, nursing, substance abuse, and vocational rehabilitation), but within the comfort of their own home and community.

It is important that any prevention- or treatment-based approach implement evidence-based practices. The term *evidence-based practice* refers to interventions for which there is consistent scientific evidence showing improved client outcomes. Standard guidelines, training materials, and toolkits can be designed using evidence-based practice to ensure consistent implementation practices and improve client outcomes (Drake et al., 2001). Guidelines are also available from organizations such as the American Psychiatric Association and other advocacy groups that are based on a mixture of scientific research and consensus of experts. Although not considered evidence-based in the strict sense, they are useful best practices to follow. Given that mental health resources are limited, people with mental health issues should be able to expect services with demonstrated effectiveness that are delivered competently and consistently.

COVID-19

In late 2019, epidemiologists from the World Health Organization identified Coronavirus disease (COVID-19), a viral infection caused by the SARS-CoV-2 virus. Though many people became infected with COVID-19, some only experienced mild to moderate respiratory symptoms, while others became extremely ill, requiring intense medical intervention. As of 2022, there have been over 6.5 million COVID-19 deaths worldwide and 1 million deaths in the United States (WHO, 2022a). Beyond the number of deaths, most of the population has been impacted by COVID-19 in multiple ways.

Stress related to COVID-19 was felt by the entire population; however, certain groups and occupations experienced more significant impacts. Single people, as opposed to those who were married or living with a significant other during the pandemic, were shown to have higher levels of stress, anxiety, and depression. In particular, people living alone in isolation and families with children reported increased stress-related psychological symptoms (Kowal et al., 2020); as well as healthcare workers who had increased risk of contracting the disease, witnessed patient deaths, and were subjected to demanding working conditions (Manchia et al., 2022.

The uncertainty, loss, and isolation experienced by many people during the course of the pandemic have also led to significant impacts on mental health across the country. Consider the statistics from the National Alliance on Mental Illness (2020b):

- 1 in 5 U.S. adults experienced a mental illness, and 1 in 15 experienced a SMI.
- 1 in 15 U.S. adults experienced a mental illness coinciding with a substance use disorder.
- More than 12 million people had thoughts of suicide.
- Of the adults receiving services for mental health, 17.7 million experienced cancellations or delays of appointments, 7.3 million encountered delays in getting prescriptions, and 4.9 million were not able to access necessary care.

The COVID-19 pandemic has also placed a unique set of mental health challenges on adolescents and young adults. Consider the additional statistics from the National Alliance on Mental Illness (2020a):

- In 2020, 1 in 6 12–17-year-olds experienced a major depressive episode, 3 million had thoughts of suicide, and there was a 31% increase in mental health-related emergency room visits.
- 1 in 3 18–25-year-olds experienced a mental illness, and nearly 4 million had serious thoughts of suicide.
- 1 in 5 young people self-reported that the pandemic had a significant, negative impact on their mental health.

Social Determinants of Mental Health

Mental health disparities exist in many subpopulations. For example, homelessness and poverty are predictive of mental health, substance abuse, and physical health issues that add to the stress of this population and complicate prevention and treatment efforts. This is particularly problematic because homelessness and poverty are on the rise in the United States. According to Poverty USA, 37 million Americans, or 11.4% of the population, are currently living in poverty, and it does not appear that poverty affects all demographics equally. For example, in 2018, 10.6% of men lived in poverty, in contrast to nearly 13% of women. Additionally, the poverty rate for individuals with a disability was 25.7%, which is about 4 million people.

Older adults also have specific mental health issues, the most common being anxiety disorders (e.g., generalized anxiety and panic disorders), severe cognitive impairment (e.g., Alzheimer's disease), mood disorders (e.g., depression and bipolar disorder), and dementia. Nearly 60% of nursing home residents have Alzheimer's or another dementia (Alzheimer's Association, 2014).

According to the Alzheimer's Association, the number of people aged sixty-five or older will grow from 58 million in 2021 to 88 million by the year 2050. People aged 65 and older are at the highest risk for developing Alzheimer's disease and other forms of dementia (Alzheimer's Association, 2022).

Lesbian, gay, bisexual, transgender, queer, and other sexual minorities (LGBTQ+) experience mental illnesses. However, it is important to be aware of unique mental health risks that LGBTQ+ people may face. Research suggests that people from sexual minorities are at higher risk for depression, anxiety, and substance use disorders (Omoto & Kurtzman, 2006). The reason for these disparities is most likely related to societal stigma and resulting prejudice and discrimination that LGBTQ+ people often face. Additional research suggests LGBTQ+ people on university campuses experience higher rates of self-harm and suicidal behaviors (Gnan et al., 2019). Factors that may reduce these risks for LGBTQ+ university students include a supportive friend group and a healthy, accepting campus community.

Although each cultural group is unique in regards to mental health, in general, racial and ethnic minorities are shown to have equal or better mental health than white Americans, yet they suffer from disparities in mental health care (Jackson, Knight, & Rafferty, 2010). These disparities are the result of a general lack of attention to the mental health needs of minorities, cost of care, fragmented services, and insufficient culturally and linguistically appropriate mental health care in racial and ethnic minority communities (US Department of Health and Human Services, 2001).

Differences also exist in the types of stressors that various racial and ethnic groups experience. Considering the multitude of issues that still confront members of various racial and ethnic groups (hate crimes, fewer educational and employment opportunities, earning less pay for the same work, higher mortality and illness rates, lower access to health care, and feelings of isolation), it is clear that being of minority status can be a source of a great deal of stress (Payne, Hahn, & Lucas, 2013).

There are many examples of innovative approaches to mental health care that can help reach underserved groups; for example, stigma and discrimination programs, free transportation services, telemedicine, at-home care, outreach, transition centers, one-on-one support, and peer mentoring programs may be particularly helpful (Mental Health Services Oversight and Accountability Commission, 2011). Other innovative approaches to mental health must focus on increasing the quality and outcomes of services, promoting community collaboration, and reducing stigma and discrimination.

Health promotion professionals must understand mental health in a wide variety of subpopulations, consider the reasons that disparities exist, and develop strategies for addressing those disparities. Improved access, quality of care, better mental health education, and a more diverse mental health workforce would go a long way toward eliminating mental health disparities.

Stress Management with Children

Stress is often considered an adult-only issue. After all, what worries could a child possibly have? Children can be seen as happy, carefree, and worry-free—and to a large extent, that perception is accurate. In most cases, children are loved, cared for, and protected from many of life's troubles. However, research tells us that children have their own set of day-to-day stressors that can have detrimental effects on their behaviors, moods, and overall health (Loy, 2010). In addition, many children can and do encounter changes or traumas that are extremely stressful, even by adult standards. Childhood stressors may be different from those encountered by adults, but they are no less detrimental. One reason that managing stress can be difficult for children is that the development of complex social and emotional understanding does not happen until about the age of 10; thus, children often have difficulty putting stress into perspective, identifying and communicating emotions, and seeking appropriate support.

Effects of Stress on Children

A child's age, personality, and coping skills affect how he or she will deal with stress and react to it (Elkind, 2001). The type of stress, how long it lasts, and how intense it is will determine how taxing it is. Some research suggests that stress in children has a synergistic rather than a cumulative effect, multiplying the negative effects of stress by as much as four times with each added stressor present in a child's life (Brenner, 1997).

Among the first indicators of stress in children are changes in behavior such as fighting, teasing, or increased hostility toward siblings, family members, or peers. Parents and teachers may notice communication problems, decreased concentration, compulsiveness, or sadness. Some children become easily tearful, whiny, anxious, demanding, fearful, and nervous. Physical symptoms may include complaints of upset stomach, headache, sore throat, or vomiting. Unusual physical behaviors such as fidgeting, stuttering, tremors, or shaking legs may arise from stress. When under stress, some older children revert to behaviors characteristic of younger children, such as baby talk, thumb-sucking, nose-picking, or wetting themselves. Stressed children may bite their nails or bite, twirl, pull, or suck their hair.

There are also long-term physical and emotional consequences of mismanaged stress among children. Stress can impair a child's self-image, self-confidence, self-esteem, academic performance, and social skills. Childhood stress can increase long-term social anxiety and insecurity, and it can contribute to substance abuse, suicidal ideation, and suicide. Unidentified and untreated stress in children contributes to physical problems ranging from lowered immune function and migraine headaches to obesity, type 2 diabetes, respiratory tract illness, asthma, and several psychiatric disorders, including depression, anxiety, chronic posttraumatic stress disorder, and developmental physical and emotional delays (Loy, 2010). Some evidence suggests that many long-term consequences persist well into adulthood (Middlebrooks & Audage, 2008) and can manifest in a range of adult emotional and physical problems such as insecurity, low self-confidence, social anxieties, substance abuse, and depression. Stress can influence everything from physical health and memory to social competence, marital success, and academic and socioeconomic attainment.

Children can appear outwardly resilient to the immediate effects of stress but, if the timing of the stress is during a critical period of personality development, they can carry the long-term effects with them for the rest of their lives. Many studies link trauma and chronic stress with poor physical and mental health over the long term (Brenner, 1997).

Stress Types Among Children

In many cases, the same things that stress adults also stress children; however, because levels of stress are influenced so strongly by one's perception and because children often perceive circumstances differently than adults do, their stressors can be unique.

Childhood stressors can be placed along a continuum beginning with normal day-to-day situations, such as keeping up with an overloaded activity calendar; mid-range stressful situations, which are usually related to change and insecurity, such as a family move or a divorce; and those highly stressful, traumatic, and chronic stressors at the far end of the continuum that are difficult to handle, such as neglect or a death in the family.

Over half of all stressors described by children come from day-to-day occurrences at home or at school (Humphrey, 2004), such as time demands, parent or school expectations, social pressures, separation from parents, and punishments. Children who have siblings often report conflicts and rivalries with siblings as frequent stressors. Stressors related to change and insecurity, although somewhat common, rank higher on the severity of stress continuum. They include divorce or family discord, remarriage, moving, decline in family income, parent alcoholism, deployment, arrival of a new sibling, and hospitalization. Most children must deal with one or more of these types of stressors sometime during their childhood.

Moderate change-related stressors can tax the individual resources of a child. At the pinnacle of the severity of the stress continuum lie traumatic and chronic stressors. They are serious, unexpected, and uncommon events, such as witnessing a death or experiencing the death of a family member. Emotional or sexual abuse, abandonment, natural disasters, and exploitation are examples of traumatic stress, as are neglect, poverty, or a major long-term illness (Courtois, 2008). All types of trauma pose serious risks to children both in their youth and in later life; in most cases, they require skillful, professional support.

During their formative years, children must deal with a multitude of stressors. Most are common and short-term, resulting in little more than short-lived poor behavior or a disagreeable mood and requiring only basic personal stress management skills and minimal support. Some stressors, especially when change and insecurity are involved, can be more taxing. If not dealt with properly, usually with the help of a skilled adult, these moderately stressful situations can lead to serious short- and long-term behavioral, emotional, or physical consequences. A few stressors involve traumas or chronic stressors that pose serious risks to children; in most cases, they just require skillful, professional support.

In any case, health promotion professionals and all adults who work with children should learn about childhood stress, be able to recognize the signs of stress in children, provide support to children when needed, and help children learn to manage stress for themselves.

Stress Among College Students

There is no shortage of stress among students on college and university campuses. According to a study from the American Addiction Centers looking at college student stress, 87.9% of students reported a stressful school life. While students majoring in teacher education and

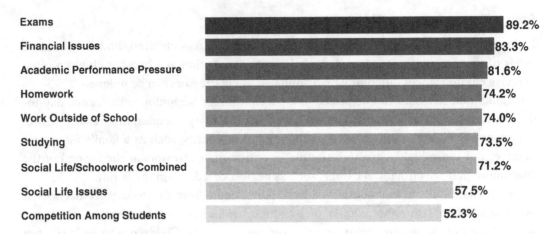

Figure 7.10   Stress Among College Students
Source: Adapted from American Addiction Centers (2022).

medicine cited the highest stress levels, elevated stress was found among students in all programs of study. Many factors contributed to college students' stress, including exams, student loans, and the pressure to perform academically. Figure 7.10 demonstrates the most stressful factors in students' lives.

In the same study, 98% of students reported that stress had an impact on their mental health. Sleep and physical exercise were cited among the most used coping mechanisms; unfortunately, not all coping was as healthy as 46.9% reported eating, 34.3% used alcohol, and 7.1% used "study drugs" like Adderall or Ritalin (American Addiction Centers, 2022).

Though college and university students are at an increased risk of experiencing stress, there are unique opportunities for student support available across most campuses. Colleges offer career counselling, tutoring, peer special interest groups, and mental health counseling with little to no cost for attending students. Of the 98% of students who said stress of college adversely affected their mental health, only 14% sought out therapy for support (American Addiction Centers, 2022) and instead ignored their stress or resorted to more risky behaviors like using drugs and alcohol. It is important for college students to not only be aware of the stress they are experiencing, but to acknowledge it, and seek appropriate help and support that may be available to them.

Stress in a Digital World

Recent literature is filled with references to stress in the digital world, calling it Digital Stress, Facebook Induced Stress, Accessibility Stress, Connection Overload, Mobile Entrapment, and Social Network Site Exhaustion (Steele, Hall, & Christofferson, 2020). Regardless of what we call it, the use of digital technologies is a primary source of stress among adolescent and college-age populations (Mihailidis, Fincham, & Cohen, 2014). In fact, social media usage has reached unprecedented levels, raising concerns that constant connectivity is causing stress and harming mental health (Reinecke et al., 2017).

In their meta-analysis of hundreds of studies across all age groups, Odgers & Jensen (2020) found many associations between social media use and stress, as well as increased rates of suicidal behaviors, depression, and loneliness (Rosenstein & Sheehan, 2018), and additional research suggesting social media use, under stressful contexts, can increase risk for type 2 diabetes, obesity, and cardiovascular disease (Everson-Rose & Lewis, 2005). However, there is ongoing debate about the impact of social media use on health, and a body of research suggests digital technologies can also offer opportunities for healthy interactions (Hunter et al., 2018). Many study participants report using social media networks to seek support and advice when they face setbacks or to seek mental health information (Kauer, Mangan, & Sanci, 2014).

Steele et al. (2020) describe four influencing factors at play with digital media's effect on peer relationships and stress. These four factors—availability stress, approval anxiety, fear of missing out, and communication overload—are described below.

- **Availability stress:** Distress, guilt, and anxiety that result from beliefs about others' expectations to be always available and responsive.

- **Approval anxiety:** Uncertainty and anxiety surrounding others' impressions, reactions, and responses to posts and digital interactions.

- **Fear of missing out:** Distress caused by real, perceived, or anticipated social consequences of being left out.

- **Connection overload:** The experience of trying to manage excessive notifications, text messages, posts, etc.

It is important for health promotion professionals to understand these and other factors that allow social media use to become a source of distress; promote awareness of relationships between reliance on social media, stress, self-esteem, and health; and promote a more mindful approach to using social media. Health promotion professionals must also keep in mind opportunities that digital tools may offer to take evidence-based interventions to scale and reduce disparities in access to effective education, resources, and intervention.

Summary

The more we learn about mental health issues and stress, in particular, the more insight we will have into the factors that influence mental health. With this in mind, there are five areas that health promotion professionals must be able to address. Health promotion professionals must: (1) understand the nature and origins of mental health-related issues and know how to respond appropriately; (2) empower individuals and communities, increasing personal control over decisions that affect mental health; (3) provide evidence-based best practices to ensure high-quality, consistent prevention, care, and treatment; (4) assist in the coordination of services that enable individuals, families, groups, organizations, and communities to play active roles in achieving, protecting, and sustaining health; and (5) practice self-care and model the use of healthy stress management in their own lives.

KEY TERMS

1. **Emotional health:** our ability to attend to our own emotional needs and the skill with which we are able to deal with everyday life

2. **Fight-or-flight response:** a human body's physiological response to stress; the response produces the energy needed to either fight back against a stressor or to flee from it

3. **Autonomic nervous system (ANS):** the part of the peripheral nervous system that regulates involuntary bodily functions such as heart rate and respiration

4. **Endocrine system:** a system of glands responsible for secreting hormones into the bloodstream

5. **Immune system:** a system of biological structures responsible for protecting the human body from infectious external agents such as bacteria and viruses and against the body's own disease-causing agents

6. **Eustress:** "good" stress; stress that can be beneficial to the experiencer

7. **Distress:** "bad" stress; stress that can be harmful to the experiencer, especially in excess amounts

8. **General adaptation syndrome (GAS):** the physical response to a stressor involving three stages: alarm, resistance, and exhaustion

9. **Mindfulness:** a way of paying attention, perceiving things as they truly are, and living in the moment

10. **Worksite stress management:** a work-site program designed to (1) create a healthier workplace and (2) build the capacity of employees to cope with stress through targeted stress management programs

REVIEW QUESTIONS

1. How would you describe the stress response?

2. How is stress linked to chronic disease?

3. How would you describe stress physiology and the three systems it affects in the body?

4. What is the difference between eustress and distress?

5. What is a coping opportunity? Identify four opportunities.

6. How would you describe the social determinants of mental health?

7. How would you describe what organizations are doing to help employees manage stress?

8. What are policies within the ACA that will improve mental health?

9. How would you describe the community mental health promotion strategy?

10. How would you describe the issues specifically affecting children's mental health?

11. How has the COVID-19 pandemic affected people's stress and mental health?

12. What factors impact stress levels in college students? What resources can college students utilize to combat high stress and poor mental health?

STUDENT ACTIVITIES

1. Prepare a twenty-minute talk for consumers on the physiology of stress.

2. Using the PRECEDE–PROCEED model of program planning, outline a process for creating a stress management program for a department on a college campus.

3. Identify the different populations in a school. Identify potential stressors for each group and describe one stress management technique that could be used to address the stressors.

4. Identify statistics that support the rising levels of stress.

Acknowledgment

I would like to thank Abigail Zoromski for skillfully reviewing and summarizing literature for this chapter and Michaela Dunn for her help in constructing several of the figures.

References

Alzheimer's Association (2014). *Special care units.* Retrieved from http://www.alz.org

Alzheimer's Association (2022). *Alzheimer's disease facts and figures. Alzheimers Dement, 2022,* 18.

American Addiction Centers (2022). *School stress for college students and unhealthy coping mechanisms.* Retrieved from https://americanaddictioncenters.org/blog/college-coping-mechanisms

American Art Therapy Association (2022). Retrieved from http://www.arttherapy.org/

American Music Therapy Association (2005). *Definition and quotes about music therapy.* Retrieved from www.musictherapy.org/about/quotes

American Psychological Association (2009). *Stress in America 2009.* Washington, DC: American Psychological Association.

American Psychological Association (2018). *Stress in America: Generation Z.* Stress in America™ Survey.

American Psychological Assocation (2022). *The American Workforce faces compounding pressure.* https://www.apa.org/pubs/reports/work-well-being/compounding-pressure-2021

Andrade, M. S., Westover, J. H., & Kupka, B. A. (2019). The role of work-life balance and worker scheduling flexibility in predicting global comparative job satisfaction. *International Journal of Human Resource Studies, 9*(2). doi:10.5296/ijhrs.v9i2.14375.

Blonna, R. (2005). *The physical basis of stress. Coping with stress in a changing world* (3rd ed., p. 117). New York: McGraw-Hill.

Brenner, A. (1997). *Helping children cope with stress.* San Francisco: Jossey-Bass.

Brown, P. B. (2006, September 2). Listen up. Know your audience. *New York Times.* Retrieved from http://www.nytimes.com/2006/09/02/business/02offline.html?_r=1&

Centers for Disease Control and Prevention (2019). *Adverse Childhood Experiences (ACEs): Preventing early trauma to improve adult health.* Vital Signs™.

Centers for Disease Control and Prevention (2022). *Facts about suicide.* Retrieved from https://www.cdc.gov/suicide/facts/index.html

Cheney, G., Christensen, L. T., Zorn, T. E., Jr., & Ganesh, S. (2011). *Organizational communication in an age of globalization: Issues, reflections and practices.* Prospect Heights, IL: Waveland Press.

Cohen, S., Janicki-Deverts, D., & Miller, G. E. (2007). Psychological stress and disease. *Journal of the American Medical Association, 298*(14), 1685–1687.

Courtois, C. A. (2008). Complex trauma, complex reactions: Assessment and treatment. *Psychological Trauma: Theory, Research, Practice, and Policy, 1*(S), 86–100.

Creswell, D. J. (2017). Mindfulness interventions. *Annual Review of Psychology, 68*, 491–516.

Daley, A. J. (2002). Exercise therapy and mental health in clinical populations: Is exercise therapy a worthwhile intervention? *Advances in Psychiatric Treatment, 8*, 262–270.

Damsgaard, J. B. & Jensen, A. (2021). Music activities and mental health recovery: Service users' perspectives presented in the CHIME framework. *International Journal of Environmental Research and Public Health, 2021*(18), 6638. doi:10.3390/ ijerph18126638.

Dasgupta, A. (2018). *The science of stress management: a guide to best practices for better well-being.* Blue Ridge Summit: Rowman & Littlefield Publishers.

Department of Mental Health and Substance Abuse (2007). *The optimal mix of services for mental health.* Geneva: World Health Organization.

Dhabhar, F. S. (2014). Effects of stress on immune function: the good, the bad, and the beautiful. *Immunol Res, 58*, 193–210. doi:10.1007/s12026-014-8517-0.

Drake, R. E., Goldman, H. H., Leff, S., Lehman, A. F., Dixon, L., Mueser, K. T., & Torrey, W. C. (2001). *Psychiatric Services.* doi:10.1176/appi.ps.52.2.179.

Elkind, D. (2001). *The hurried child growing up too fast too soon* (3rd ed.). Cambridge, MA: Perseus Publishing.

Everson-Rose, S. A. & Lewis, T. T. (2005). Psychosocial factors and cardiovascular diseases. *Annual Review of Public Health., 26*, 469–500.

Girdano, D. A., Dusek, D. E., & Everly, G. S., Jr. (2009). *Controlling stress and tension: A holistic approach* (8th ed.). San Francisco, CA: Pearson Benjamin Cummings.

Gnan, G. H., Rahman, Q., Ussher, G., Baker, D., West, E., & Rimes, K. A. (2019). General and LGBTQ-specific factors associated with mental health and suicide risk among LGBTQ students. *Journal of youth studies, 22*(10), 1393–1408.

Goetzel, R. Z., Anderson, D. R., Whitmer, R. W., Ozminkowski, R. J., Dunn, R. L., Wasserman, J., & The Health Enhancement Research Organization (HERO) Research Committee (1998). The relationship between modifiable health risks and health care expenditures: An analysis of the multi-employer HERO health risk and cost database. *Journal of Occupational and Environmental Medicine, 40*(10), 843–854.

Greenberg, J. (2009). *Occupational stress comprehensive stress management* (11th ed., pp. 310–343). New York: McGraw-Hill.

Herriot, P. (2002). Selection and self: Selection as a social process. *European Journal of Work and Organizational Psychology, 11*, 385–402. doi:10.1080/135943 20244000256.

Hesson, O. (2010). *The science of stress. Stress management for life* (2nd ed., p. 34). Clifton Park, NY: Cengage Learning.

Holmes, T. H. & Rahe, R. H. (1967). The social readjustment rating scale. *Journal of Psychosomatic Research, 11*(2), 213–218.

Howard, J. (2007). Foreword. In M. A. Bond, A. Kalaja, P. Markkanen, D. Cazeca, S. Daniel, L. Tsurikova, & L. Punnett (Eds.), *Expanding our understanding of the psychosocial work environment: A compendium of measures, discrimination, harassment and work-family issues* (p. 3). Washington, DC: Department of Health and Human Services.

Humphrey, J. H. (2004). *Childhood stress in contemporary society* (11th ed.). Binghamton, NY: Haworth Press.

Hunter, R. F., Gough, A., O'Kane, N., McKeown, G., Fitzpatrick, A., Walker, T., . . . Kee, F. (2018). Ethical issues in social media research for public health. *American Journal of Public Health., 108*(3), 343–348.

Jablin, F. M. & Krone, K. J. (1994). Task/work relationships: A life-span perspective. In M. L. Knapp & G. R. Miller (Eds.), *Handbook of interpersonal communication*. Thousand Oaks, CA: Sage.

Jackson, J. S., Knight, K. M., & Rafferty, J. A. (2010). Race and unhealthy behaviors: Chronic stress, the HPA axis, and physical and mental health disparities over the life course. *American Journal of Public Health, 100*(5), 933–939.

Karasek, R. A. (1979). Job demands, job decisions latitude, and mental strain: Implications for job redesign. *Administrative Science Quarterly, 24*(2), 285–308.

Karasek, R. A. & Theorell, T. (1990). *Healthy work: Stress, productivity, and the reconstruction of working life*. New York: Basic Books.

Kauer, S. D., Mangan, C., & Sanci, L. (2014). Do online mental health services improve help-seeking for young people? A systematic review. *J med Internet Res., 16*(3), 66.

Kelley, D. (2009). The effects of exercise and diet on stress. *Nutritional Perspectives: Journal of the Council on Nutrition, 32*(1), 37–39.

Kowal, M., Coll-Martín, T., Ikizer, G., Rasmussen, J., Eichel, K., Studzińska, A., . . . Ahmed, O. (2020). Who is the most stressed during the COVID-19 pandemic? Data from 26 countries and areas. *Applied Psychology: Health and Well-Being, 12*(4), 946–966.

de Lange, A. H., Taris, T. W., Kompier, M. A., Houtman, I. L., & Bongers, P. M. (2003). "The very best of the millennium": Longitudinal research and the demand-control-(support) model. *Journal of Occupational Health Psychology, 8*(4), 282–305.

Loy, M. (2001). Combining heart and work: A prescription for a stress-free career. *The Communication Connection, 15*(3), 5–7.

Loy, M. (2010). *Children and stress: A handbook for parents, teachers, and therapists*. Duluth, MN: Whole Person Associates.

Manchia, M., Gathier, A. W., Yapici-Eser, H., Schmidt, M. V., de Quervain, D., van Amelsvoort, T., . . . Vinkers, C. H. (2022). The impact of the prolonged COVID-19 pandemic on stress resilience and mental health: A critical review across waves. *European Neuropsychopharmacol, 55*, 22–83.

Masiero, G., Mazzonna, F, Steinbach, S. (2020). Happy Pills? Mental Health Effects of the Dramatic Increase of Antidepressant Use. *IDEAS Working Paper Series from RePEc.*

McKenzie, J. F., Pinger, R. R., & Kotecki, J. E. (2008). *An introduction to community health* (5th ed.). Sudbury, MA: Jones & Bartlett.

Mental Health Services Oversight and Accountability Commission (2011). *Prevention and early intervention: Trends report 2011.* Sacramento, CA: Mental Health Services Oversight and Accountability Commission.

Middlebrooks, J. S. & Audage, N. C. (2008). *The effects of childhood stress on health across the lifespan.* Atlanta: Centers for Disease Control and Prevention, National Center for Injury Prevention and Control.

Mihailidis, P., Fincham, K., & Cohen, J. (2014). Toward a media literate model for civic engagement in digital culture: Exploring the civic habits and dispositions of college students on Facebook. *Atlantic Journal of Communication, 22*(5), 293–309.

Morey, J. N., Boggero, I. A., Scott, A. B., & Segerstrom, S. C. (2015). Current directions in stress and human immune function. *Current Opinion in Psychology, 5*, 13–17.

National Alliance on Mental Illness (2020a). *Recognizing the Impact.* Mental Health by the Numbers.

National Alliance on Mental Illness (2020b). *Youth and Young Adults.* Mental Health by the Numbers.

National Alliance on Mental Illness (2022a). *Mental Health by the Numbers.* Retrieved from https://nami.org/mhstats

National Institute of Mental Health (2022b). *Statistics.* Retrieved from https://www.nimh.nih.gov/health/statistics/mental-illness

Odgers, C. L. & Jensen, M. R. (2020). Annual Research Review: Adolescent mental health in the digital age: facts, fears, and future directions. *The Journal of Child Psychology and Psychiatry., 61*(3), 336–348.

Olpin, M. & Hesson, M. (2016). *Stress management for life: A research-based, experiential approach* (4th ed.). Boston, MA: Cengage Learning.

Omoto, A. M. & Kurtzman, H. S. (2006). *Sexual orientation and mental health: Examining identity and development in lesbian, gay and bisexual people.* Washington, DC: APA Books.

Payne, W. A., Hahn, D. B., & Lucas, E. B. (2013). *Understanding your health* (12th ed.). New York, NY: McGraw-Hill.

Proctor, T. & Doukakis, I. (2003). Change management: The role of internal communication and employee development. *Corporate Communications, 8*(4), 268–277. doi:10.1108/13563280310506430.

Reinecke, L., Aufenanger, S., Beutel, M. E., Dreier, M., Quiring, O., Stark, B., . . . Müller, K. W. (2017). Digital stress over the life span: The effects of communication load and internet multitasking on perceived stress and psychological health impairments in a German probability sample. *Media Psychology, 20*(1), 90–115.

Rosenstein, B. & Sheehan, A. (2018). Open letter from JANA partners and CALSTRS to Apple Inc. *Think differently about kids.* Retrieved from https://thinkdifferentlyaboutkids.com/letter/

Seaward, B. L. (2004). The physiology of stress. In *Managing stress* (4th ed., p. 38). Sudbury, MA: Jones & Bartlett.

Seaward, B. L. (2011). *Managing stress: Principles and strategies for health and well-being.* Sudbury, MA: Jones & Bartlett.

Selye, H. (1956). *The stress of life* (Vol. 5). New York: McGraw-Hill.

Steele, R. G., Hall, J. A., & Christofferson, J. L. (2020). Conceptualizing digital stress in adolescents and young adults: Toward the development of an empirically based model. *Clinical Child and Family Review, 23,* 15–26.

Sypniewska, B. A. (2014). Evaluation of factors influencing job satisfaction. *Contemporary Economics., 8*(1), 57–72. doi:10.5709/ce.1897-9254.131.

The American Institute of Stress (2022). *Workplace Stress.* Retrieved from https://www.stress.org/workplace-stress

US, Department of Health and Human Services (2001). *Mental health: Culture, race, and ethnicity.* Rockville, MD: US Department of Health and Human Services, Substance Abuse and Mental Health Services Administration, Center for Mental Health Services.

Whyte, D. (1994). *The heart aroused: Poetry and the preservation of the soul in corporate America.* New York: Currency and Doubleday.

World Health Organization (2010). *Mental health and development: Targeting people with mental health conditions as a vulnerable group.* Geneva: WHO Press.

World Health Organization (2022a). *United States of America Situation.* Retrieved from https://covid19.who.int/region/amro/country/us

World Health Organization. (2022b). *World mental health report: transforming mental health for all.*

Yerkes, R. M. & Dodson, J. D. (1908). The relation of strength of stimulus to rapidity of habit-formation. *Journal of Comparative Neurology and Psychology, 18,* 459–482.

CLINICAL PREVENTIVE SERVICES

Trends, Access, Promotion, and Guidelines

Casey Korba

It is empowering to realize that it is possible to have tremendous control over many aspects of our health—our genetics and family history do not always completely determine our fate. The social determinants of health—the environment in which we are born, live, work, worship, and age, also play a major role in our health. They affect what we eat; how often we exercise; our sleep habits; social habits; coping mechanisms; and our access to clinical preventive services. All of these factors and services influence our chances of developing certain illnesses and conditions, and in the case of clinical preventive services, give us the ability to potentially diagnose conditions and intervene at an earlier disease stage. Not every health risk can be avoided, but we can reduce our chances of developing many debilitating health conditions and contracting certain diseases while improving our overall health prognosis when we develop healthy habits and behaviors, including the provision of recommended clinical preventive services.

Through screening and other clinical preventive services that individuals receive at their primary care doctor's office, at their local pharmacy, or increasingly, at a work site or community-based health fair, individuals can detect certain conditions while they are asymptomatic, often leading to improved health outcomes (see Table 8.1). Complications from chronic conditions and diseases such as cardiovascular disease and related risk factors, type 2 diabetes, certain types of cancer, and certain infectious diseases can be prevented by following evidence-based recommendations for specific preventive services based on age and gender.

Research demonstrates linkages between certain unhealthy behaviors, such as tobacco use, a sedentary lifestyle, and a high-fat, high-calorie diet, with chronic health conditions, which include heart disease, type 2 diabetes,

LEARNING OBJECTIVES
After reading this chapter, the student will be able to:

- Define clinical preventive services.

- Describe how clinical preventive services are linked to promoting health.

- Identify aged-related clinical services for chronic disease.

- Describe the barriers and opportunities for accessing clinical preventive services.

- Identify what actions healthcare companies, communities, and work sites are doing to encourage preventive services.

- Describe how the Affordable Care Act incorporates clinical services into health care.

Introduction to Health Promotion, Second Edition. Edited by Anastasia Snelling.
© 2024 John Wiley & Sons Inc. Published 2024 by John Wiley & Sons Inc.
Companion Website: www.wiley.com/go/snelling2e

Table 8.1   Select Preventive Screenings Examinations

Screening Test	What the Test Is For	When It Should Be Conducted*
Blood pressure (BP)	High blood pressure Desirable blood pressure is <120/80	Screening annually in adults forty years and older and for adults at increased risk for hypertension (such as Black persons, persons with high-normal blood pressure, or persons who are overweight or obese)every two years with BP < 120/80 Screening less frequently (every three to five years) for adults aged eighteen to thirty nine years not at increased risk and with prior normal BP reading every year with systolic BP of 120–139 mmHg or diastolic BP of 80–90 mmHg
Statin use for the primary prevention of cardiovascular disease in adults	Preventive medication to control cholesterol	The USPSTF recommends that clinicians prescribe a statin for the primary prevention of CVD for adults aged forty to seventy five years who have one or more CVD risk factors (i.e., dyslipidemia, diabetes, hypertension, or smoking) and an estimated 10-year risk of a cardiovascular event of 10% or greater
Mammography	Breast cancer	Every two years between the ages of fifty and seventy-four
Colonoscopy	Colorectal cancer	Beginning at age fifty and continuing every ten years until age seventy-five
Weight loss to prevent obesity-related morbidity and mortality in adults	Behavioral interventions	The USPSTF recommends that clinicians offer or refer adults with a body mass index (BMI) of 30 or higher (calculated as weight in kilograms divided by height in meters squared) to intensive, multicomponent behavioral interventions

* If no other risk factors are present, such as family history

and certain cancers. Changing or controlling these unhealthy behaviors can improve health outcomes. For example, most risk factors for heart disease and stroke—specifically high blood pressure, high cholesterol, smoking, and obesity—are preventable and controllable. Yet heart disease is currently the number one cause of death in the United States, bringing about approximately seven hundred thousand deaths each year in this country (Centers for Disease Control and Prevention (CDC), 2022a). Regular physical activity, controlling high blood pressure and high cholesterol, healthy eating, not smoking, and weight management could reduce the risk of heart attack or stroke by more than 80% (CDC, 2018).

Benefits of Evidence-based Clinical Preventive Services

Clinical preventive services include screening tests, immunizations, counseling, and preventive medications; many of these services are highly effective at extending and improving health and well-being. Screening tests, through the timely identification of reversible or treatable conditions, can prevent disease progression and costly outcomes (American Journal of Managed Care, 2019). Immunization practices have eliminated many infectious diseases and dramatically reduced the rates of others. Effective health behavior counseling can reduce a significant percentage of deaths attributable to physical inactivity and unhealthy diet, and problem drinking (Nelson, 2020).

clinical preventive services

Services provided at one's primary care physician's office, local pharmacy, or health fairs to detect and reduce the risk of specific health conditions from progressing; examples include screening tests, immunizations, counseling, and preventive medications.

Recommended Levels of Preventive Services

Encouraging the use of certain clinical preventive services will save lives. The CDC estimates that 250,000 lives could be saved from heart disease, cancer, stroke, chronic obstructive lung disease, and unintentional injuries if all states performed as well as the best ones in reducing mortality.

Patient Protection and Affordable Care Act

The Patient Protection and Affordable Care Act (ACA), otherwise known as the healthcare reform bill, was enacted in 2010. It included many new policies around clinical and community preventive services and set the stage for an increase in regulations regarding clinical and community preventive health services.

The ACA included the creation of the National Prevention, Health Promotion, and Public Health Council (National Prevention Council), which was tasked with developing a national prevention strategy. The goal of the **National Prevention Strategy** is to move the nation from an emphasis on illness and disease to one based on prevention and wellness. The strategy's framework aims to guide the federal government and the nation on the most effective and achievable means for improving the health of the nation through prevention and health promotion policies and programs. The National Prevention Strategy has four strategic directions, which include a focus on healthy environments, clinical and community preventive services, empowered people, and the elimination of health disparities. The National Prevention Strategy's 2011 framework states,

> Clinical and Community Preventive Services: Ensure that prevention-focused health care and community prevention efforts are available, integrated, and mutually reinforcing. The provision of evidence-based clinical and community preventive services and the integration of these activities are central to improving and enhancing physical and mental health. Certain clinical preventive services have proven to be both effective and cost-saving through decades of practice and research; The ACA reduces barriers to people receiving many clinical preventive services. Clinical preventive services can be supported and reinforced by community prevention efforts that have the potential to reach large numbers of people (US Department of Health and Human Services, 2011).

National Prevention Strategy
The National Prevention Strategy aims to guide our nation in the most effective and achievable means for improving health and well-being. The Strategy prioritizes prevention by integrating recommendations and actions across multiple settings to improve health and save lives.

History of Preventive Services

It is hard for many of us to believe that smoking in a hospital room used to be an accepted practice, that people drove in cars without seat belts, and that babies were held in laps rather than car seats. Through research, we have learned how to better keep people safe and healthy. Clinical preventive services have evolved over the years as growing evidence has demonstrated what works most effectively to improve the health and well-being of diverse populations. Science has guided public and private policies, as well as medical practices, influencing social norms.

Because clinical preventive services are typically addressed during a primary care office visit, clinicians have to make decisions about what services are feasibly covered in each office visit. As science evolves, these recommendations change over time. In the 1970s, pediatricians had fewer vaccines to provide, and childhood obesity was not as prevalent. In 2022, pediatricians are focused on the increase in developmental disorders such as autism and an increase in the number of vaccines available, as well as increased focus on mental health in children. It is likely that pediatricians do not spend time counseling parents of young children regarding motor vehicle safety, as they may have been twenty-five years ago, considering that car seat use is addressed by state law, and social norms encourage parents to regularly use appropriate child safety restraints.

Health Resources and Services Administration (HRSA)
It is the primary federal agency for improving access to health care services for people who are uninsured, isolated, or medically vulnerable.

The **Health Resources and Services Administration (HRSA)**, the primary federal agency for improving access to health care services for people who are uninsured, isolated, or medically vulnerable, was formed in 1982. In 1984, the federal government formally established the US Preventive Services Task Force (USPSTF), which now serves as the gold standard in evidence-based clinical preventive services recommendations for physicians and clinicians, public health experts, government agencies, and health insurance plans.

The federal government's involvement in the public's health goes back to the earliest roots of our nation, with the passage of various bills to help the sick and disabled and protect the public from the spread of infectious diseases. In 1953, the Cabinet-level Department of Health, Education, and Welfare was created under President Eisenhower. In 1979, the Department of Education Organization Act was signed into law, providing for a separate Department of Education. Health, Education, and Welfare became the Department of Health and Human Services in 1980 (US Department of Health and Human Services, 2014)

The US Preventive Services Task Force (USPSTF)

US Preventive Services Task Force (USPSTF)
The USPSTF is an independent panel of national experts in prevention and evidence-based medicine composed of practicing doctors and nurses in the fields of family medicine, general internal medicine, gynecology-obstetrics, nursing, pediatrics, and preventive medicine, as well as health behavior specialists.

Since it was first convened in 1984 by the US Public Health Service, the **USPSTF** has worked to fulfill its mission of doing the following:

- Assessing the benefits and harms of preventive services in people asymptomatic for the target condition, based on age, gender, and risk factors for disease.

- Making recommendations about which preventive services should be incorporated routinely into primary care practice.

The Task Force makes recommendations based on rigorous reviews of the scientific evidence to help primary care professionals and patients decide together whether a preventive service is right for a patient's needs (USPSTF, 2022d). The Task Force does not conduct research studies but reviews and assesses the existing peer-reviewed evidence to make recommendations.

The Task Force chooses topics to review and makes recommendations based on the following criteria:

- Public health importance (i.e., burden of suffering and expected effectiveness of the preventive service to reduce that burden).

- Potential for the recommendation to have an impact on clinical practice.

- New evidence that may change prior recommendations.

- The need for a balanced portfolio of topics in clinical preventive services.

Table 8.2   US Preventive Services Task Force (USPSTF) Grading System

Grade	Definition
A	The USPSTF recommends the service. There is high certainty that the net benefit is substantial.
B	The USPSTF recommends the service. There is high certainty that the net benefit is moderate or there is moderate certainty that the net benefit is moderate to substantial.
C	The USPSTF recommends selectively offering or providing this service to individual patients based on professional judgment and patient preferences. There is at least moderate certainty that the net benefit is small.
D	The USPSTF recommends against the service. There is moderate or high certainty that the service has no net benefit or that the harms outweigh the benefits.
I Statement	The USPSTF concludes that the current evidence is insufficient to assess the balance and benefits and harms of the service. Evidence is lacking, of poor quality, or conflicting, and the balance of benefits and harms cannot be determined.

The Task Force does not consider the costs of a preventive service when making recommendations. The recommendations apply only to people who have no signs or symptoms of the specific disease or condition under evaluation, and the recommendations address only services offered in the primary care setting or services referred by a primary care clinician.

Although the primary audience of the Task Force recommendations is the primary care clinician, recommendations are also relevant to and widely used by policymakers, health insurance companies, public and private payers, quality improvement organizations, research institutions, and patients and consumers. Since 2010, the ACA requires that all new (non-grandfathered) health insurance plans cover USPSTF recommendations graded A or B, without cost-sharing or copays. Services graded A or B are those services for which the Task Force has determined that the potential benefit of the preventive service outweighs its potential harms. The grading system of the USPSTF is presented in Table 8.2.

USPSTF Recommendations for Asymptomatic People

The recommendations are on preventive services for asymptomatic people (people without signs or symptoms of the conditions the recommendation targets). The recommendations are intended to prevent or delay the onset, spread, or complications of disease and are focused on three types of services:

- Screening tests, such as screening for colorectal cancer and blood pressure or cholesterol measurement.

- Preventive medications, such as aspirin for preventing stroke or heart disease.

- Counseling about healthy behaviors, such as quitting smoking, eating a healthy diet, or staying active.

Although immunizations are considered a preventive service, the Task Force defers to another expert panel to make recommendations on immunizations. This group is called the ACIP and is described later in this chapter.

Member Composition

Originally convened in 1984 by the US Public Health Service, since 1998, the Agency for Healthcare Research and Quality (AHRQ) has been authorized by the US Congress to convene the Task Force and to provide ongoing scientific, administrative, and dissemination support to the Task Force. AHRQ provides ongoing scientific, administrative, and dissemination support to the USPSTF. Currently, the Task Force has sixteen members, serving four-year terms. appointed on a rolling basis for four years, with the possibility of a one- or two-year extension. Members are appointed by the director of AHRQ with assistance from the Task Force chairs and vice chair (USPSTF, 2022c). Members serve on a voluntary basis and are national experts in prevention and evidence-based medicine. They are screened to ensure they do not have substantial conflicts of interest that could cloud the recommendations' integrity. Task Force members are practicing doctors and nurses in the fields of family medicine, general internal medicine, gynecology-obstetrics, nursing, pediatrics, and preventive medicine, as well as health behavior specialists.

Identifying Evidence-based Preventive Services

The USPSTF is widely recognized as having one of the most rigorous and consistent methodologies for choosing, reviewing, and rating evidence. Its first step in undergoing a review of the evidence is to set a work plan and appropriately scope the topic, which means deciding what research questions are important to answer and what evidence (usually studies published in peer-reviewed journals) should be examined. Once the review is complete, the evidence is synthesized and the Task Force uses established rules to make a recommendation.

Grading System

Letter grades are assigned according to the strength of the evidence regarding the harms and benefits of a specific preventive service (USPSTF, 2022b).

An "A" Recommendation   Screening for hypertension is an example of an A recommendation from the Task Force. In its review of the evidence, the Task Force weighed the benefits versus harms of this screening and recommended screening for hypertension in adults 18 and older with office blood pressure measurement. The Task Force recommends obtaining blood pressure measurements outside of the clinical setting for diagnostic confirmation before starting treatment. In the final assessment, the USPSTF concluded that there is high certainty that the net benefit of screening for high blood pressure in adults is substantial (USPSTF, 2021).

Other Recommendations   Services graded with a B are also recommended, but the evidence suggests the net benefit to be moderate rather than substantial. In general, the USPSTF states a C recommendation is when a service is offered or provided to individual patients based on professional judgment and patient preferences. There is at least moderate certainty that the net benefit is small. For example, the USPSTF recommendation for statin use for the prevention of heart disease in adults contains both a B and C recommendation. For adults between the ages of 40 and 75 who have at least one risk factor for heart disease and an estimated 10% or greater risk for heart disease in the next decade, the Task Force gives a B recommendation for this population to be prescribed statins. For adults in this same age group with at least one risk factor but with less than a 10% risk of heart disease in the next decade, the recommendation is a C. In that population, the clinician might prescribe a statin (USPSTF, 2022b).

A D recommendation indicates evidence proves the risks outweigh the benefits and clinicians should not perform this intervention. An example of this would be screening for pancreatic cancer. The Task Force recommends against this screening in asymptomatic adults (USPSTF, 2019a). When the evidence is insufficient, the Task Force will give an I recommendation. In 2022, the Task Force found there was insufficient evidence to screen for obstructive sleep apnea in adults (USPSTF, 2022d).

Benefits and Harms

The concept of benefits and harms is an important one for preventive services and one that is easily misunderstood by the public. It can sometimes be difficult for patients to understand that screening may cause harm. Many times harm occurs after the screening, not during the screening itself. For example, some screening tests have a high rate of false positives, incorrectly identifying patients as having a risk for a condition they do not have. Or, the test maybe so sensitive that it identifies a few cancerous cells that may not cause a problem in a person's lifetime. In these cases, patients may undergo a series of additional tests and procedures that can be harmful, either physically or psychologically. Psychological harms include the anxiety resulting from the uncertainty regarding a patient's condition or the anxiety caused by undergoing certain tests.

The Advisory Committee on Immunization Practices (ACIP)

Established under section 222 of the Public Health Service Act (42 USC § 217a), as amended and given a statutory role under section 13631 of the Omnibus Budget Reconciliation Act of 1993, the **ACIP** consists of fifteen experts in fields associated with immunization who have been selected by the secretary of the US Department of Health and Human Services to provide advice and guidance to the secretary, the assistant secretary for health, and the CDC on the control of vaccine-preventable diseases. In addition to the fifteen voting members, the ACIP includes eight ex officio members who represent other federal agencies with responsibility for immunization programs in the United States and thirty nonvoting representatives of liaison organizations that bring related immunization expertise. The role of the ACIP is to provide advice that will lead to a reduction in the incidence of vaccine-preventable diseases in the United States and an increase in the safe use of vaccines and related biological products. The ACIP is responsible for determining the vaccine schedule for children and adults. It is recommended that children receive several vaccines before they turn two.

Advisory Committee on Immunization Practices (ACIP) Consists of fifteen experts in fields associated with immunization who have been selected by the secretary of the US Department of Health and Human Services to provide advice and guidance to the secretary, the assistant secretary for health, and the CDC on the control of vaccine-preventable diseases.

Vaccines: Myths and Misinformation

Vaccines are a major public health success story. Most children growing up today will rarely hear about the types of diseases that were common when their grandparents were growing up, including polio, measles, mumps, and many diseases. However, the viruses and bacteria that cause vaccine-preventable disease and death still exist and can be passed on to people who are not protected by vaccines.

Polio is a serious, life-threatening, and debilitating disease that can be prevented through vaccination; because the polio vaccination has been routine in the United States for many decades, until 2022 it rarely occurred in the United States or anywhere in the Western hemisphere. Public health experts have warned that because it is endemic in Afghanistan, India, Nigeria, and Pakistan, if US vaccinations were to stop, polio would return. In the summer of 2022, the state of New York declared a public health emergency due to the discovery of poliovirus circulating in the wastewater and the diagnosis of a resident of Rockland, New York with paralytic polio. According to the World Health Organization, widespread use of the measles vaccine in the United States has led to a greater than 99% reduction in measles compared with the prevaccine era. In 2019, there were more than 1,200 reported cases of measles across thirty-one states, the highest recorded number since 1992 (CDC, 2022c). Experts believe the disease is spreading more easily as pockets of unvaccinated communities contract the disease from travelers. Again, without immunization, measles eventually would increase to prevaccine levels.

Current issues surrounding vaccination policy are described in the following sidebar.

Unfortunately, in recent years, a small percentage of parents have opted to forego certain or all recommended vaccines for their children or to delay some vaccinations. The ACIP makes recommendations on the vaccination schedule to protect babies and children as early as possible from vaccine-preventable diseases. When parents opt to alter the recommended course of vaccines, they create their own schedule. They may receive guidance from their pediatricians, some of whom prefer the parents to space them out or delay them if the alternative would be forgoing the vaccines. However, most pediatricians do not have the expertise and have not reviewed the evidence as thoroughly as the ACIP; any schedule that modifies the CDC schedule is not based on the best available evidence.

Why do some parents delay or forgo all or selected vaccines, and why is this dangerous? Vaccines work because of herd immunity—when large numbers of people are vaccinated, it is more difficult for the chain of infection to continue (APIC, 2021). There always will be people who cannot be vaccinated, such as people with compromised immune systems, very young infants, or people who are allergic to certain vaccine components. For most vaccine-preventable diseases, the disease can be kept at bay if between 80% and 95% of the population is vaccinated. When that percentage drops, the rates of disease will begin to increase.

COVID-19: A RECENT EXAMPLE OF VACCINE HESITANCY

Likely everyone reading this book has been affected by the COVID-19 pandemic and has had to make a decision on whether to get a COVID-19 vaccine and boosters. Vaccine hesitancy is not new, but in recent years, it has escalated and gained more attention. Social media has been one contributor, as has the introduction of new vaccines like COVID-19, which by 2022 was recommended for everyone aged six months and older.

The COVID-19 pandemic caused major disruptions to American life, with school and business closures and many people staying home for periods of time in 2020 when the virus began to emerge in the US. When the vaccine rollout began in late 2020 and 2021, some people thought the vaccine was rushed, not well-tested, caused too many side effects, or was not necessary (Johns Hopkins, 2022). By late 2022, about 79% of the US population have received at least one shot (USA Facts, 2022). The top federal scientific agencies including the CDC state that hundreds of millions of people have received the available COVID-19 vaccines in the US under the most intense safety monitoring in our country's history, and continue to recommend the vaccines for everyone six months and older (CDC, 2022b).

Vaccine hesitancy increases an individual and the community's risk of contracting disease. It is a complex issue that will require continued research and many different strategies to address.

Health Resources and Services Administration (HRSA)

In addition to requiring new health insurance plans to cover A and B recommendations of the USPSTF and routine recommendations of the ACIP, the ACA also included a requirement that new health insurance plans cover evidence-informed preventive care and screenings for infants, children, and adolescents identified in guidelines supported by the HRSA and evidence-informed preventive services for women identified in guidelines supported by HRSA. For children, these guidelines include well-baby and well-child visits, and for women, the services include well-woman visits, screening and counseling for sexually transmitted infections including HIV, screening for domestic violence, breastfeeding support and services, contraception counseling, and services, and screening for gestational diabetes in pregnant women.

Promoting the Use of Preventive Services

In recent years, the federal government has continued to support, promote, and encourage the use of clinical and community preventive services. In addition, new media outlets and advancements in science and medicine are successfully promoting and encouraging the use of preventive services. A few of these efforts are described in the following sections.

Healthcare Coverage of Evidence-based Preventive Services

The ACA has several sections related to prevention and wellness. Section 2713 of the act states that new (non-grandfathered) health plans offering coverage in the group and individual markets are required to cover certain services without cost-sharing (e.g., a copayment, coinsurance, or deductible). These services include the following:

- Evidence-based services that have a graded A or B in the current recommendations of the USPSTF
- Routine immunizations for children, adolescents, and adults as recommended by the ACIP
- Evidence-informed preventive care and screenings for infants, children, and adolescents identified in guidelines supported by HRSA
- Evidence-informed preventive services for women identified in guidelines supported by HRSA

For the USPSTF, this provision means that recommendations once intended for primary care clinicians are now also required by law to be covered by health insurance plans (this applies only to the A and B recommendations). Increased attention and scrutiny of the Task Force has led to increased transparency and communication initiatives to ensure that the public understands and has input into Task Force processes. The Task Force invites public comment at all major steps of the recommendation process (see Figure 8.1).

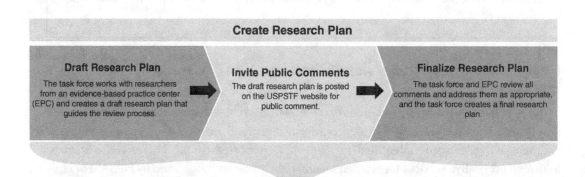

Create Research Plan

Draft Research Plan
The task force works with researchers from an evidence-based practice center (EPC) and creates a draft research plan that guides the review process.

Invite Public Comments
The draft research plan is posted on the USPSTF website for public comment.

Finalize Research Plan
The task force and EPC review all comments and address them as appropriate, and the task force creates a final research plan.

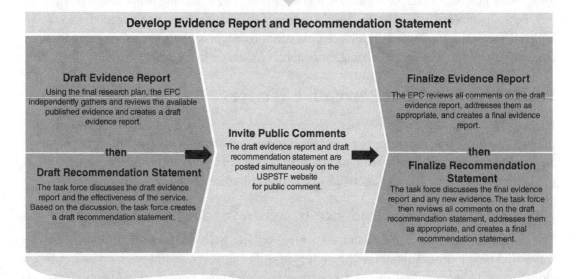

Develop Evidence Report and Recommendation Statement

Draft Evidence Report
Using the final research plan, the EPC independently gathers and reviews the available published evidence and creates a draft evidence report.

then

Draft Recommendation Statement
The task force discusses the draft evidence report and the effectiveness of the service. Based on the discussion, the task force creates a draft recommendation statement.

Invite Public Comments
The draft evidence report and draft recommendation statement are posted simultaneously on the USPSTF website for public comment.

Finalize Evidence Report
The EPC reviews all comments on the draft evidence report, addresses them as appropriate, and creates a final evidence report.

then

Finalize Recommendation Statement
The task force discusses the final evidence report and any new evidence. The task force then reviews all comments on the draft recommendation statement, addresses them as appropriate, and creates a final recommendation statement.

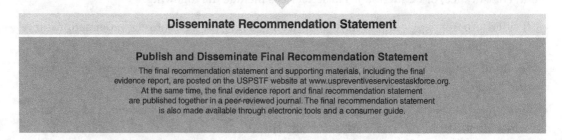

Disseminate Recommendation Statement

Publish and Disseminate Final Recommendation Statement
The final recommendation statement and supporting materials, including the final evidence report, are posted on the USPSTF website at www.uspreventiveservicestaskforce.org. At the same time, the final evidence report and final recommendation statement are published together in a peer-reviewed journal. The final recommendation statement is also made available through electronic tools and a consumer guide.

Figure 8.1   USPSTF Recommendation Process
Source: Adapted from US Preventive Services Task Force (2013c).

With the passage of the act, the Task Force is committed to making its work as transparent as possible so it can continue to serve as an open, credible, independent, and unbiased source of clinical recommendations. It has made substantial efforts to ensure that the public and the media have a clear understanding of its recommendations and processes. The public has the opportunity to comment on and help shape the research plan for each topic and comment on the evidence report that results from the research plan. The evidence report that results from the research plan and a draft recommendation statement are posted simultaneously for public comment. Typically comment periods of thirty days at both stages of the process are established for input. In addition, members of the public can also nominate new members to the Task Force and nominate new topics or request an update on an existing topic.

The Task Force produces plain language fact sheets for each of its final recommendations, designed to help the media and the public understand what the recommendation means for them. The plain language sheets provide information describing why the topic area is important for the public's health, providing specific information about the recommendation and what population(s) it applies to, explaining what the recommendation means, and listing resources for more information.

Other Preventive Services Provisions

In addition to rules established for new group and individual plans in the private insurance market, there are specific preventive services provisions established for individuals enrolled in **Medicare** and **Medicaid**.

Section 4103 of the act requires that Medicare cover an annual wellness visit for individuals that results in a "personalized prevention plan" describing services recommended for that individual patient. Personalized prevention plan services include a health risk assessment and may include services such as updating family history, listing providers that regularly provide medical care to the individuals, screening for cognitive impairment, and other screenings and services. Section 4104 of the ACA requires Medicare to waive coinsurance requirements for many preventive services, including those graded A or B by the USPSTF.

Section 4106 is a provision that incentivizes states to cover USPSTF-graded A and B recommendations as well as ACIP-recommended immunizations with no cost-sharing by providing them with an increased federal medical assistance percentage or one percentage point for these services. Under section 4107, states will be required to provide Medicaid coverage with no cost-sharing for tobacco cessation services for pregnant women (Centers for Medicare and Medicaid Services (CMS), 2013).

Challenges to the ACA's coverage of clinical preventive services, while the ACA's provision to ensure that most health plans cover USPSTF A and B recommendations has been in effect for more than a decade, there is no guarantee the provision will forever be law. A group of six people and two businesses in the state of Texas have challenged the provision in court, citing concerns about providing employer-sponsored health insurance coverage for pre-exposure prophylaxis (PrEP) medications, used to prevent the transmission of HIV. The group argues that requiring coverage of these medications violates religious freedom. In 2022, a District Court judge agreed with the plaintiff, Braidwood Management. The case

Medicare
Federally funded healthcare services provided to individuals beginning at the age of sixty-five years.

Medicaid
Federally funded healthcare services provided to individuals living below the poverty line or those who are disabled.

will go to a higher court. Critics are alarmed that the entire USPSTF process and the provision enabling copays and cost-sharing to be waived for recommended clinical preventive services are in jeopardy (Kaplan & Davidson, 2022).

Million Hearts Initiative

A major initiative to prevent heart disease through targeting risk factors is Million Hearts, launched in 2011 by the Department of Health and Human Services under the joint leadership of the CDC and the CMS. This initiative is a public–private partnership with a goal to prevent one million heart attacks and strokes in five years. Million Hearts brings together communities, health systems, nonprofit organizations, federal agencies, and private-sector partners from across the country to fight heart disease and stroke (US Department of Health and Human Services, 2022).

- Million Hearts: Convenes healthcare and public health champions.
- Facilitates impactful collaboration and resource sharing.
- Promotes implementation of evidence-based strategies to prevent heart disease.
- Addresses health inequity through specific policies, processes, and practices.

The initiative focuses on optimizing care through improving appropriate aspirin or anticoagulant use, improving blood pressure control, cholesterol management, smoking cessation, and increase use of cardiac rehabilitation. Examples of Million Hearts programs and more information about the initiative can be found at www.millionhearts.hhs.gov.

Nontraditional Sites of Care

Nontraditional sites of care that enable people to access clinical services outside the traditional primary care clinic are becoming more prevalent. Many employers host company-wide health fairs where employees can participate in a variety of screenings and gather information regarding a variety of important health topics. Some employers are building on-site clinics at the work site, encouraging employees to improve their health and making primary care services as convenient as possible for employees. Retail clinics are now prevalent in pharmacies and grocery stores around the country and are helping to expand access to care, preventive screenings, and other services. Millions of Americans are accessing mental healthcare as well as services to manage chronic conditions or acute conditions such as respiratory infections through telehealth, either through their employer, health plans, or a direct-to-consumer vendor.

Genetic Testing

Genome sequencing and genetic testing is a rapidly growing field that will continue to shape the prevention and early diagnosis of diseases. Genetic tests are tests on blood and other tissue to identify genetic disorders. Physicians use genetic tests to identify possible genetic diseases in unborn babies, determine if people carry a gene for a disease that maybe genetically passed on, diagnose adults with genetic diseases prior to the appearance of symptoms, and to confirm a diagnosis of a disease in a person who is presenting symptoms (US National Library of Medicine, 2013).

Currently, the USPSTF has one recommendation for genetic risk assessment. The USPSTF recommends that women whose personal or family history is associated with an increased risk for certain common mutations in breast cancer BRCA1 or BRCA2 genes be referred for genetic counseling and evaluation to test for these gene mutations. The USPSTF recommends against routine referral for genetic counseling or routine breast cancer susceptibility gene testing for women whose family history is not associated with an increased risk for these common mutations in breast cancer (USPSTF, 2019a).

As research evolves, whole-genome sequencing, a process that determines the complete DNA sequence of an organism's genome, will offer more information about what diseases individuals maybe susceptible to and ideally help identify diseases early while providing information on the best target treatment. However, not all results will be straightforward and there is the risk that ambiguous results will lead to increased worry, frequent screenings, and potentially unnecessary procedures—for diseases they might never develop or that we may not know how to treat. Dr. Francis Collins, a pioneer in the field for his work in discovering the gene that causes cystic fibrosis and the former director of the National Institutes of Health, spoke about the potential future of genetic testing combined with wearables and other health assessments: "One of the things that I'm excited about in that regard is the All of Us study, which is in the process of enrolling a million Americans, following them prospectively, many of them currently healthy. They share their electronic health records, they have blood samples taken that measure all kinds of things, including their complete genome sequences; they answer all kinds of questionnaires, and they walk around with various kinds of wearable sensors. That's going to be a database that gives us information about exactly what's happened to the health of our nation and what could we do about it" (Simmons-Duffin, 2021).

Advances in Behavioral Science

Behavioral science is another area that will continue to evolve and shape the evidence base for clinical and community preventive services. Although we have some information on what preventive services most benefit which individuals and research findings regarding what behaviors and habits can help keep us healthy, there is still more to learn about what motivates people to make decisions that influence their health-related behaviors. Advances in behavioral science can help us better understand how we can increase participation in recommended preventive services and what motivates people to make healthier eating choices or stop smoking. Research on how to engage consumers on health and healthcare will continue to inform program development, policies, and social norms.

Barriers to Increase the Use of Evidence-based Preventive Services

Although we have made great strides in building the evidence base for clinical and community preventive services and promoting and encouraging the use of evidence-based preventive services, challenges remain. These challenges consist of educating the public and sharing accurate medical and health information with patients, medical research limitations, as well as healthcare barriers. The Centers for Medicare & Medicaid Services is looking for ideas on how to increase certain high-value healthcare services that Medicare beneficiaries should be receiving but for a variety of reasons, are not. In 2022, CMS issued a Request for Information to understand barriers and potential solutions Medicare beneficiaries face around high-value, underused services, including the preventive services discussed in this chapter. While the healthcare system recognizes these services as high value, it can be harder to convince patients they need these services, for many reasons. Prevention is tough because many of us when we are not having an acute episode or are not feeling sick, can find reasons not to schedule a doctor's appointment. Lack of time, transportation, and financial concerns are common barriers to why people might not get these services.

Educating the Public About Preventive Services

The media play a significant role in how scientific findings are shared with the public. Unfortunately, facts and accurate, consistent information often get lost in the message. Reporters do not always understand the science on which they report, and editors often condense stories to make them easier to read or to create controversy. News stories often present controversial topics as if there are two, equally relevant sides to the story. In the age of social media, anyone can have a blog, and frequently opinion gets passed on as fact. One issue is that the media and bloggers do not always adequately capture the methodological difference between high-quality studies or the nuances between different kinds of studies that should not be compared or given equal weight. For example, laboratory studies and epidemiological studies serve different purposes. A vaccine laboratory study may involve studying the effects of a vaccine or vaccine component on a small group of animals or humans. Epidemiological studies show the effect of the vaccine on an entire population of people. An example of this is early studies examining the link between cigarette smoking and lung cancer. In 1939, a cancer surgeon was the first to propose the link between smoking and lung cancer, but results from laboratory studies on animals were inconclusive. A large epidemiological study in the 1950s clearly demonstrated the link and the dose response (the more people smoked, the greater their risk of lung cancer) (Doll & Hill, 1950). Similarly, several epidemiological studies have been helpful in demonstrating the safety of the US vaccine program.

Research Limitations

Sometimes, the USPSTF does a thorough review of the literature, only to find there is insufficient evidence to make a recommendation. The ACA requires the USPSTF to provide an annual report to Congress that outlines critical evidence gaps regarding clinical preventive services, as well as gaps in the evidence that exists for certain populations and age groups. Recent examples of USPSTF-identified high-priority topics with evidence gaps include screening for type 2 diabetes in children, and screening for atrial fibrillation in asymptomatic adults (USPSTF, 2022e).

Not all evidence reviews yield the same conclusions. Sometimes, recommendations from different groups may conflict or not completely align. For example, if you look up osteoporosis screening recommendations or certain cancer screening recommendations, you will find conflicting recommendations of when to start screening based on age and gender from different organizations.

Though there maybe differences in clinical guidelines from various organizations, the USPSTF is widely recognized as the gold standard because of its methodology and rigor. In 2011, the Institute of Medicine (IOM) published a report, commissioned by the US Congress, called *Clinical Practice Guidelines We Can Trust* (IOM, 2011). Because of the large number of clinical practice guidelines made by various organizations and expert panels, Congress called for the IOM to undertake a study on the best methods used in developing clinical practice guidelines to cut down on the confusion for practitioners and patients when determining, which guidelines are of high quality. The aim of the IOM report was to provide a mechanism to immediately identify high-quality, trustworthy clinical practice guidelines and ultimately improve decision making—potentially improving healthcare quality and health outcomes. In the report, the IOM outlined eight standards for developing rigorous, trustworthy clinical practice guidelines. The standards are summarized as follows:

- Guideline issuers should have a transparent process (it should be clear who is making the recommendations and how the conclusions are made).

- Guideline issuers should appropriately manage conflicts of interest.

- The group issuing the guidelines should be balanced and multidisciplinary, and the public should be engaged on some level.

- The systematic reviews conducted should follow certain quality standards.

- The recommendations issued should be rated based on the strength of the evidence.

- Recommendations should be articulated in a standardized form.

- An external review process should be in place.

- There should be a plan in place for updating the recommendations (National Research Council, 2011).

The methodology and processes of the USPSTF are supported by the IOM in this document because they incorporate many of these best practices.

Alternatively, some clinical services maybe overused or misused, meaning some populations may get a service that is not recommended for them. The Choosing Wisely initiative brings together different medical specialty societies that have examined the evidence and found that many services are overused ABIM Foundation, 2018). The group came together to identify twelve common services that are commonly overused. These include use of antibiotics for respiratory infections, DEXA scans, and routine annual cervical cancer screening.

Healthcare Service Barriers

Any obstacle that prevents individuals from receiving the preventive services recommended for them including time, cost of travel, and lack of available services in their area.

Summary

Clinical preventive services are screenings, counseling, and related interventions including immunizations that individuals receive at their primary care doctor's office, at their local pharmacy, or at a health fair that aim to detect certain conditions when they are asymptomatic, often leading to improved health outcomes. Recommended clinical preventive services are based on age and gender. The USPSTF, the ACIP, and the Health Resource and Services Administration are the sources of recommended clinical preventive services authorized by the ACA. Physicians, health insurance plans, employers, and communities promote recommended clinical preventive services with the goal of improving health outcomes. The promotion of preventive services includes educating individuals on what services they need, encouraging them to talk to their healthcare provider about these services, and increasing access to these services by offering them at work sites and retail clinics.

KEY TERMS

1. **Clinical Preventive Services:** services provided at one's primary care physician's office, local pharmacy, or health fairs to detect and reduce the risk of specific health conditions from progressing; examples include screening tests, immunizations, counseling, and preventive medications

2. **National Prevention Strategy:** guidelines developed as a result of the ACA; provides guidance to the federal government and the nation regarding the most effective and achievable means for improving health through prevention and health promotion policies and programs

3. **Health Resources and Services Administration (HRSA):** the primary federal agency for improving access to health care services for people who are uninsured, isolated, or medically vulnerable

4. **US Preventive Services Task Force (USPSTF):** an independent panel of nonfederal experts in prevention and evidence-based medicine composed of primary care providers such as internists, pediatricians, family physicians, gynecologists and obstetricians, nurses, and health behavior specialists

5. **Advisory Committee on Immunization Practices (ACIP):** consists of fifteen experts in fields associated with immunization who have been selected by the secretary of the US Department of Health and Human Services to provide advice and guidance to the secretary, the assistant secretary for health, and the CDC on the control of vaccine-preventable diseases

6. **Medicare:** federally funded healthcare services provided to individuals over the age of sixty-five years

7. **Medicaid:** federally funded healthcare services provided to individuals living below the poverty line or those who are disabled

8. **Healthcare Service Barriers:** any obstacle that prevents individuals from receiving the preventive services recommended for them including time, cost of travel, and lack of available services in their area

REVIEW QUESTIONS

1. What are common conditions or health risks that can be detected early or prevented through recommended clinical preventive services?

2. What are some barriers to individuals getting recommended clinical preventive services?

3. Why are some clinical preventive services recommended for some populations and not for others?

4. What are the entities that recommend evidence-based clinical preventive services identified by the ACA?

5. Describe the rating system for preventive care and give examples of A–D ratings.

6. Why does the US government invest in preventive care services?

7. Why, as a health promotion professional, are preventive services important?

STUDENT ACTIVITIES

1. Create a campaign to promote a recommended clinical preventive service for a certain population, keeping in mind the barriers that this population might face.

2. Debate whether families should be allowed to opt out of required vaccinations.

3. Create a chart that details the life stage and the appropriate clinical service needed during that stage.

References

ABIM Foundation (2018). *Choosing wisely*. Retrieved from https://www.choosingwisely.org/resources/updates-from-the-field/the-top-12-recommendations-that-are-reducing-overuse/

American Journal of Managed Care (2019). *Population health screenings for the prevention of chronic disease progression*. Retrieved from https://www.ajmc.com/view/population-health-screenings-for-the-prevention-of-chronic-disease-progression

Association for Professionals in Infection Control and Epidemiology (2021). *Herd immunity*. Retrieved from https://apic.org/monthly_alerts/herd-immunity/

Centers for Disease Control and Prevention (2018). *Preventing 1 Million Hearts and Strokes*. Retrieved from https://www.cdc.gov/vitalsigns/million-hearts/index.html

Centers for Disease Control and Prevention (2022a). *Heart disease facts*. Retrieved from www.cdc .gov/heartdisease/facts.htm

Centers for Disease Control and Prevention (2022b). *Safety of COVID-19 vaccines.* Retrieved from: https://www.cdc.gov/coronavirus/2019-ncov/vaccines/safety/safety-of-vaccines.html

Centers for Disease Control and Prevention (2022c). Measles (Rubeola). https://www.cdc.gov/measles/cases-outbreaks.html

Doll, R. and Hill, A.B. (1950). Smoking and carcinoma of the lung. *British Medical Journal 2* (4682): 739–748.

Institute of Medicine (2011, March). *Clinical practice guidelines we can trust*. Retrieved from https://www.uspreventiveservicestaskforce.org/uspstf/sites/default/files/inline-files/Clinical%20Practice%20Guidelines%202011%20Insert_0.pdf

Johns Hopkins Medicine (2022). COVID-19 Vaccines: Myths vs. Facts.

Kaplan, R.M. & Davidson, K.W.. 2022, November 2 The USPSTF process is in jeopardy. *Medpage*. Retrieved from https://www.medpagetoday.com/opinion/second-opinions/101544?xid=nl_mpt_DHE_2022-11-02&eun=g1911982d0r&utm_source=Sailthru&utm_medium=email&utm_campaign=Daily%20Headlines%20Evening%202022-11-02&utm_term=NL_Daily_DHE_dual-gmail-definition

National Research Council (2011). Clinical practice guidelines we can trust. Washington, DC: National Academies Press. Retrieved from www.ion.edu/Reports/2011/Clinical-Practice-Guidelines-We-Can-Trust

Nelson, H. (2020). Chronic disease prevention linked to patient engagement, counseling. *Patient Engagement HIT*. Retrieved from https://patientengagementhit.com/news/chronic-disease-prevention-linked-to-patient-engagement-counseling

Simmons-Duffin, S. (2021). The NIH director on why Americans aren't getting healthier, despite medical advances. *NPR*. Retrieved from https://www.npr.org/sections/health-shots/2021/12/07/1061940326/the-nih-director-on-why-americans-arent-getting-healthier-despite-medical-advanc

US Coronavirus Vaccine Tracker (2022). USA Facts, https://usafacts.org/visualizations/covid-vaccine-tracker-states

US Department of Health and Human Services (2011). *National Prevention Strategy*. Retrieved from https://www.hhs.gov/sites/default/files/disease-prevention-wellness-report.pdf

US Department of Health and Human Services (2014, February 12). *What is the history of HHS? When did it get started? What years were the most important in its history?* Retrieved from http://answers.hhs.gov/questions/3049

US Department of Health and Human Services (2022). Million hearts. Retrieved from: https://millionhearts.hhs.gov/index.html

US National Library of Medicine. (2013) *Genetic testing*. Retrieved from www.nlm.nih.gov/medlineplus/genetictesting.html

US Preventive Services Task Force. (2019a) *Pancreatic cancer screening*. Retrieved from https://www.uspreventiveservicestaskforce.org/uspstf/recommendation/pancreatic-cancer-screening

US Preventive Services Task Force. (2019b) *BRCA-related cancer: Risk assessment, genetic counseling and genetic testing*. Retrieved from https://www.uspreventiveservicestaskforce.org/uspstf/recommendation/brca-related-cancer-risk-assessment-genetic-counseling-and-genetic-testing

US Preventive Services Task Force. (2013c). Genetic risk assessment and BRCA mutation testing for breast and ovarian cancer susceptibility. Retrieved from www.uspreventiveservicestaskforce.org/uspstf/uspsbrgen.htm

US Preventive Services Task Force. (2021) *Hypertension in adults: Screening.* Retrieved from https://www.uspreventiveservicestaskforce.org/uspstf/recommendation/hypertension-in-adults-screening

US Preventive Services Task Force. (2022a) *About the USPSTF.* Retrieved from https://uspreventiveservicestaskforce.org/uspstf/about-uspstf

US Preventive Services Task Force. (2022b) *Grade definitions.* Retrieved from https://uspreventiveservicestaskforce.org/uspstf/about-uspstf/methods-and-processes/grade-definitions

US Preventive Services Task Force. (2022c) *Our members.* Retrieved from https://uspreventiveservicestaskforce.org/uspstf/about-uspstf/current-members

US Preventive Services Task Force. (2022d) *Obstructive sleep apnea in adults.* Retrieved from https://www.uspreventiveservicestaskforce.org/uspstf/recommendation/obstructive-sleep-apnea-in-adults-screening

USPSTF (2022e). High 12th Annual Report to Congress. https://www.uspreventiveservicestaskforce.org/uspstf/sites/default/files/inline-files/2022-annual-report-to-congress.pdf

PART THREE

HEALTH PROMOTION IN ACTION

CHAPTER 9

NATIONAL AND STATE INITIATIVES TO PROMOTE HEALTH AND WELL-BEING

Jennifer Childress and Jill Dombrowski

Throughout the nation, Americans are experiencing declining levels of health. How is this determined? What measurements are used, and who measures them? What programs have been developed to address declining health levels? Partnerships and data are key to improving the health of Americans where we live, work, and play throughout all life stages.

Healthy People: 1979–2030

Since 1979, the **US Department of Health and Human Services (HHS)** has been setting ten-year national health objectives for Americans called **Healthy People**. By establishing benchmarks and monitoring progress over time, Healthy People's aims are to do the following:

- Encourage collaboration across communities and sectors.
- Empower individuals toward making informed health decisions.
- Measure the impact of prevention activities.

Since the 1980s, the HHS Healthy People initiatives have built on their predecessors and addressed new areas of importance related to the health of the nation. Given the comprehensiveness and pervasiveness of health, the development of Healthy People goals involves input from multiple sectors and stakeholders.

The goals identified in Healthy People 2030 are broad and include objectives for areas that were included in prior Healthy People goals, such as nutrition and physical activity, immunizations, cancer, heart disease, medical insurance coverage, mental health, environmental quality, and substance abuse. In addition, Healthy People 2030 has been expanded to include new

LEARNING OBJECTIVES
After reading this chapter, the student will be able to:

- Discuss the history of the Department of Health and Human Services' Healthy People initiative with an emphasis on Healthy People 2030

- Describe the work of key federal government agencies to support research, share findings, and develop guidelines for healthy living.

- Identify government programs that promote health.

- Recognize key surveillance surveys and activities that monitor the health of the US population.

- Summarize state-level programs that use national guidelines to promote health.

Introduction to Health Promotion, Second Edition. Edited by Anastasia Snelling.
© 2024 John Wiley & Sons Inc. Published 2024 by John Wiley & Sons Inc.
Companion Website: www.wiley.com/go/snelling2e

US Department of Health and Human Services (HHS)

the US government's principal agency tasked with protecting the health of all Americans and providing essential human services

Healthy People

ten-year national health objectives for Americans released by the US Department of Health and Human Services

areas of focus such as housing and homes and the built environment, as well as emerging issues such as opioid use disorder and adolescents' use of e-cigarettes.

HISTORY OF HEALTHY PEOPLE

- 1979 surgeon general's report, *Healthy People: The Surgeon General's Report on Health Promotion and Disease Prevention*

- Healthy People 1990: Promoting Health/Preventing Disease: Objectives for the Nation

- Healthy People 2000: National Health Promotion and Disease Prevention Objectives

- Healthy People 2010: Objectives for Improving Health

- Healthy People 2020: A society in which all people live long, healthy lives.

- Healthy People 2030: Building a Healthier Future for All.

Healthy People 2030

The majority of deaths among Americans are the result of chronic diseases that are preventable through lifestyle and behavior modifications. On August 18, 2020, Healthy People 2030 was released with the vision of building a healthier future for all. (USDHHS, ODPHP) https://health .gov/news/202008/healthy-people-2030-here#:~:text=On%20August%2018%2C%20 ODPHP%20released,most%20critical%20public%20health%20priorities. This iteration of Healthy People is more focused, with less objectives than previous versions and allows users to build a list of objectives relevant to their work. The vision of Healthy People 2030 is "A society in which all people can achieve their full potential for health and well-being across the lifespan." The mission of Healthy People 2030 is "To promote, strengthen, and evaluate the nation's efforts to improve the health and well-being of all people." (USDHHS, ODPHP) https://health .gov/healthypeople/about/healthy-people-2030-framework#:~:text=Healthy%20People%20 2030%27s%20overarching%20goals,and%20well%2Dbeing%20of%20all

The overarching goals of Healthy People 2030 are:

- Attain healthy, thriving lives and well-being free of preventable disease, disability, injury, and premature death.

- Eliminate health disparities, achieve health equity, and attain health literacy to improve the health and well-being of all.

- Create social, physical, and economic environments that promote attaining the full potential for health and well-being for all.

- Promote healthy development, healthy behaviors, and well-being across all life stages.

- Engage leadership, key constituents, and the public across multiple sectors to take action and design policies that improve the health and well-being of all.

There are 350 core or measurable objectives in Healthy People 2030. These indicators are being tracked, measured, and reported regularly throughout the decade to better

Table 9.1   Healthy People 2030 Leading Health Indicators

All ages*

- Children, adolescents, and adults who use the oral health care system (2+ years)

- Consumption of calories from added sugars by persons aged 2 years and over (2+ years)

- Drug overdose deaths

- Exposure to unhealthy air

- Homicides

- Household food insecurity and hunger

- Persons who are vaccinated annually against seasonal influenza

- Persons who know their HIV status (13+ years)

- Persons with medical insurance (<65 years)

- Suicides

- *except where noted

Infants

- Infant deaths

Children and adolescents

- 4th grade students whose reading skills are at or above the proficient achievement level for their grade

- Adolescents with major depressive episodes (MDEs) who receive treatment

- Children and adolescents with obesity

- Current use of any tobacco products among adolescents

Adults and older adults

- Adults engaging in binge drinking of alcoholic beverages during the past 30 days

- Adults who meet current minimum guidelines for aerobic physical activity and muscle-strengthening activity

- Adults who receive a colorectal cancer screening based on the most recent guidelines

- Adults with hypertension whose blood pressure is under control

- Cigarette smoking in adults

- Employment among the working-age population

- Maternal deaths

- New cases of diagnosed diabetes in the population

Source: U.S. Department of Health and Human Services/https://health.gov/healthypeople/objectives-and-data/leading-health-indicators/last accessed February 09, 2023.

evaluate the nation's progress toward meeting Healthy People 2030 goals. Leading health indicators (LHIs) are a smaller subset, composed of 23 objectives that reflect high-priority issues and associated actions to address them (see table 9.1). The LHIs are divided into categories by lifestage: all ages, infants, children and adolescents, and adults and older adults.

The website also allows users to track specific LHIs over the decade (https://health .gov/healthypeople/objectives-and-data/leading-health-indicators). Although the large number of indicators and associated data may seem overwhelming, HHS has created easy-to-use web-based applications to quickly access this data. With easy access to relevant data, health professionals can better assist Americans where they live, work, and learn.

Also included in Healthy People 2030 is a focus on Social Determinants of Health, which are "the conditions in the environments where people are born, live, learn, work, play, worship, and age that affect a wide range of health, functioning, and quality-of-life outcomes and risks." (https://health.gov/healthypeople/prieority-areas/social-determinants-health). Social determinants of health include economic stability, education access and quality, healthcare access and quality, neighborhood and built environment, and social and community context.

US Department of Health and Human Services (HHS)

"The mission of the U.S. Department of Health and Human Services (HHS) is to enhance the health and well-being of all Americans by providing for effective HHS and by fostering sound, sustained advances in the sciences underlying medicine, public health, and social services." (https://www.hhs.gov/about/index.html). HHS works with state and local governments to provide HHS through state or county agencies and through private-sector grantees. HHS programs are administered by twelve operating divisions, comprising nine agencies in the US Public Health Service and three human services agencies.

As a department within the federal government, the secretary of HHS sits on the president's cabinet and is a presidential appointee. Every four years, the secretary of HHS is responsible for updating a five-year strategic plan that defines the department's missions and goals and the means by which progress will be measured. The most recent strategic plan (2022–2026) is available on the HHS website and is designed to be a living, vital document that is updated frequently to reflect progress. The last update to the strategic plan was on March 28, 2022 (US Department of Health and Human Services, 2022). https://www.hhs .gov/about/strategic-plan/2022-2026/message/index.html

---

HHS STRATEGIC GOALS

- Protect and Strengthen Equitable Access to High Quality and Affordable Health Care
- Safeguard and Improve National and Global Health Conditions and Outcomes
- Strengthen Social Well-being, Equity, and Economic Resilience
- Restore Trust and Accelerate Advancements in Science and Research for All
- Advance Strategic Management to Build Trust, Transparency, and Accountability.

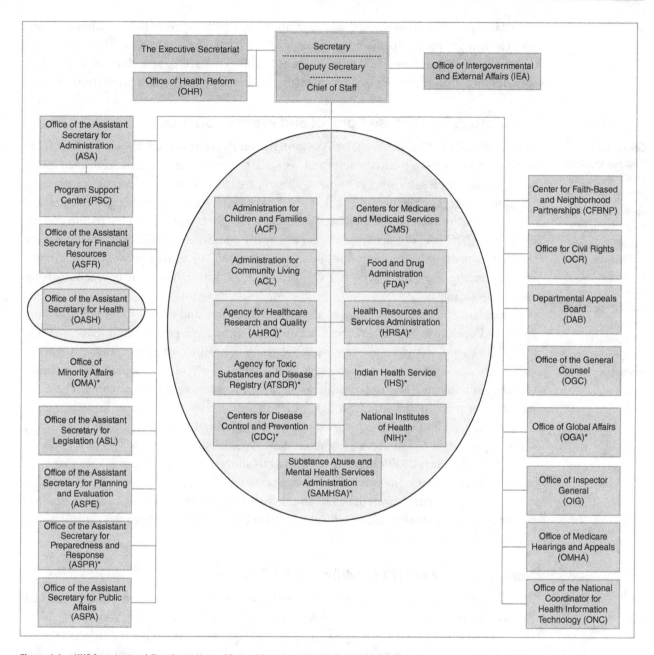

Figure 9.1   HHS Organizational Chart https://www.hhs.gov/about/agencies/orgchart/index.html
Note: *Designates that it is a component of the US Public Health Service.
Source: US Department of Health and Human Services (n.d-c).

The organizational chart in figure 9.1 identifies the twelve operating divisions and nine agencies under HHS (www.hhs.gov). When visiting the HHS website, you can click on the organizational chart to be directed to the division or agency website and view the sublayers that exist in addition to those pictured in figure 9.1.

HHS-operating divisions and agencies are tasked with carrying out initiatives to support Healthy People 2030 objectives. Many of the initiatives discussed in this textbook fall under one of the entities of HHS in figure 9.1. Following are descriptions of some HHS agencies or divisions that are of particular interest in the field of health promotion.

The Centers for Disease Control and Prevention (CDC)

Centers for Disease Control and Prevention (CDC)
a federal agency under the US Department of Health and Human Services responsible for the public health of the nation; works to protect the public health and safety of people in the United States by tracking, detecting, and responding to threats

The mission of the **Centers for Disease Control and Prevention (CDC)** is to "work 24/7 to protect America from health, safety, and security threats, both foreign and in the United States. Whether diseases start at home or abroad, are chronic or acute, curable, or preventable, human error or deliberate attack, CDC fights disease and supports communities and citizens to do the same" (CDC, 2022). Working with partners throughout the nation and the world, the CDC seeks to accomplish its mission by conducting critical science, providing health information that protects our nation against expensive and dangerous health threats, and responding when these arise (CDC, April 29, 2022) https://www.cdc.gov/about/organization/mission.htm.

The CDC is composed of various centers, an institute, and offices to meet its mission, goals, and objectives, share resources, and effectively address public health concerns. On the CDC website, viewers may examine the plethora of health-related topics addressed. The CDC provides information, publications, multimedia, and tools to support experts, individuals, communities, and organizations as they act to address health concerns. The CDC strives to provide information through various mediums to its audience; for example, in addition to print and online, information is available through podcasts. To address a larger audience, many CDC resources are also available in Spanish.

During the years 2020–2022, the CDC had to address criticism of guidelines that were put forth regarding the emerging infectious disease COVID-19.

Information sharing from the CDC about seasonal influenza remains a solid example of the types of detailed information typically provided by the CDC for both the general public and healthcare professionals.

Seasonal Influenza (Flu) Addressed by CDC

The CDC provides information to the general public regarding flu activity and surveillance. The website provides maps and information through the weekly Flu View. Viewers can identify areas of flu outbreaks throughout the United States or customize the information to generate state-specific reports. Information includes the proportion of people visiting health care providers for influenza-like illness (ILI) (see figure 9.2), influenza-related mortality rates, the geographic spread of influenza, and hospitalizations related to influenza.

> The CDC Influenza Application for Clinicians and Health Care Professionals (available in the App Store) provides information on the latest recommendations and flu activity updates, videos from subject matter experts, and products to print out and post in the workplace or distribute to patients.

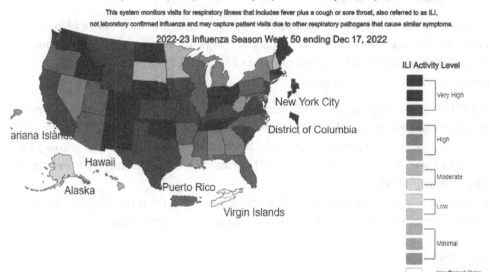

Figure 9.2   CDC flu view webpage: ILI activity indicator map

Source: Centers for Disease Control and Prevention (2022).

In addition to tracking influenza patterns, the CDC also provides information and facts regarding prevention and treatment of the flu. Through the CDC Seasonal Influenza Resource Center, the agency provides infographics and social media graphics to encourage three actions to prevent and fight the flu. The campaign outlines these three actions, along with steps and research supporting each one:

- Take time to get the flu vaccine.
- Take everyday preventive actions to stop the spread of germs.
- Take flu antiviral drugs if your doctor prescribes them.

(CDC, 2022). https://www.cdc.gov/flu/resource-center/toolkit/index.htm.

National Institutes of Health (NIH)

The **National Institutes of Health** (NIH) is the nation's medical research agency, composed of 27 institutes and centers supporting scientific studies with the theme of turning discovery into health (www.nih.gov).

> NIH's mission is to seek fundamental knowledge about the nature and behavior of living systems and the application of that knowledge to enhance health, lengthen life, and reduce illness and disability. National Institutes of Health, (2017) https://www.nih.gov/about-nih/what-we-do/mission-goals

The NIH is the leading supporter of biomedical research in the world, with an impact that reaches beyond health to job creation and the US economy. The NIH states that the thirty-year increase in life expectancy of a baby born in the United States today, compared to one born in 1900, is due in large part to NIH research (NIH, n.d.) https://www.nia.nih.gov/about/budget/introduction-4.

The areas of research covered by NIH are broad, ranging from the lifelong impact of acute kidney injury to wonders of the brain to the landscape of genomics.

Clinical Center

The NIH Clinical Center, "America's Research Hospital," is the home of NIH clinical research trials and is devoted entirely to clinical research. The Clinical Center facilitates the rapid translation of scientific observations and laboratory discoveries into medical approaches to diagnose, treat, and prevent disease. Findings from clinical trials are communicated to the public through the website, traditional news channels, and social media. Examples of recently successful clinical trial research projects include combination anti-HIV infusions that suppress the virus for prolonged periods and clinical trials on monoclonal antibodies to prevent malaria in US adults (NIH, December 14, 2022) https://clinicalcenter.nih.gov/ocmr/mediaclips.html

Chronic Disease Institutes

Health promotion professionals benefit from work conducted by the National Heart, Lung, and Blood Institute (NHLBI) (www.nhlbi.nih.gov) and the National Institute of Diabetes and Digestive and Kidney Diseases (NIDDK) (www.niddk.nih.gov). The NHLBI's Heart Truth program is widely recognized by the red dress logo during American Heart Month (February). The aim of Heart Truth is to unite women in the fight against their number one killer: heart disease. The campaign increases awareness of risk factors and empowers women and their families to take steps to reduce their risks. NHLBI provides resources and tools for the public on heart disease, cholesterol, heart attacks, high blood pressure, and sleep disorders.

> NIDDK conducts and supports research on many of the most common, costly, and chronic conditions to improve health. https://www.niddk.nih.gov/

The conditions include diabetes, digestive diseases, kidney disease, weight management, liver disease, urologic diseases, endocrine diseases, and diet and nutrition. For health professionals, the Institute offers clinical practice tools, patient management, and education materials.

NIDDK offers community health and outreach programs that are useful resources for health promotion professionals, communities, and individuals. "Kidney Sundays" is a toolkit that encourages African American faith-based organizations to promote kidney health at their services, programs, and events. The Kidney Sundays Toolkit includes a Youtube video about how to host a Kidney Sundays Event, and can be supplemented with the Family Reunion Healthguide. The program recommends that website users do the following:

- **Hold conversations with your congregation** about kidney health using our talking points.

- **Share materials** that highlight useful kidney facts and tips.

- **Partner with a health facility or organization** to host a health screening, or review our list of potential partners for your upcoming event.

(NIDDK, March 2020) https://www.niddk.nih.gov/health-information/community-health-outreach/kidney-sundays-toolkit.

U.S. Department of Agriculture (USDA)

The **U.S. Department of Agriculture (USDA)** (usda.gov) is responsible for the development and dissemination of the Dietary Guidelines for Americans, the cornerstone of federal nutrition policy and nutrition education activities. Every five years, USDA and HHS jointly update and issue these guidelines, which are centered on reducing caloric intake, making informed food choices, and being physically active for individuals aged two years and older. The most recent guidelines were issued in 2020 and will be updated again in 2025 (see table 9.2).

The Dietary Guidelines recognize that many Americans do not eat foods that are adequately nutritious, even though they are available. The Guidelines provide recommendations based on two major concepts:

- Maintain calorie balance over time to achieve and sustain a healthy weight.

- Focus on consuming nutrient-dense foods and beverages (e.g., limiting sodium, solid fats, added sugars, and refined grains while emphasizing fruits, vegetables, whole grains, low-fat or fat-free milk products, seafood, lean meats, poultry, eggs, beans, peas, nuts, and seeds).

Recommendations are provided for the general public and for specific populations (e.g., pregnant or breastfeeding women and individuals over fifty). The Dietary Guidelines for Americans 2020–2025, Make Every Bite Count, is the first Guidelines document to provide guidance by life stage (USDA & USDHHS, 2020). The Guidelines are a "customizable framework" that people can tailor to make affordable choices based on their cultural and

U.S. Department of Agriculture (USDA)
The US government's primary agricultural agency responsible for supporting America's agriculture and providing safe and nutritious foods to the US public; responsible for the development and dissemination of the Dietary Guidelines for Americans

Table 9.2 Examples of Tests Included in The National Health and Nutrition Examination Survey (NHANES)

Health Measurements by Participant Age and Gender

- Physician's exam—all ages
- Blood pressure—ages 8 years and older
- Liver Ultrasound—ages 12 years and older
- Condition of teeth and gums—ages 1 year and older
- Hearing test—ages 6–19 years and 70 years and older
- Height, weight, and other body measures—all ages

Lab Tests on Urine: (3 years and older)

- Kidney function tests—ages 6 years and older
- Sexually transmitted diseases (STD)
  - chlamydia and gonorrhea—ages 14–39
  - Trichomonas—ages 14–59
- Exposure to environmental chemicals such as Arsenic and Nickel—selected persons ages 6 and older
- Pregnancy test—females 12 years and older

Lab Tests on Blood: (1 year and older)

- Anemia—all ages
- Total Cholesterol and HDL—ages 6 years and older
- Triglycerides and LDL—selected participants, ages 12 and older
- Glucose measures—ages 12 years and older
- Infectious diseases—ages 2 years and older
- Kidney function tests—ages 12 years and older
- Lead—1 year and older
- Cadmium—1 year and older
- Mercury—ages 1 year and older
- Liver function tests—ages 12 years and older
- Nutrition status—1 year and older
- Exposure to environmental chemicals—selected persons ages 6 and older
- Infectious Diseases
  - Hepatitis B virus (ages 2 and up)
  - Hepatitis C viruses (ages 6 and up)
  - Cytomegalovirus—ages 1-5 years
  - Genital Herpes—ages 14-49 years
  - Human immunodeficiency virus (HIV)—ages 18–49 years

Other Lab Tests

- Vaginal swabs (self-administered)—females ages 14–59years
- Penile swabs (self-administered)—males ages 14–59 years

Private Health Interviews

- Health status—ages 12 years and older
- Questions about drug and alcohol use—ages 12 years and older (No drug testing will be done)
- Nutrition—all ages
- Reproductive health—females ages 12 years and older
- Questions about sexual experience—ages 14–69 years
- Tobacco use—ages 12 years and older

After the Visit to the NHANES Examination Center

- Persons asked about the foods they eat will receive a phone call 3–10 days after their exam for a similar interview, all ages.
- Then participants, or an adult for participants 1–15 years old, will be asked about food shopping habits.

Source: Centers for Disease Control and Prevention (2017).

traditional preferences. This information is also addressed in chapter 5 about nutrition. The USDA focuses on four major recommendations:

1. Follow a healthy dietary pattern at every life stage.

2. Customize and enjoy nutrient-dense food and beverage choices to reflect personal preferences, cultural traditions, and budgetary considerations.

3. Focus on meeting food group needs with nutrient-dense foods and beverages, and stay within calorie limits.

4. Limit foods and beverages higher in added sugars, saturated fat, and sodium, and limit alcoholic beverages.

Monitoring the Nation's Health

The CDC and other HHS divisions use multiple federal datasets to monitor the nation's health. Using these data, federal departments, agencies, and divisions with health-related responsibilities produce reports, publications, and recommendations to address specific areas of focus. CDC surveillance systems collect data on chronic diseases and their risk factors. These systems—often the only source of such data—are vital for understanding how chronic diseases affect people in the United States. Without them, our prevention and control efforts would be guesswork. Surveillance data guide us in putting our resources to the best use. (National Center for Chronic Disease Prevention and Health Promotion, 2021) (figure 9.3).

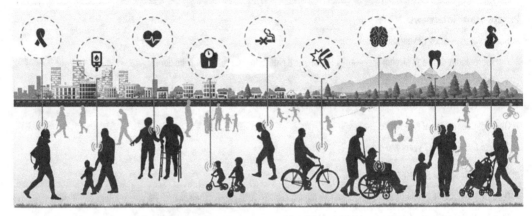

CDC'S NATIONAL CENTER FOR CHRONIC DISEASE PREVENTION AND HEALTH PROMOTION

Using Surveillance Systems to Prevent and Control Chronic Diseases

Figure 9.3   Using surveillance systems to prevent and control chronic diseases
Source: Image from: https://www.cdc.gov/chronicdisease/data/surveillance.htm.

Behavioral Risk Factor Surveillance System (BRFSS)

Behavioral Risk Factor Surveillance System (BRFSS)
the world's largest, ongoing telephone health survey system, tracking and reporting on health conditions and risk behaviors in the United States on an annual basis

The **Behavioral Risk Factor Surveillance System** (BRFSS) (http://www.cdc.gov/brfss) is the nation's premier system of health-related telephone surveys that collect state data about U.S. residents regarding their health-related risk behaviors, chronic health conditions, and use of preventive services. Established in 1984 with 15 states, BRFSS now collects data in all 50 states as well as the District of Columbia and three U.S. territories. BRFSS completes more than 400,000 adult interviews each year, making it the largest continuously conducted health survey system in the world.

With technical and methodological assistance from CDC, state health departments use in-house interviewers or contract with telephone call centers or universities to administer the BRFSS surveys continuously throughout the year. The states use a standardized core questionnaire, optional modules, and state-added questions. The survey is conducted using random digit dialing (RDD) techniques on both landlines and cell phones.

BRFSS collects state data about U.S. residents regarding their health-related risk behaviors and events, chronic health conditions, and use of preventive services. BRFSS also collects data on important emerging health issues such as vaccine shortages and influenza-like illnesses. For example, since September 2009, federal, state, and local health agencies have used BRFSS to monitor the prevalence rates of influenza-like illness to help with pandemic planning. Interviewers administer the annual BRFSS surveys continuously throughout the year. (National Center for Chronic Disease Prevention and Health Promotion, Division of Population Health, 2022)

THE BEHAVIORAL RISK FACTOR SURVEILLANCE SYSTEM (BRFSS)

CDC works with state and territorial partners to collect uniform, state-specific information about health risk behaviors, chronic health conditions, use of preventive services, and other factors that affect the health of US adults, such as:

- Physical activity
- Nutrition
- Alcohol and commercial tobacco use
- Diabetes
- Heart disease
- Immunizations
- Injuries
- Health care access
- Use of health care services

Currently, all states collect BRFSS data to help them establish and track state and local health objectives, plan health programs, implement disease prevention and health promotion activities, and monitor trends. Nearly two-thirds of states use BRFSS data to support health-related legislative efforts.

Adults 18 years of age or older are asked to take part in the survey. Participants are not compensated monetarily but should know that they are taking part in a rewarding endeavor that helps improve the health of U.S. residents. The number of interviews within each state will vary based on funding and the size of regions, such as health districts, within each state.

Annual questionnaires dating back to 1984 are available on the BRFSS website. Examples of questions included in the 2021 BRFSS Core Section, include:

Section	Question Text	Responses
Health Status	Would you say that in general, your health is _____.	Read: 1 Excellent 2 Very Good 3 Good 4 Fair 5 Poor Do not Read: 7 Don't know/Not sure 9 Refused
Healthy Days (Physical Health)	Now thinking about your physical health, which includes physical illness and injury, for how many days during the past 30 days was your physical health not good?	___ number of days (01-30) 88 None 77 Don't know/not sure 99 refused

Section	Question Text	Responses
Healthy Days (Mental Health)	Now thinking about your mental health, which includes stress, depression, and problems with emotions, for how many days during the past 30 days was your mental health not good?	___ number of days (01-30) 88 None 77 Don't know/not sure 99 refused
Healthy Days (Poor Health)	During the past 30 days, for about how many days did poor physical or mental health keep you from doing your usual activities, such as self-care, work, or recreation?	___ number of days (01-30) 88 None 77 Don't know/not sure 99 refused
Hypertension Awareness (BP High)	Have you ever been told by a doctor, nurse, or other health professional that you have high blood pressure?	1 Yes 2 Yes, but female told only during pregnancy 3 No 4 Told borderline high or pre-hypertensive or elevated blood pressure 7 Don't know/Not sure 9 Refused
Hypertension Awareness (BP Meds)	Are you currently taking prescription medicine for your high blood pressure?	1 Yes 2 No 7 Don't know/Not sure 9 Refused
Tobacco Use	Have you smoked at least 100 cigarettes in your entire life?	1 Yes 2 No 7 Don't know/Not sure 9 Refused
Tobacco Use (Smoke Day)	Do you now smoke cigarettes every day, some days, or not at all?	1 Every day 2 Some days 3 Not at all 7 Don't know/Not sure 9 Refused
Tobacco Use (Use Now)	Do you currently use chewing tobacco, snuff, or snus every day, some days or not at all?	1 Every day 2 Some days 3 Not at all 7 Don't know/Not sure 9 Refused
Tobacco Use (E-Cigarette)	Do you now use e-cigarettes or other electronic vaping products every day, some days, or not at all?	1 Every day 2 Some days 3 Not at all 7 Don't know/Not sure 9 Refused

Data from the BRFSS may be displayed in different formats, including maps, graphs, and tables. Below is a map showing the 2021 data for when people reported having more than 14 days when their physical health was not good (https://www.cdc.gov/brfss/brf ssprevalence/) (figure 9.4).

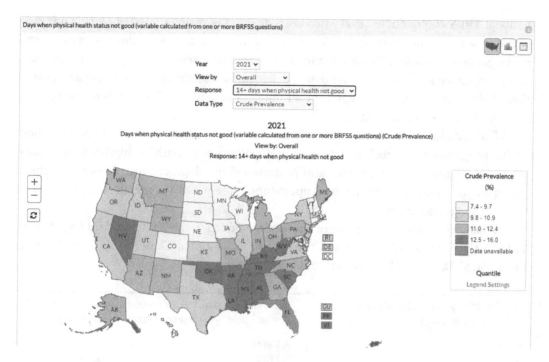

Figure 9.4 Example of BRFSS question: Days when physical health not-good

Youth Risk Behavior Surveillance System (YRBSS)

The YRBSS was developed in 1990 to monitor health behaviors that contribute markedly to the leading causes of death, disability, and social problems among youth and adults in the United States. These behaviors, often established during childhood and early adolescence, include

- Behaviors that contribute to unintentional injuries and violence.

- Sexual behaviors related to unintended pregnancy and sexually transmitted infections, including HIV infection.

- Alcohol and other drug use.

- Tobacco use.

- Unhealthy dietary behaviors.

- Inadequate physical activity.

In addition, the YRBSS monitors the prevalence of obesity, asthma, and other health-related behaviors plus sexual identity and sex of sexual contacts.

Similar to the BRFSS for adults, YRBSS data are used to track progress toward meeting health goals and objectives, identify trends, and develop relevant legislation, policy, and programming. YRBSS data may also be used to seek funding to support new initiatives. The

Youth Risk Behavior Surveillance System (YRBSS) a survey conducted among middle and high school students in the United States to monitor health-risk behaviors that contribute to the leading causes of death and disability among youth and adults

national YRBSS is conducted every two years during the spring semester. During one class period, a survey administrator distributes survey materials and reads directions to the students. Students complete the questionnaire in one class period. Participation is voluntary and anonymous; local parental permission procedures are followed prior to the administration of the YRBSS. The data represent all public and private school students in the fifty states and the District of Columbia.

YRBS data have proven useful to help develop programs and policies, including school health programs and policies, programs and policies for youth in high-risk situations, instructional guides and materials, and professional development programs for teachers. And data are a valuable resource to support funding requests to federal, state, and private agencies and foundations.

In the table below are examples of questions included in the 2021 Standard High School YBRFSS (Division of Adolescent and School Health, National Center for HIV/AIDS, Viral Hepatitis, STD, and TB Prevention, 2022):

How often do you wear a seat belt when riding in a car driven by someone else?	During the past 30 days, how many times did you ride in a car or other vehicle driven by someone who had been drinking alcohol?
A. Never	A. 0 times
B. Rarely	B. 1 time
C. Sometimes	C. 2 or 3 times
D. Most of the time	D. 4 or 5 times
E. Always	E. 6 or more times
During the past 30 days, on how many days did you text or e-mail while driving a car or other vehicle?	Have you ever used an electronic vapor product?
	A. Yes B. No
A. I did not drive a car or other vehicle during the past 30 days	
B. 0 days	
C. 1 or 2 days	
D. 3 to 5 days	
E. 6 to 9 days	
F. 10 to 19 days	
G. 20 to 29 days	
H. All 30 days	
How old were you when you had your first drink of alcohol other than a few sips?	During your life, with how many people have you had sexual intercourse?
A. I have never had a drink of alcohol other than a few sips	A. I have never had sexual intercourse
B. 8 years old or younger	B. 1 person
C. 9 or 10 years old	C. 2 people
D. 11 or 12 years old	D. 3 people
E. 13 or 14 years old	E. 4 people
F. 15 or 16 years old	F. 5 people
G. 17 years old or older	G. 6 or more people

Below are figures showing national results from select questions from the 2019 YBRFSS (Centers for Disease Control and Prevention, 2020).

(https://www.cdc.gov/healthyyouth/data/yrbs/pdf/2019/su6901-H.pdf)

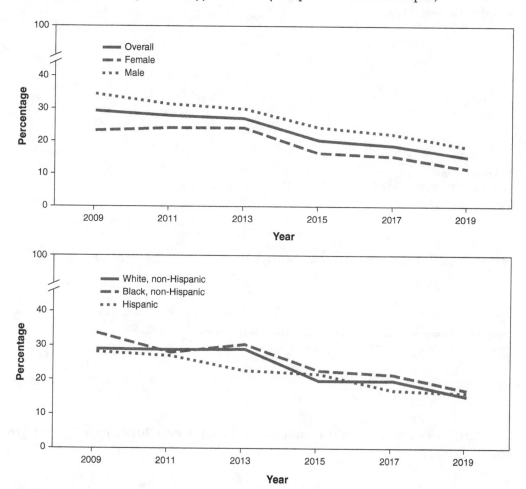

* During 2009–2019, a significant linear decrease was observed in the percentage of students who had drunk sugar-sweetened soda or pop ≥1 time/day overall and among female, male, white, black, and Hispanic students. Based on trend analyses by using a logistic regression model controlling for sex, race/ethnicity, and grade (p<0.05).

(https://www.cdc.gov/healthyyouth/data/yrbs/pdf/2019/su6901-H.pdf)

					Percentages										Trend from 1991–2019[1]	Change from 2017–2019[2]
1991	1993	1995	1997	1999	2001	2003	2005	2007	2009	2011	2013	2015	2017	2019		
Drank alcohol before age 13 years (had their first drink other than a few sips)																
32.7	32.9	32.4	31.1	32.2	29.1	27.8	25.6	23.8	21.1	20.5	18.6	17.2	15.5	15.0	Decreased 1991–2019 No change 1991–1999 Decreased 1999–2019	No change
Current alcohol use (at least one drink of alcohol on at least 1 day during the 30 days before the survey)																
50.8	48.0	51.6	50.8	50.0	47.1	44.9	43.3	44.7	41.8	38.7	34.9	32.8	29.8	29.2	Decreased 1991–2019 Decreased 1991–2007 Decreased 2007–2019	No change
Reported that the largest number of drinks they had in a row was 10 or more (within a couple of hours, during the 30 days before the survey)																
—[3]	—	—	—	—	—	—	—	—	—	—	6.1	4.3	4.4	3.1	Decreased 2013–2019	Decreased

(https://www.cdc.gov/healthyyouth/data/yrbs/factsheets/2019_alcohol_trend_yrbs .htm)

National Health and Nutrition Examination Survey (NHANES)

National Health and Nutrition Examination Survey (NHANES) a program of studies, including interviews and physical examinations, to assess the health and nutritional status of adults and children in the United States

The **National Health and Nutrition Examination Survey (NHANES)** (https://www.cdc .gov/nchs/nhanes/about_nhanes.htm) is a program of studies designed to assess the health and nutritional status of adults and children in the United States. The survey is unique in that it combines interviews and physical examinations. NHANES is a major program of the National Center for Health Statistics (NCHS). NCHS is part of the Centers for Disease Control and Prevention (CDC) and has the responsibility for producing vital health statistics for the nation.

The NHANES program began in the early 1960s and has been conducted as a series of surveys focusing on different population groups or health topics. In 1999, the survey became a continuous program that has a changing focus on a variety of health and nutrition measurements to meet emerging needs. The survey examines a nationally representative sample of about 5,000 persons each year. These persons are located in counties across the country, 15 of which are visited each year.

The NHANES interview includes demographic, socioeconomic, dietary, and health-related questions. The examination component consists of medical, dental, and physiological measurements, as well as laboratory tests administered by highly trained medical personnel.

Findings from this survey will be used to determine the prevalence of major diseases and risk factors for diseases. Information will be used to assess nutritional status and its association with health promotion and disease prevention. NHANES findings are also the basis for national standards for such measurements as height, weight, and blood pressure. Data from this survey will be used in epidemiological studies and health sciences research, which help develop sound public health policy, direct and design health programs and services, and expand the health knowledge for the nation.

Tests included in the health exam are listed in table 9.2.

State Initiatives

In addition to federal health initiatives, states have their own initiatives aimed at improving the health of their citizens. State health departments primarily provide data-based information and resources to their citizens. During the COVID-19 pandemic, many people became more familiar with their state health departments, which provided weekly updates (including number of cases, related hospitalizations, and vaccination rates), as well as information on where people could get tested and vaccinated.

In addition to infectious disease information, public health departments also provide programs, resources, and information to help reduce chronic diseases.

Examples of specific state initiatives and activities are provided in the following sections.

Arizona

Arizona's Health Improvement Plan (AzHIP) is a five-year roadmap bringing together partners to align resources and efforts, focusing on priorities underlying multiple health issues and disparities. The 2021–2025 AzHIP Priorities are centered on health equity, and include:

- Mental well-being
- Health in all policies/social determinants of health
- Rural & urban underserved health
- Pandemic recovery/resiliency

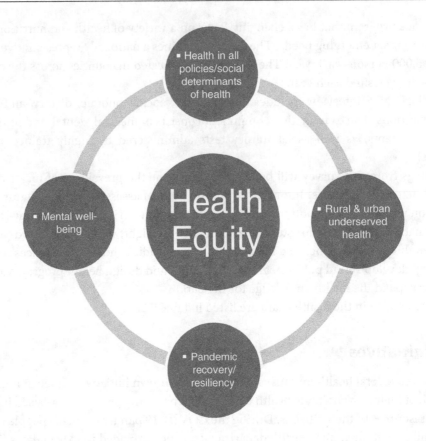

SOCIAL DETERMINANTS OF HEALTH: THE IMPACT OF "PLACE" ON HEALTH

The social determinants of health are defined by the CDC as the "conditions in the places where people live, learn, work, and play that affect a wide range of health and quality of life risks and outcomes."

The social determinants of health include five key areas, each of which reflects a multitude of issues:

- Economic stability
- Education
- Social and community context
- Health and health care
- Neighborhood and built environment

A wide range of public and private partners, including the list below, will implement the AzHIP.

- State agencies
- Local health departments

Table 9.3   Health Services to increase healthcare access

Behavioral Health	**CNHS Eyeglass Program**	**Emergency Medical Services**
Behavioral health includes outpatient mental health services, substance abuse treatment, and community-based programs promoting mental health.	The Eyeglass Program is designed to provide funding to eligible patients who have received eye exams from an eye care provider with the CNHS.	Emergency Medical Services is a state-licensed paramedic-level ambulance service owned and operated by the Cherokee Nation.
HIV and Hep C Services	**Patient Benefit Coordinators**	**Rehabilitation Services**
CNHS offers HIV and Hepatitis C services that work to eliminate the viruses through screening, treatment, and education.	Patient Benefit Coordinators: Learn about the role of PBCS and their locations.	In the outpatient setting, CNHS offers Physical Therapy, Occupational Therapy, and Speech-Language Pathology Services.

* Community-based organizations
* Employers and private organizations
* Universities
* Local nonprofits
* Other local agencies and organizations

Cherokee Nation Health Services (Tahlequah, Oklahoma)

The Cherokee Nation Health Services (CNHS) (https:health.cherokee.org) provides information on a variety of care through programs with the help of grants and partnerships (table 9.3). The services featured below allow the health system to increase access to care for patients and improve quality of life. (Cherokee Nation, 2022)

Utah

The Utah Department of Health and Human Services (www.dhhs.utah.gov/services) believes in ensuring all individuals and communities in Utah have access to a system of services. Its services promote fair and equitable opportunities to live safe and healthy lives (Utah Department of Health and Human Services, 2022). Among the services featured are (table 9.4):

The health of our nation is influenced by public health policies. Examples of health policies include vaccination laws, and requirements for children in schools and daycares, college/university students, healthcare workers, and patients in certain facilities. State laws also affect who can give vaccinations (e.g., doctors, nurses, and pharmacists). Another area included under health policy is the protection of health information (such as your medical records) and who has access to them and how they can be shared. Other examples of policies include menu labeling, and where tobacco-related products may be consumed.

National Nonprofit Organizations

National organizations provide policy information on the public health system, a few examples are described below.

Table 9.4   Family and Child Services to increase healthcare access

Family Services	Family services provide and promote resources and services to children and families through departmental agencies. Services assist with disabilities, mental and behavioral health, child support, financial stability, and more.
	• Adoption
	• Child support
	• Disability services (DSPD)
	• Foster care
	• Kinship Care
	• Report child abuse or neglect
	• Stabilization and Mobile Response
Youth Services	The Youth Services model is a "no wrong door" approach to early intervention. Through this model, Utah delivers evidence-based individualized youth and family plans with early screening, assessment, plan management, and comprehensive access to services, all driven by the youth and family strengths and needs.
	• Education
	• High Fidelity Wraparound
	• Juvenile competency
	• Juvenile Justice
	• Mental health resources and services for youth
	• Stabilization and Mobile Response
	• Youth in foster care
	• Youth Services Referral
	• Vaccine for Children Program
Adult Services	Adult Services is a link between the national Administration on Aging and local programs to provide home- and community-based services to millions of older persons. Utah Adult Protective Services has the responsibility and authority to investigate abuse, neglect, and exploitation of vulnerable adults.
	• Abuse, neglect, and exploitation
	• Caregiver support
	• Disability services (DSPD)
	• Governor's Century Club
	• Guardianship
	• Healthy aging classes
	• Long-term care ombudsman
	• Meals on Wheels
	• Mental Health Resources and Services for Adults
	• Senior centers
	• Senior events

Health Services	Health services protect the public's health by preventing avoidable illness, injury, disability, and premature death; assuring access to affordable, quality health care; and promoting healthy lifestyles.

- Adult Autism Treatment Account Program
- Baby Watch Early Intervention
- Baby Your Baby
- Cancer screenings
- Children's Health Insurance Program (CHIP)
- Developmental Center
- Emergency Medical Services and Preparedness
- Fostering Healthy Children Program
- Health Clinics of Utah
- HIVandMe
- Integrated Services Program
- Kurt Oscarson Children's Organ Transplant Fund
- Medicaid
- Medicaid Recovery
- Medical cannabis
- Medical Examiner
- Mental health
- Mother To Baby
- Naloxone
- Newborn screening
- Prevention, Treatment, and Care
- Substance abuse
- TBI Fund
- Tobacco Cessation
- Utah State Hospital
- Youth Vaping

Association of State and Territorial Health Officials (ASTHO)

From an association perspective, the **Association of State and Territorial Health Officials (ASTHO)** (www.astho.org) is a nonprofit organization committed to supporting the work of state and territorial public health officials and furthering the development and excellence of public health policy nationwide.

ASTHO's membership is comprised of 59 chief health officials from each of the 50 states, Washington, D.C., five U.S. territories, and three Freely Associated States. ASTHO also supports peer communities of state and territorial health leaders and senior executives

Association of State and Territorial Health Officials (ASTHO) a national nonprofit organization representing state-level public health agencies in the United States, the US territories, and the more than one hundred thousand public health professionals these agencies employ

in health departments who work with the over 100,000 public health professionals employed at state and territorial public health agencies.

ASTHO's primary functions are to:

- Develop strong and effective public health leaders.

- Improve public health through capacity building, technical assistance, and thought leadership.

- Advocate for resources and policies that improve the public's health and well-being.

ASTHO supports, equips, and advocates for state and territorial health officials in their work of advancing the public's health and well-being by providing capacity-building and technical assistance in a variety of areas (Association of State and Territorial Health Officials, 2022). Topics include (table 9.5):

Trust for America's Health

The Trust for America's Health (TFAH) (www.tfah.org) is a nonprofit, non-partisan health policy advocacy organization. TFAH focuses on addressing the social determinants of health and correcting health inequities.

TFAH works with partners in a broad range of sectors to advance evidence-based policies and programs that improve health and well-being of people and communities. These initiatives convene experts and policymakers and partner with states and communities to improve health and well-being. They seek and report on evidence and innovation. They generate ideas for new federal, state, and local policies, and they help build support to advance programs and policies that work.

Examples of TFAH's work include (Trust for America's Health, 2022):

- Age-Friendly Public Health Systems—TFAH is partnering with state and local health departments to implement a public health framework to improve the health and well-being of older adults.

- Health Equity/Social Determinants of Health—Health equity is the equal opportunity for all Americans to enjoy optimal health. TFAH creates and supports community-based initiatives, evidence-based recommendations, and a policy agenda that promotes health equity.

- Healthy Students, Promising Futures—The Healthy Students, Promising Futures Learning Collaborative provides educators and other student health advocates opportunities for structured peer-to-peer learning, formal technical assistance, strategic advice, and the sharing of best and emerging practices across sectors and states. Trust for America's Health and the Healthy Schools Campaign co-led the collaborative between 2016 and 2019. TFAH is now a Collaborative national partner.

- Promoting Health and Cost Control in States (PHACCS)—focuses on state-level policies that can be adopted and implemented to promote health and control cost growth.

Table 9.5   Capacity building and technical assistance for public health initiatives

Data Modernization and Informatics	Leadership and Workforce Development
Environmental Health	**Population Health and Prevention**
• Climate and Health	• Chronic Disease Prevention and Health Improvement
• Food and Water Safety	• Healthy Aging and Brain Health
• Vector-Borne Diseases	• Healthy People 2030
	• Heart Disease and Stroke Prevention
	• Tobacco Control and Cessation
	• Healthcare Access
	• Community Health Workers
	• Medicaid and Public Health Partnerships
	• Primary Care and Public Health
	• Telehealth
	• Social and Behavioral Health
	• Adverse Childhood Experiences
	• Injury, Suicide, and Violence Prevention
	• Overdose Prevention
	• Women, Infant, and Family Health
	• Breastfeeding and Early Life Nutrition Support
	• Early Brain Development
	• Increasing Access to Contraception
	• Maternal Morbidity and Mortality
	• Risk Appropriate Care
Health Equity	**Public Health Infrastructure**
• Disability Inclusion	• Public Health Assessment
• Health in All Policies	• Public Health Finance
• Operationalizing Equity	• Public Health Planning
• Social Determinants of Health	
• Tribal Health	
Infectious Disease	**Preparedness**
• Antimicrobial Resistance	• Natural Disasters
• COVID-19	• Pandemics
• Healthcare-Associated Infections	• Radiation
• Immunization	
• Influenza	
• Sexually Transmitted Infections	
• Syndemic-Related Infections	

WomenHeart
WomenHeart (www
.womenheart.org) is a
nonprofit organization
with a mission to improve
the lives of women with
or at risk for heart disease
while fighting for equity
in heart health. Access
to affordable health
insurance, heart disease
research, ensuring
women are included
in medical research,
and more are all made
possible through laws
and public policies.
WomenHeart works
to advance federal
policies that support
women living with or
at risk of heart disease,
and we train and
encourage women to be
advocates for themselves
(WomenHeart, 2022).

WomenHeart empowers advocates by providing resources and tools to communicate with lawmakers about matters that impact women with heart disease. Policy priorities include:

- Access to health coverage and care
- Access to cardiac rehabilitation
- Increased representation of women in clinical trials and medical research
- Full funding for heart and stroke research
- Awareness and support around pregnancy and heart disease

Local Programs

Programs established in communities through organizations such as YMCAs or Jewish community centers support healthier individuals and communities by providing resources, which may include space, information, and activities for community members. Chapter 6 provides detailed information regarding community-level physical activity initiatives sponsored by the YMCA. Other local programs supporting the health of communities include local farmers' markets and food cooperatives, as well as local health advocacy nonprofits. One example of such an organization is DC Greens (www.dcgreens.org), an organization based in Washington, DC, whose mission is to advance health equity by building a just and resilient food system by focusing on transformational changes at the systems-level; building bridges between government, private sector, communities, and nonprofits; developing advocacy channels to amplify marginalized voices; curating best practices and leveraging existing infrastructure.

In conjunction with state health departments, cities and districts often implement programs directed to specifically address health issues within a defined area. For example, in Richmond, Virginia, the Richmond City Health Department offers programs that address adolescent health and teen pregnancy prevention.

The Richmond and Henrico Health District has partnered with a variety of organizations across the region to promote food justice and increase food access through innovative projects, including mobile markets, other nonprofits, and the Richmond Public School Health Advisory Board (Virginia Department of Health, 2022).

> Food justice is about more than whether our communities have enough to eat. It is about growing community and reclaiming power and choice. Working toward food justice means answering questions like: How can we ensure that people in every community can access, afford, buy, cook, grow, and sell food of their choice? How do we change the way we think, talk, act, and invest in food and power in Richmond if we want to support real growth and healing?

CityHealth (www.cityhealth.org) is an initiative of the de Beaumont Foundation and Kaiser Permanente, which rates the nation's 40 largest cities based on their progress in adopting an evidence-based policy package that provides city leaders with a pragmatic, achievable, yet aspirational policies that could align with their city priorities and needs.

The CityHealth 2.0 Policy Package includes 12 tried and tested policy solutions that will help cities provide access for everyone to have a safe place to live, a healthy body and mind, and a thriving environment (CityHealth, 2021).

The policies include:

- Affordable Housing Trusts
- Complete Streets
- Earned Sick Leave
- Eco-Friendly Purchasing
- Flavored Tobacco Restrictions
- Greenspace
- Healthy Food Purchasing
- Healthy Rental Housing
- High-Quality, Accessible Pre-K
- Legal Support for Renters
- Safer Alcohol Sales
- Smoke-Free Indoor Air

Summary

Using data collected by federal organizations such as the CDC can help health promoters and policymakers identify leading health threats. Health issues facing communities affect the nation. HHS has developed the Healthy People 2030 goals as a guidepost for the nation to meet certain levels of health. Using these goals, health promotion professionals can develop plans, policies, and programs to help improve the health of individuals, businesses, churches, schools, communities, states, and, ultimately, the health of all Americans.

KEY TERMS

1. Behavioral Risk Factor Surveillance Survey (BRFSS): the world's largest, ongoing telephone health survey system, tracking and reporting on health conditions and risk behaviors in the United States on an annual basis

2. Youth Risk Behavior Surveillance Survey (YRBSS): a survey conducted among middle and high school students in the United States to monitor health-risk behaviors that contribute to the leading causes of death and disability among youth and adults

3. National Health and Nutrition Examination Survey (NHANES): a program of studies, including interviews and physical examinations, to assess the health and nutritional status of adults and children in the United States

REVIEW QUESTIONS

1. In addition to showing the status of health and health behaviors, how else is national data used?

2. What are social determinants of health?

3. What are the differences in the way data is collected for the Risk Behavior Surveillance Survey and the National Health and Nutrition Examination Survey?

4. What are some examples of organizations that health departments can partner with to address health within their states?

5. What were some services that you were interested to learn were provided by state health departments?

STUDENT ACTIVITIES

1. Review Youth Risk Behavior Surveillance Fact Sheets showing trends from 1991–2019 (https://www.cdc.gov/healthyyouth/data/yrbs/yrbs_data_summary_and_trends.htm). What trends do you find most interesting? What factors do you attribute to the change (or lack thereof) in certain behaviors? Compare the national rates to those of the state that you grew up in. What are the similarities and differences?

2. Based on the BRFSS data for your state, identify a program or service offered by your home state's health department that addresses one of the areas of most need.

3. What area of health are you most interested in? Research to find related federal, state, and local policies. Is there a way that you can become an advocate?

4. Check out CityHealth and review 3 of the policy solutions. How are the cities featured in the policy briefs associated with each of the solutions for implementing policies to improve health?

References

Association of State and Territorial Health Officials (2022). Our Work. Retrieved from https://www.astho.org/topic/

Centers for Disease Control and Prevention. (2017). National Center for Health Statistics. https://www.cdc.gov/nchs/nhanes/index.htm

Centers for Disease Control and Prevention (2020). Youth Risk Behavior Surveillance – United States, 2019. *MMWR Suppl* 2020: 69. Retrieved from https://www.cdc.gov/healthyyouth/data/yrbs/pdf/2019/su6901-H.pdf.

Centers for Disease Control and Prevention (2022). Mission of CDC. Retrieved from: https://www .cdc.gov/about/organization/mission.htm

Centers for Disease Control and Prevention (2022). Behavioral Risk Factor Surveillance System. Retrieved from: https://www.cdc.gov/brfss/index.html

Cherokee Nation (2022). *Health Services.* Services and Programs: Retrieved from https://health .cherokee.org/.

CityHealth (2021). 2.0 Policy Package. Retrieved from https://www.cityhealth.org/our-policy-package/2-0-policy-package/

Division of Adolescent and School Health, National Center for HIV/AIDS, Viral Hepatitis, STD, and TB Prevention (2022). *YRBSS Questionnaires.* Retrieved from https://www.cdc.gov/healthyy outh/data/yrbs/questionnaires.htm

National Center for Chronic Disease Prevention and Health Promotion (2021). *Using Surveillance Systems to Prevent and Control Chronic Diseases.* Retrieved from https://www.cdc.gov/chronicdis ease/resources/infographic/surveillance-systems.htm

National Center for Chronic Disease Prevention and Health Promotion, Division of Population Health (2022). *Behavioral Risk Factor Surveillance System.* Retrieved from https://www.cdc.gov/ brfss/index.html

National Institute of Health (nd). https://www.nia.nih.gov/about/budget/introduction-4

National Institutes of Health (2017). About NIH. Retrieved from www.nih.gov/about/mission.htm

National Institute of Diabetes and Digestive and Kidney Diseases (2020). About NiDDK. https:// www.niddk.nih.gov/about-niddk

Trust for America's Health (2022). Issues. Retrieved from https://www.tfah.org/issues/

US Department of Agriculture and Department of Health and Human Services (2020). Make every bite count. Retrieved from: https://www.usda.gov/media/press-releases/2020/12/29/ make-every-bite-count-usda-hhs-release-dietary-guidelines-american

Utah Department of Health and Human Services (2022). Services. Retrieved from https://dhhs.utah .gov/services/

US Department of Health and Human Services. (n.d-c). HHS organizational chart. Retrieved from www.hhs.gov/about/orgchart

Virginia Department of Health (2022). *Working Toward Food Justice in Richmond and Henrico.* Retrieved from https://www.vdh.virginia.gov/richmond-city/food-justice/

WomenHeart (2022). *Advocate for Women with Heart Disease.* Retrieved from https://www.women heart.org/your-heart-journey/advocate-for-women-with-heart-disease/.us/LHD/richmondcity/ programs.htm

CHAPTER 10

SETTINGS FOR HEALTH PROMOTION

David Stevenson

Inspirational and effective health promotion programs and services may be offered in many different settings where healthy lifestyle habits can be developed, nurtured, and sustained. The unique characteristics and strengths of environments where people live, learn, work, relax, recover, and worship can be used in teaching, modeling, and supporting positive health behaviors. Although settings may be very different, characteristics common to all effective health promotion programs include competent and enthusiastic leadership, a feeling of being welcome and safe, camaraderie among participants and with staff, involvement, and adherence to proven programs and services, and measures of success leading to a sense of achievement. Health promotion programs and settings also offer excellent opportunities for professional and volunteer leaders to make a positive impact on the health and well-being of others. Let's explore diverse settings where healthy lifestyles can be developed, promoted, and supported (Breckon, Harvey, & Lancaster, 1998; Floyd & Allen, 2004).

The Home

An individual's place of residence is likely to be the most important setting for the development of positive health behaviors. Prior to the COVID-19 pandemic, most individuals spent eight of their waking hours at home each day. During and following the pandemic, that number has increased to 10 waking hours each day. (U.S. Department of Labor, 2011). The development of new technology including improved access to information (the Internet), expanded opportunities for entertainment (cable television), and new opportunities to interact with others using social media have led to more time being spent in the home. Also contributing to this trend is an expanded use of business technology and home-based offices, enabling individuals to work from home while reducing costs for

LEARNING OBJECTIVES
After reading this chapter, the student will be able to:

- Identify the major settings where health promotion occurs.

- Describe each setting and the opportunities where health promotion professionals can promote health.

- Discuss how the major settings reach people in different places.

- Explain how the settings complement each other.

- Describe how the targeted behaviors are uniquely incorporated into the settings.

- Summarize opportunities for employment and volunteerism in various health promotion settings.

employees and employers (Matthews et al., 2008). It is also known that more individuals are using their homes as a place to exercise. In fact, the Sport and Industry Fitness Association (www.SGMA.com) reports that the purchase of home exercise equipment far outpaces the purchase of exercise equipment by commercial health clubs and other institutions.

In 2020, the US Department of Health and Human Services launched Healthy People 2030 (www.HealthyPeople.gov) presenting new objectives for improving the health of all Americans. Many of the health promotion settings and concepts presented in this chapter, such as early childhood centers, schools, worksites, physical activity, policies, and structural environments, are included in the new national objectives for improving health and well-being.

Family

Relationships with those held most closely in a person's life can have a profound effect on one's health and wellness. It is understood, therefore, that an individual's family or those whom they live with will play a vital role in their well-being (Umberson, 1987). To explore this concept, we must recognize that society's understanding of the word *family* has changed dramatically since the 1950s. In addition to the traditional family of parents and children, today's home often supports a new definition of family. Multigenerational families, foster homes, same-sex families, group homes, and homes supporting individuals with disabilities are a few examples of the diversity in the composition of today's modern family.

In families led by adults, the modeling and leadership offered by a parent, guardian, or caregiver is critical to the healthy development of the child (Golan & Crow, 2004). Children who live in a household where healthy foods are served, where fun physical activity is modeled and encouraged, where access to screen time (television, computers, hand-held devices) is limited, and where the day begins after a good night's sleep will have a solid foundation for lifelong well-being. Inversely, living in a home with easy access to unhealthy foods, where little physical activity takes place, where family members are glued to screens in a motionless state for many hours each day, and where family members start the day without proper rest can have a devastating effect on the health and well-being of all in the home.

Physical Space

Physical Space
The physical makeup of the home, office, or other environments; changes to one's personal space can make daily activities easier to complete, but require less physical movement, making exercise a task to be intentionally pursued

The **physical space** of the home may also support or detract from an individual's pursuit of a healthy lifestyle. Modern inventions designed to minimize physical exertion have achieved their goal. Conveniences such as the power garage door opener, washing machine, TV remote, and self-propelled lawn mower facilitate the completion of life's daily chores, often with just the lift of a finger. The physical requirements of daily chores for many in modern American society have been reduced to such an extent that exercise must be intentionally pursued to maintain health and wellness. Many leading health experts have pointed to this physical inactivity crisis as a major contributor to the epidemic of overweight and obesity taking place in developed countries (van Sluijs, McMinn, & Griffin, 2007).

According to the National Association of the Remodeling Industry (www.NARI.com), adding or renovating a home exercise space offers the owner a major advantage – convenience. As the number of home exercisers continues to grow, the dedication of space for fitness activities in the American home is becoming more common.

Personal Training

Services provided by a **personal trainer** in the home or other venues can offer the encouragement, support, and guidance necessary for improvement of an individual's health and wellness. Experienced and sought after personal trainers possess sound **interpersonal communication skills**, knowledge of exercise science, and understand how to inspire individuals to adopt and maintain healthy living habits. Personal trainers should be certified in emergency response including cardiopulmonary resuscitation and often possess certification through the American College of Sports Medicine (www.ACSM.org), National Strength and Conditioning Association (www.NSCA.com), YMCA (www.YMCA.net), National Academy of Sports Medicine (www.NASM.org), or other certifying organizations. Chapter 11 provides more detail on personal training certifications and other health promotion-related certifications.

Personal Trainer
A fitness professional proficient in exercise prescription and instruction; motivates clients by setting goals and providing feedback and accountability

Interpersonal Communication Skills
The process by which people exchange information, feelings, and meaning through verbal and nonverbal messages; message content can be seen as equally important as how it is said, including the tone of voice, facial expressions, gestures, and body language

Physical Safety

Serious accidents can take place in the home, particularly involving young children and older adults. Special precautions can be employed to minimize safety risks in the home by installing adequate lighting and skid protection, removing tripping hazards, limiting access to stairways, securing hazardous chemicals, and ensuring safe access and use of ladders, appliances, and swimming pools. Safety measures in homes where older adults live may include walking surfaces free of obstructions such as extension cords, grab bars in bathrooms enabling safe use, access to handrails and other support around stairways, and communications systems that can be easily accessed in case of an emergency. Useful home safety tips are offered by organizations such as the American Association of Retired Persons (AARP) and the National Association of Home Builders (NAHB).

Communities

Defined as families and individuals living or working in close proximity and who share common services, **communities** serve as a natural setting for the promotion of health. Grassroots community health initiatives have proven to be very effective in reducing health risks and promoting healthy lifestyles (Kaiser Permanente, 2008). Strategies and programs developed by not-for-profit organizations, schools, healthcare providers, and local government agencies have led to community-wide health promotion opportunities including the following:

Communities
Defined as families and individuals living or working in close proximity and who share common services

- Health education through community health fairs and seminars

- New opportunities for physical activity through community walks and fun runs, expanded green spaces, bike lanes, and better sidewalks

- Easier access to healthy foods grown in community gardens or sold at local farmers' markets

We have also learned that comprehensive community wellness initiatives developed and offered by organizations working in partnership will expand and strengthen the outcomes desired in improved community health (Perkins, 2002). Not-for-profits, schools, healthcare providers, and government agencies each bring unique and complementary strengths to providing a comprehensive and collaborative approach to address community health and wellness. When working together, these organizations can have a powerful impact on the lives of many. Funding for community health programming can be particularly challenging because few health and wellness initiatives generate revenue from the users. Local health departments wishing to develop and implement health promotion strategies and programs are often able to secure necessary funding through government grants and support from generous foundations wishing to improve community health. One such organization is the Robert Wood Johnson Foundation (www.RWJF.org), which has funded many community health promotion initiatives throughout the United States.

Health Fairs

Health Fair
An educational and interactive event designed for outreach to provide basic preventive medicine and medical screening to people in the community or employees at a worksite

A community **health fair** offers an excellent example of organizations coming together to assess the health of local residents and to offer educational services to improve health and well-being.

Local hospitals often play a leadership role in organizing health fairs, which can be held in community gathering places such as senior centers, shopping malls, recreation centers, libraries, employee cafeterias, and schools, to name a few. In addition to local hospitals, partners in community health fairs often include physician groups, physical therapy and chiropractic groups, public health departments, weight management groups, and educational and research organizations including the American Heart Association and American Cancer Society among others. Working in an open-space setting where individuals can move from booth to booth, health fair participants can visit with providers in a relaxed and more comfortable environment that contributes to a sense of community.

Targeted Community Initiatives

The Young Men's Christian Association (the Y) offers an evidence-based model aimed at improving community health through the Diabetes Prevention Program (www.ymca.net/diabetes-prevention) supported by local Y staff leadership and in partnership with a national health insurer. The goal of the program is to identify and coach those at risk for type 2 diabetes through education and coaching programs over the course of one year. The program is multifaceted because local Ys work with healthcare providers and other local organizations to encourage participation and program adherence.

Another example of an excellent community health initiative can be found in urban biking programs through which physical activity is increased and the use of automobiles is decreased, thereby reducing traffic congestion and carbon emissions. Effective collaborations among biking enthusiasts, local government, bicycle manufacturers, and local bike shops have led to improved biker safety including new bike lanes, the availability of bikes for rent at convenient locations, and improved awareness and acceptance of bicycles in cities and towns.

Farmers' Markets and Community Gardens

Farmers' markets and community gardens are great examples of settings for health promotion. This is especially true in urban areas that may be struggling to provide residents with easy access to healthy foods. Growers who bring their harvest and other goods to a local community serve many purposes in addition to providing a variety of healthy food at reasonable prices. The opportunities to learn about the health benefits of different foods, for socialization (also a component of good health!), and to stimulate the local economy are all positive benefits of farmers' markets. Community gardens also expand a community's healthy food choices, promote socialization, and increase physical activity.

Volunteer Opportunities

Programs and services designed to strengthen community health and wellness offer exciting opportunities for volunteerism. Offering one's time to work at health fairs, lead a community wellness initiative, or support a farmers' market or community garden can lead to personal satisfaction and program success, and can positively affect the program's financial position. National health organizations, including the American Heart Association (www.Heart.org), American Lung Association (www.Lung.org), American Cancer Society (www.Cancer.org), and many others, offer outstanding volunteer development opportunities.

Early Childhood Centers

It is well accepted that a significant portion of an individual's development takes place in the early years of life. Bonding with loved ones, learning how to socialize with other children, and developing learning skills are all characteristics of healthy development at a young age. The early childhood setting, which can include full and part-day childcare as well as nursery or prekindergarten programs, also offers an excellent opportunity to teach, model, and provide opportunities for healthy activities that can lead to positive lifetime habits. Characteristics of early childhood programs that offer high-quality health promotion components include the following:

- Validation of a child's current health status before entering a program including health history, preenrollment physician clearance, and proper immunizations
- Leadership from staff members who teach and model positive health behaviors including proper hygiene and safety
- Opportunities for physical play that are embedded in the early childhood program experience
- Offerings of healthy and flavorful foods
- Opportunities for health examinations including vision and hearing assessments

Hygiene and Safety Habits

Quality-based not-for-profit and for-profit early childhood centers, including nationwide providers such as the Y and KinderCare, incorporate intellectual, physical, social, and emotional development into their curriculum for preschool children. In most states, childcare teachers and support staff are required to meet stringent certification requirements in all areas of child development and administration including components of healthy development through physical activity, nutrition, and proper safety practices. Quality-based childcare organizations encourage modeling by their staff in proper hygiene, such as hand washing, proper handling of food, and how to protect others when sneezing or coughing. Staff members are required to follow safety practices thereby demonstrating to children how to avoid accidents. Special attention is given to the safe use of sharp objects such as scissors, toys, arts and crafts supplies, and the proper use of equipment including playgrounds, sports gear, bicycles, and tricycles.

Physical Activity

Quality-based childcare programs will include scheduled times for structured physical activity and free-play time for children throughout the day. Organized programs are led by trained professionals and may include activities ranging from group games to swimming lessons. Fair play, sportsmanship, safety, and the joy of physical activity are modeled and rewarded by staff leaders. Equally important to a child's well-being and development is time spent in free play (Ginsburg, 2007). Also referred to as free-range play or recess, unstructured playtime enables children to have fun and enjoy physical activity while expressing themselves, building new relationships, exploring new environments, and developing new skills and abilities.

Nutrition and Healthy Eating Habits

Proper nutrition and healthy eating are vital components of the early childhood experience. Many children enrolled in a full-day childcare program will eat two to three meals and one or more snacks during their time at the center. To ensure a healthy diet, special care should be given to developing a menu that is well balanced, flavorful, and age appropriate. Serving food to young children that tastes good including fruits and vegetables will begin good eating habits that can last for a lifetime. For those children who bring food to the center, staff members are encouraged to educate parents and guardians about proper nutrition for a developing child. Serving an occasional meal to the entire family at the early childhood center will enable families to spend time together while enjoying a healthy meal and reinforcing good health habits. It will also give staff time to interact with parents and guardians on a more relaxed basis (other than drop off or pickup). Serving food also presents opportunities to teach children about safe ways in which to handle and store food and the postmeal procedures for cleanup and dishwashing.

Health Assessments
A plan of care that identifies the specific needs of the client and how these needs will be addressed by the healthcare system or skilled nursing facility; in an early childhood setting may include annual onsite examinations for general health, vision, hearing, dental, and speech

Health Assessments

Early childhood programs serving low-income families, such as Head Start (www.acf.hhs.gov/programs/ohs), offer important opportunities to assess the health and wellness of the preschooler. Often required by the organization's curriculum or licensing agency, **health assessments** may include annual on-site examinations for general health, vision, hearing, dental, and speech. These services offer a valuable benefit to the child and the family who may be uninsured, underinsured, or may not have the funds to pay for or the ability to schedule regular health assessments.

Schools

The use of the elementary, middle, and high school settings to positively impact health habits and future success holds tremendous potential for students, as well as faculty, staff, and members of the community. It is well established that early development of positive health behaviors will likely lead to better health and well-being as an adult and that good health and physical fitness benefit children in many ways including their ability to learn and perform academically (Chomitz et al., 2009).

Quality-based health promotion in a school setting involves far more than what traditional physical education classes typically address. Characteristics of an effective school-based health promotion program include the following:

- Support from the school principal and governing board who are committed to each child's health, education, and development through health and wellness policy development, curriculum structure, and program funding

- Guidance and support from faculty members and staff to teach and reinforce positive health habits throughout the school day

- Opportunities throughout the day for children to get up and move their bodies; special emphasis is based on progressive physical education programs that teach lifetime fitness skills and daily recess when children can physically play in an unstructured environment

- Offerings of healthy and flavorful foods in the school cafeteria

- Active involvement by the school nurse or healthcare team to ensure that children have received appropriate exams and screenings, and have been identified for follow-up based on their health history or physical exams

- Celebration of improvements in individual and group health, wellness, and fitness with a special emphasis on participation

- Use of school buildings and grounds after traditional school hours (evenings and weekends) to support public recreation, exercise, and other wellness programs

Academics and Health

Elementary and secondary schools are experiencing significant challenges because many of the demands of modern society are placed at their doorsteps. Funding support, increased costs, curriculum demands, political pressures, student performance, the education achievement gap, graduation rates, and aging facilities are but a few of the problems facing today's school boards and administrators. Although improved health and wellness are known to strengthen academic performance, many school systems have reduced or eliminated time dedicated to physical education, health, wellness, and other time for physical activity including recess (National Association for Sport and Physical Education, 2009). Part of this challenge relates to the fact that teachers and administrators are accountable for student *academic* performance and not necessarily for the health and well-being of the student. Time, therefore, is spent on curriculum, classes, and programs that will improve academic test scores. There are exceptions to this trend, and many school districts fully recognize the value of health promotion in the school setting. These schools offer daily physical education, well-developed health education curriculum and programs, and free time for physical activity (recess). Sadly, many school districts have reduced time devoted to these important components of elementary and secondary student development.

School Policy Supporting Health

School Wellness Policies
An important tool for parents, local educational agencies, and school districts in promoting student wellness, preventing and reducing childhood obesity, and providing assurance that school meal nutrition guidelines meet the minimum federal school meal standards

Schools that offer well-developed health, physical education, and health promotion curricula and programs to their students typically enjoy professional and elected leaders who understand the relationship between investment in student health and well-being and the resulting positive impact on academic performance. These school superintendents and boards have developed and adopted **school wellness policies** designed to strengthen student health and wellness, and have worked hard to maintain adequate funding for these important programs. In fact, federal law enacted in 2006 requires all public school districts to adopt and implement a wellness policy including goals for nutrition education, nutrition guidelines, physical activity, parental and community involvement in policy development and review, and a plan to measure the implementation of the wellness policies. Although modest progress has been made, only 46% of students attended schools in 2010–2011 with a wellness policy that included all of the required elements (Robert Wood Johnson Foundation, 2013). The negative impact of the pandemic has brought challenges caused by school closures and staffing shortages resulting in learning loss that have required schools to re-commit to a robust-school wellness policy. Experienced school administrators understand that student health and wellness mean more than athletics and sports teams. Curriculum addresses current-day health challenges facing youth including overweight and obesity, physical inactivity, poor eating habits, and substance abuse, to name a few. Comprehensive school-based health promotion programs also offer physical activity programs designed for *all* students, not just the select few on the competitive sports teams.

Teacher's Roles

Schools offering excellent student health promotion programs have also gained the enthusiastic support of faculty members and staff who model, teach, and encourage healthy behaviors and activities within their student populations. Oftentimes, these teachers do more than simply talk about health and well-being; they are personally committed to living a healthy lifestyle and use the greatest teaching tool known – personal example. In fact, many progressive school districts have implemented comprehensive health promotion programs for faculty members and staff based on the philosophy that an investment in an individual's health and well-being will lead to improved performance in the workplace – in this case, the classroom.

Healthy Food Choices

Offering healthy and flavorful foods that students want to eat is a vital component of an effective school-based health promotion program. The often-maligned school lunch has endured many negative stereotypes in which children have shunned the bland and tasteless food offered by the school in favor of sweet or salty items such as snack foods and dessert items available in the cafeteria. Sadly, some administrators view their cafeteria or food service as a profit center to generate revenue through the sale of popular yet often unhealthy foods. Doughnuts in the morning, vending machines selling high-sugar drinks, and ice cream bars may add to a school's bottom line, but they do not contribute to students' health and wellness. In response to growing concerns from parents and others about healthy food choices, and youth overweight and obesity, the Healthy Hunger-Free Kids Act was passed in 2010 to improve school nutrition standards. Many school districts have reinvented the school meal offerings to include foods lower in fat and calories, higher in complex carbohydrates, and use locally grown produce (often coming from the school garden!), colorful food choices, and foods that are prepared using healthy cooking techniques. Enlightened school administrators, nutritionists, and cafeteria managers are creating a healthy school meal experience that kids enjoy and that contributes to student well-being.

School Healthcare Services

The role played by the school nurse and healthcare team has become more than simply making sure that students have gotten their shots and that the medical forms are filled out properly. Efficient administration is still required, but many school districts have expanded the role of the school nurse to include identification of students who may exhibit serious health concerns and developing programs targeted toward students based on health challenges. Working as a team, the school nurse, principal, health and physical education teacher, and classroom teacher can develop individualized health plans for students aimed at addressing specific concerns. Many schools have adopted plans to identify students with high **body mass index** (BMI) and have developed programs in partnership with hospitals, Ys, and others in an effort to help students gain and maintain ideal body weight. A popular initiative used by many school districts is the **5210 program** in which on a daily basis students strive to eat five servings of fruits and vegetables, limit screen time to two hours, be physically active for one hour, and consume zero sugared drinks (www.letsgo .org). Programs such as the 5210 Club are strengthened when families are invited to participate.

Body Mass Index (BMI)
A weight-to-height ratio, calculated by dividing one's weight in pounds by the square of one's height in inches; then multiplying by 703; it is used as an indicator of overweight, obesity, ideal weight, and underweight status

5210 Program
program in which on a daily basis students strive to eat five servings of fruits and vegetables, limit screen time to two hours, be physically active for one hour, and consume zero sugared drinks

Health Promotion Initiatives

Recognition and celebration inspire students to continue in the pursuit of healthy living and can come in many forms. Simple recognition for student or class success can include a mention of goal achievement in the morning announcements, and more formal celebrations can include certificates or other awards or prizes during formal ceremonies such as graduation. Schools with innovative health promotion programs are always finding new and exciting ways to regularly celebrate success and inspire adherence to healthy living practices.

School After-hours

School districts committed to health promotion often recognize the opportunity to contribute to community health and wellness by making school buildings and grounds available to the public and not-for-profit organizations who offer recreation, exercise, and wellness programming. Communities that have access to low or no-cost evening and weekend activities and programs held in the school gym, all-purpose room, or on the athletic field enjoy interesting and fun opportunities to strengthen individual and family health and wellness.

Coordinated School Health

The Centers for Disease Control and Prevention (www.cdc.gov) offers an excellent resource for the development of comprehensive health promotion programs in the school setting. The CDC's Whole Schook, Whole Community, Whole Child (WSCC) Program addresses school-based physical education and activity, nutrition environment and services, health education, social and emotional climate, physical environment, health services, counseling, psychological services, employee wellness, community involvement, and family engagement.

Professional Opportunities

Elementary, middle, and high school settings offer many opportunities for the professional wishing to make a positive impact on the health and wellness of young people. Most school-based teaching positions will require a four-year bachelor's degree in disciplines such as health education or physical education, and a school nurse position will often require a bachelor's degree as well as certification as a school nurse (National Association of Registered School Nurses, n.d.).

Colleges and Universities

Many public and private institutions of higher education, including two-year community colleges and four-year colleges and universities, now offer formal health promotion programs, services, and facilities to their students, faculty, and staff. Students entering colleges or universities face many new opportunities including decisions about their personal health and wellness, and college administrators recognize their responsibility and the opportunity to guide students toward positive lifestyle choices. Characteristics of quality-based comprehensive health promotion programs in the college and university setting include the following:

- Commitment from administrators to develop, fund, implement, and evaluate health promotion programs and services

- Recognition of all aspects of campus life including the student health center, dining hall, clubs and activities, and sports and recreation in developing a collaborative approach to improving and supporting healthy habits within the college or university community

- Development of the college campus to encourage physical activity through new or renovated recreation, fitness and sports facilities, safe sidewalks, and bike lanes

Safe and Healthy Environment

Students entering college often enjoy many new freedoms that they had not experienced during their high school years. The ability to use time as one wants, to move about freely regardless of the time of day, to make decisions without parental oversight, and to have access to foods, alcohol, drugs, and other substances that may range from unhealthy to dangerous create many crossroads for the college student. Administrators understand that although these new freedoms are part of a student's individual development, an environment must be developed and maintained that will lead students toward safe and healthy choices. Experienced and thoughtful college presidents will lead a regular dialogue (speeches, social media, student newspapers, small groups, etc.) about student health and safety including responsibilities held by students and the college or university. Campus communication systems, interpersonal relationships and dating, student counseling and support groups, and policies regarding alcohol and drugs are but a few of the topics that are continually addressed by higher education administrators. Funding necessary to develop and support these efforts will be included in the yearly budget and regular evaluation will be completed to ensure that initiatives and programs are effective and are meeting the safety, health, and wellness needs of the college student.

Coordinated Health Promotion

Comprehensive high-quality **coordinated health promotion programs** offered in the college and university setting use all of the resources of the institution through a well-coordinated offering of programs and services. Campus leaders meet to share how their departments are contributing to student health and well-being and discuss ways in which they may be able to work together to strengthen the college-wide health promotion experience. In addition to caring for students who are ill, the student health center should offer proactive educational programs, including ways to avoid diseases and disorders, and can serve as a resource for preventive services such as flu shots. Dining halls will offer healthy and delicious foods when students want to eat. Clubs and college event planners should consider student safety, health, and well-being as criteria when developing new activities. Student intramurals, club sports, and other physical activities will be viewed as fun and safe and should be developed to encourage participation by all students.

Coordinated Health Promotion Programs
Programs that use all of the resources of the institution through a well-coordinated offering of programs and services

Physical Environment

College and university campuses have experienced explosive growth in athletic and recreation facilities over the past few decades (Bogar, 2008). Major universities have built huge stadiums and arenas to support their teams, especially for football and basketball. As colleges and universities strive to attract the best students, campus facilities such as classrooms, labs, libraries, dormitories, dining halls, and health centers have also been built or updated. This trend in campus redevelopment has created opportunities to enhance the wellness experience by improving and encouraging pedestrian and biker safety, as well as constructing new fitness, wellness, and intramural sports centers for all students.

Professional Opportunities

The diversity of college life creates many opportunities to positively impact the health and wellness of students, faculty, and staff. Healthcare professionals, including physicians, physician assistants, and nurses, work in the campus health center offering prevention and care for illnesses and injuries. Many campus-based wellness and fitness centers and intramural programs are led by degreed and certified professionals and are often staffed by college students earning degrees in health, physical education, recreation, or related fields.

The Worksite

A large portion of adult life is devoted to professional pursuits; thus, the worksite offers a special opportunity to positively affect health and wellness. An employer's commitment to investing in programs and activities that strengthen wellness and minimize job-related health hazards can produce excellent results for the employee and the employer. From a human relations perspective, employers who offer health promotion programs are often perceived as caring leaders who are interested in the well-being of their workers. Additionally, organizations that invest in employee health through proven programs will strengthen their company's bottom line. In fact, a review of the research shows that for every $1 invested in quality-based health promotion leadership, programs, and facilities, $3-$5 will be saved through reduced employee healthcare costs (Linnan, 2010). Beyond the return on investment, many professionals are connecting health and human capital and encouraging worksite health promotion professionals to expand the benefits to quality of life (Chenoweth, 2007).

The continued evolution of the worksite, including varied full-time and part-time work schedules, telecommuting, and remotely based staff, poses new challenges for the effective delivery of health promotion programs and services. Quality-based worksite health promotion has adapted rapidly to the constantly changing nature of the workplace with a solid health promotion strategy and flexible delivery of services that are meaningful to employees at their place of work.

Worksite health promotion has evolved dramatically since the 1940s. At that time, business leaders recognized the benefit of staying fit and began to develop gymnasiums and fitness facilities primarily for executives. With the explosion of the fitness industry in the 1970s, worksite wellness grew through many businesses as well as deeper into employee populations. Recognizing the benefit to the employee *and* the organization, companies began to develop comprehensive wellness and recreation programs for all in their workforce.

Characteristics of an effective worksite health promotion include the following:

• Ongoing support from the organization's leadership, including the clear identification of employee health and wellness as a priority, and allocation of leadership, funds, space, and other resources to operate an effective health promotion program

- The creation of a culture that promotes health and one that minimizes health risks in the workplace (industrial accident prevention, protection against exposure to unhealthy work environments and materials, opportunities for periodic activity breaks for those in sedentary jobs, etc.)

- Opportunities to participate in evidence-based programs and activities such as exercise, nutrition counseling, smoking cessation, stress management, and low back injury prevention

- An assessment system including guidance by a health coach to ensure targeted programming that will lead to regular participation and measurable results

- The use of technology, electronic media, and the Internet to educate, inspire, and provide continuous feedback on success, thereby improving program adherence

- An incentive system through which participation is rewarded by meaningful recognition or other more tangible means such as reduced healthcare insurance premiums

Leadership

Regardless of mission or profit motives, excellent employers understand the benefit of a healthy workforce. For-profit companies, not-for-profit organizations, government agencies, schools, and other strong organizations demonstrating solid employee productivity share a commitment to employee health and wellness, including leadership and support from the chief executive officer. For a new business, product, or company initiative to be successful, leadership from the top of the organization is vital, and comprehensive and effective employee health promotion programs are no exception. Often leading by example, chief executives will dedicate the time, personnel, funds, space, equipment, and other resources necessary to promote, develop, and maintain good health and well-being within the employee population.

Results-driven worksite health promotion programs can range from offering basic health screenings and wellness education programs to highly developed strategies including sophisticated health assessments and comprehensive wellness facilities. Worksite health promotion programs that are well-resourced often provide fitness facilities and equipment to their employees, and many organizations have integrated employee wellness incentives and improvement into their strategic plans and measures of overall organizational success.

NATIONAL COMMITTEE FOR QUALITY ASSURANCE (NCQA)'S 2020 WELLNESS STANDARDS

1. Client Organization Engagement

2. Data Exchange and Integration

3. Privacy and Confidentiality

4. Engage the Population

5. Health Appraisal

---

6. Identification and Targeting

7. Self-Management Tools

8. Health Coaching

9. Rights and Responsiblities

10. Measuring Effectiveness - Accreditation

11. Incentive Management

12. Reporting WHP Performance

13. Measuring Effectiveness - Certificatiions

14. Delegation of WHP Activities

Source: www.ncqa.org

Worksite Safety

An important component of an employee health promotion program can be found in the commitment of many healthcare providers to their patients, "First, do no harm." Responsible employers create a culture of safety and protect their employees from potentially hazardous or unhealthy environments. This is especially true for manufacturing and construction organizations, where employees may work with and be exposed to heavy equipment and tools, chemicals, building materials, and harsh weather. To prevent workers from being killed or seriously harmed at work, the Occupational Safety and Health Act was passed in 1970. The law created the Occupational Safety and Health Administration (OSHA), which established and enforces protective safety and health standards in the workplace. OSHA also provides employers and their workers with information, training, and assistance to improve workplace safety.

An employer's first responsibility to the health and well-being of its workforce is to ensure that risks are identified and that reasonable safeguards are in place to protect workers. After identification, the next step is to educate all employees about the potential hazards they may face in the workplace. Ensuring that employees fully understand the potential dangers of the tools or machines they work with, the chemicals and materials that they are exposed to, and the history and type of accidents that can happen on the job will serve as a solid foundation in protecting employee safety, health, and well-being. Basic cautionary measures, such as wearing protective gear (safety glasses, proper clothing, protective footwear, etc.) and periodic breaks to ensure that employees are rested and alert, are well accepted in most workplaces. More advanced safeguards may include regular safety reviews and inspections, drug and alcohol screening, fall protection, and driving training and tests. To prevent accidents and other chronic injuries or disorders in the workplace, employers will strive to develop the physical conditioning and strength of their employees as well as educating their employees about the importance of performing certain physical tasks properly (e.g., lifting). By developing a culture of safety, employers can minimize health risks, reduce and eliminate accidents, contribute to employee morale and productivity, and increase profits.

Health Promotion

Employers fully committed to comprehensive health promotion will offer a wide range of programs and services designed to target specific health concerns and strengthen employee health and well-being. Program offerings may address topics such as healthy eating and weight loss, smoking cessation, stress management, type 2 diabetes prevention, as well as programs targeting injury prevention. A program can be as simple as a brown bag lunch talk when a fifteen to thirty-minute program is offered during the lunch break or it can be a more in-depth exploration over the course of weeks or months learning about the causes of an unhealthy behavior and specific steps that can be adopted for improvement.

Quality-based employee health promotion programs will also use a variety of opportunities to encourage, monitor, and celebrate employee participation in physical activities and fitness programs. Many well-resourced companies offer a full range of fitness facilities, including gymnasiums, swimming pools, group exercise centers, athletic fields, locker rooms, and wellness centers that offer a variety of cardiovascular exercise and strength-training equipment. Organizations that are not able to offer these kinds of facilities and equipment must be creative in identifying and developing other opportunities for physical activity and exercise. Organizing groups within the workforce that share common interests such as walking, running, hiking, and biking is a great way to promote physical activity either on company time or on personal time. Many organizations including the Y, Jewish Community Centers (JCCs), public recreation centers, and for-profit fitness centers offer employee wellness programs and group rates.

Health Coaches

Facilities and equipment can be terrific resources for the employee health promotion program. More important, however, is the guidance and counsel provided by a health promotion professional. Often referred to as **health coaches**, the health promotion professional provides programs and services at the worksite and offers advice and support that will inspire employees to improve and maintain a good level of health, physical conditioning, and well-being. Effective coaches develop a personal relationship with employees through an understanding of the individual's background, work requirements, and motivations, which can be used in building adherence to healthy lifestyle practices. Through this relationship, the coach and the employee can focus on particular areas for improvement and can track and celebrate milestones and achievements together. The coach builds a solid level of trust with employees and can be counted on to protect confidential information. Excellent coaches have received education in the health sciences and psychology and always demonstrate a caring, enthusiastic, and outgoing personality and attitude.

Health Coaches Provide programs and services at the worksite and offer advice and support that will inspire employees to improve and maintain a good level of health, physical conditioning, and well-being; effective coaches develop a personal relationship with employees through an understanding of the individual's background, work requirements, and motivations, which can be used in building adherence to healthy lifestyle practices

Employee Assistance Programs

Employee assistance programs (EAPs) are offered by many employers to help workers and their families manage issues in their personal lives. Originally established in the 1950s to support workers struggling with alcohol dependency, EAPs have evolved to help employees address issues such as substance abuse, emotional distress, major life events, healthcare concerns, personal financial problems, and family and personal relationships to name a few. EAPs typically use counselors to provide assessment, support, and referrals to employees and family members facing serious challenges. In many cases, employers work through a third party to provide EAP services. Confidentiality must be maintained during the process of seeking and gaining guidance and support, and EAPs can serve as an important benefit to workers and their employers.

Technology and Social Media

The use of technology and social media offers a great tool supporting the improvement and maintenance of good employee health and wellness (see "The Internet"). Special company websites for employees can be used to promote new health promotion programs and services and can serve as a platform to track group progress and to announce and celebrate achievements. Tools such as e-mail and text messaging, and social media including Instagram, Facebook, and Threads can be sued by coaches and employees to communicate with each other. Technology providers Apple Fitness, Nike Training Club, and Fitbit offer excellent applications that will enable participants to record, track, and celebrate fitness milestones including the use of cardiovascular exercise and strength-training equipment.

Measuring and Celebrating Success

Tracking, evaluating, and celebrating success are hallmarks of a comprehensive quality-based worksite health promotion program. During times when organizations are challenged to show a return on investment, employee health promotion programs must continually demonstrate a positive benefit to the workforce and to the organization's bottom line. Employee feedback should be collected using in-house surveys or evaluations administered by third-party professionals and analyzed to measure the qualitative and quantitative benefits of the worksite health promotion program. Through use of this data, organizations can focus resources on areas in which the greatest impact can be made. Historically, these areas have included increased employee productivity and morale and decreased healthcare use, sick leave, and accidents. Recognition and reward systems can also be developed using data. Some employers will recognize participation and improvement of individual health and wellness through financial rewards such as bonuses or decreased health insurance costs for employees. Others may use the powerful tools of praise or public recognition to celebrate success and encourage continued participation and growth.

Professional Opportunities

Health promotion professionals serving in a worksite–based wellness program will often possess a hybrid of skills, abilities, and certifications. In addition to possessing skills and certification in the field of health promotion, including wellness assessment, exercise programming, and nutrition counseling, worksite wellness professionals must possess business acumen and solid communication skills. By fully understanding the mission and culture of the organization where they are working, professionals can relate to, communicate with, and support the employees they are serving.

Healthcare Providers

The opportunities for healthcare providers, such as physicians in offices and hospitals, therapists in physical therapy and rehabilitation centers, and those who work in long-term care centers, to positively affect health and wellness are boundless. This is especially true for those healthcare organizations that have adopted preventive healthcare as a primary focus. Unique opportunities for health promotion exist in healthcare settings because most clients and patients are searching for care or treatment to combat disease, disorder, or discomfort. In other words, individuals are seeking help and are motivated to improve their health.

A major obstacle to improving an individual's health and well-being is the requirement for change. Changing one's lifestyle can be daunting and is often looked upon negatively. The advantage held by healthcare organizations or professionals is that they are usually viewed favorably and are held in high regard because of their reputation, training, expertise, and sincere interest in the patient's health and well-being. This perception positions professional healthcare organizations or providers very well in leading and supporting positive change in a patient's health.

Physicians

The physician may have the greatest opportunity to inspire improvement in an individual's health and well-being. People usually like and respect their doctor and will take action based on the advice he or she offers. The challenge for the physician is to move beyond treating a specific disease or disorder by educating patients about the benefits of healthy lifestyle habits and then helping their patients through the process of making positive changes. Simply *telling* a patient to lose weight (most patients already know this!) will rarely lead to successful weight loss. Successful weight loss is more likely to occur if the physician and support staff show the patient *how* to lose weight through education, guidance, support, and regular follow-up.

Other Healthcare Providers

Other healthcare and long-term care providers, including hospitals, rehabilitation centers, chiropractic centers, assisted-living homes, and nursing homes, can make significant contributions to an individual's health and well-being through the unique strengths possessed by each organization. Hospitals enjoy a wide range of complementary programs and services that can be offered onsite. In fact, hospitals that have rebranded as healthcare organizations or systems often offer preventive services and facilities, including fitness centers, rehabilitation centers, and health promotion programs such as nutrition education and smoking cessation. Long-term care centers, such as assisted living and nursing homes, can lead and support residents on their journeys toward healthier living by serving nutritious foods, encouraging physical activity, and building social relationships centered on positive health habits.

Faith-based Centers

Health promotion programs and services offered in a faith-based setting can provide meaningful benefits to participants, particularly those seeking spiritual growth or the improvement of the whole person in spirit, mind, and body. Research suggests there can be a benefit to the inclusion of faith or spiritual growth as a contributing component to the improvement of whole-person wellness initiatives (Powell, Shahabi, & Thoreson, 2003). Faith-based settings such as religious institutions hold characteristics that have contributed to strong success in improving wellness:

- A belief that strengthening the spirit, mind, and body is part of the religion that one practices

- Offering a setting where people feel comfortable and may gather with others who share common beliefs

- The development of wellness facilities, including gymnasiums and fitness centers, as part of a religious institution's physical facilities

Many religions recognize the relationship among healthy spirit, mind, and body and take proactive steps to strengthen these three core components of total health and wellness. Churches, synagogues, mosques, and other centers of worship often provide educational, wellness, physical fitness, and other health promotion programs to their followers in comfortable and nonthreatening environments. Other faith-based organizations, including the Y and the JCC, were founded to promote spiritual beliefs and have grown to offer many educational and wellness programs, services, and facilities. A study of the Y's history shows the evolution of the organization from one that simply proclaimed the teachings of Jesus Christ to an organization that developed and promotes the concept of fulfillment of the whole person through growth in spirit, mind, and body, and is exemplified in the Y triangle. Today, with a mission "to put Christian principles into practice through programs that build a healthy spirit, mind, and body for all" (Young Men's Christian Association, 2014), the Y is one of the largest not-for-profit organizations in the United States.

The Internet

Recognition of the Internet (websites, search engines, social media, blogosphere, e-mail, texting, etc.) as a setting for health promotion invites interesting discussion. Although the Internet is not characterized as a physical space, it does serve as a tool through which we can be inspired and entertained, gather information, communicate with others, store data, and track progress. In fact, the Internet, now available to most US citizens, has, arguably, changed the way Americans lead their lives. How, then, is the Internet used as a setting to positively affect health and well-being?

Access to Information and Data

An important characteristic of any quality-based setting for health promotion is the opportunity to gather information and learn. The Internet provides limitless opportunities for access to information regarding wellness topics such as physical activity, healthy eating, stress management, substance abuse prevention, spiritual wellness, and safety. A key strength of the Internet is instantaneous access to information through hand-held devices such as cellular telephones, tablets, and laptop computers. Using search engines such as Google and Bing, we simply enter keywords or phrases such as *fitness, nutrition, preventive screening,* or *stress management* and can begin to learn about all of the components of healthy living. The use of an incredible variety of websites can also be helpful in educating ourselves about health and well-being. Most health and wellness organizations in America have well-developed websites that offer information about their mission, programs, and services and may include interactive tools to help educate the visitor. These tools can be as simple as entering a few numbers to receive a basic health measure such as BMI or more sophisticated systems that would accept comprehensive biometric information that may produce a complete profile identifying health risks and areas for improvement.

Although the Internet offers incredible tools for the promotion of health, the health seeker and professional must emphasize the importance of confidentiality and the quality of information being gathered. One must exercise caution in storing and sharing data as well as viewing information. Using multiple sources to validate information is prudent, particularly when an individual's health is being addressed.

Tracking Personal Health Data

Many health and wellness websites also offer opportunities to store and track personal health data. Wellness centers will use technology to enable the participant to enter physical activity information including type of exercise, intensity, and minutes and will provide feedback on ways to improve the participant's program to achieve desired results more effectively. Sophisticated programs offer websites that include personal coaching from trained professionals who maintain regular contact with the participant through messaging tailored to the individual's goals and objectives. Weight loss programs such as Jenny Craig (www .JennyCraig.com), Nutrisystem (www.Nutrisystem.com), and Weight Watchers (www .WeightWatchers.com) make excellent use of their websites and other communication technologies to educate their clients about effective weight loss, track progress, and celebrate success.

Social Media

The use of social media can be very powerful in the pursuit of a healthy lifestyle and holds special opportunities for health promotion leaders and organizations. Progressive health promotion organizations have recognized the value of maintaining a presence on Instagram, Facebook, LinkedIn, Threads, Twitter, and other social media because an increasing number of individuals use social media as a primary form of communication. Organizations use these media to attract new clients, disseminate information in a timely manner, and inspire clients and the public with messages of encouragement, praise, and recognition. Social media is a powerful tool to connect individuals with each other based on common characteristics such as shared health challenges, activity preferences, geographic locations, and so on. The use of tools that help to connect people holds special value because we understand the benefit of positive personal relationships and the feeling of belonging to like-minded groups of people striving to develop and maintain healthy lifestyles.

Summary

Settings where we live, learn, work, relax, recover, and worship each present unique and powerful opportunities to positively impact the health and wellness of individuals and groups. Although varied in location, structure, and offerings, environments supporting and contributing to healthy lifestyles are most effective when they become part of our daily life. Those individuals who enjoy a healthy home, school, workplace, and other positive settings are likely to experience the compounding effect of continued wellness education, inspiration, and support throughout the day. The health promotion setting also offers exciting opportunities for employment and volunteerism through which committed leaders can positively affect the health and wellness of others by providing ongoing encouragement, education, coaching, and evaluation. Outstanding health promotion settings enable individuals to learn, build healthy and positive relationships, inspire us to move our bodies, eat healthy foods, and foster a sense of achievement and growth.

KEY TERMS

1. **Physical space:** the physical makeup of the home, office, or other environments; changes to one's personal space can make daily activities easier to complete, but require less physical movement, making exercise a task to be intentionally pursued

2. **Personal trainer:** a fitness professional proficient in exercise prescription and instruction; motivates clients by setting goals and providing feedback and accountability

3. **Interpersonal communication skills:** the process by which people exchange information, feelings, and meaning through verbal and nonverbal messages; message content can be seen as equally important as how it is said, including the tone of voice, facial expressions, gestures, and body language

4. **Communities:** defined as families and individuals living or working in close proximity and who share common services

5. **Health fair:** an educational and interactive event designed for outreach to provide basic preventive medicine and medical screening to people in the community or employees at a worksite

6. **Health assessments:** a plan of care that identifies the specific needs of the client and how these needs will be addressed by the healthcare system or skilled nursing facility; in an early childhood setting may include annual on-site examinations for general health, vision, hearing, dental, and speech

7. **School wellness policies:** important tools for parents, local educational agencies, and school districts in promoting student wellness, preventing and reducing childhood obesity, and providing assurance that school meal nutrition guidelines meet the minimum federal school meal standards

8. **Body mass index (BMI):** a weight-to-height ratio, calculated by dividing one's weight in pounds by the square of one's height in inches; then multiplying by 703; it is used as an indicator of overweight, obesity, ideal weight, and underweight status

9. **5210 Program:** program in which on a daily basis students strive to eat five servings of fruits and vegetables, limit screen time to two hours, be physically active for one hour, and consume zero sugared drinks

10. **Coordinated health promotion programs:** programs that use all of the resources of the institution through a well-coordinated offering of programs and services

11. **Health coach:** provides programs and services at the worksite and offers advice and support that will inspire employees to improve and maintain a good level of health, physical conditioning, and well-being; effective coaches develop a personal relationship with employees through an understanding of the individual's background, work requirements, and motivations, which can be used in building adherence to healthy lifestyle practices

12. **Employee assistance programs (EAPs):** offered by many employers to help workers and their families manage issues in their personal lives; originally established in the 1950s to support workers struggling with alcohol dependency, EAPs have evolved to help employees address issues such as substance abuse, emotional distress, major life events, healthcare concerns, personal financial problems, and family or personal relationships, to name a few

REVIEW QUESTIONS

1. How can elementary, middle, and high schools promote health?

2. What health issues are of concern on college and university campuses?

3. What are the guidelines for health promotion at the worksite?

4. How does a worksite evaluate its health promotion programs?

5. What guidelines would you provide to someone when searching for health information on the Internet?

STUDENT ACTIVITIES

1. Describe what a health-promoting community would offer its residents.

2. Health issues are many times age specific. Identify the health issues a health promotion program would target for the following settings:

    a. Worksite

    b. College campus

    c. Daycare setting

3. Identify one setting you believe is important for individuals and then find one example of this setting in the literature that can be used as a model program for a similar setting.

4. Track the life span of a person and describe health promotion opportunities as the person ages.

References

Bogar, C.T. (2008). Trends in college recreation facilities. *The Sport Journal 11* (4).

Breckon, J., Harvey, J.R., and Lancaster, R.B. (1998). *Community health education: Settings, roles, and skills for the 21st century.* Gaithersburg, MD: Aspen Publishers.

Centers for Disease Control and Prevention (CDC). (2010). *Components of coordinated school health.* Retrieved from www.cdc.gov?HealthyYouth/CSHIP

Chenoweth, D.H. (2007). *Worsksite health promotion*, 2e. Champaign, IL: Human Kinetics.

Chomitz, V.R., Slining, M.M., McGowan, R.J. et al. (2009). Is there a relationship between physical fitness and academic achievement? Positive results from public school children in the northeast United States. *Journal of School Health 79*: 30–37.

Floyd, P.A. and Allen, B.J. (2004). *Careers in health, physical education and sport.* Belmont, CA: Wadsworth-Thompson Learning.

Ginsburg, K.R. (2007). The importance of play in promoting healthy child development and maintaining strong parent-child bonds. *Pediatrics 119* (1): 182–191.

Golan, M. and Crow, S. (2004). Parents are key players in the prevention and treatment of weight-related problems. *Nutrition Reviews 62* (1): 39–50.

Kaiser Permanente. (2008, December). *Kaiser Permanente community health initiative: Interim report.* Retrieved from http://share.kaiserpermanente.org/media_assets/pdf/communitybenefit/assets/pdf/our_work/global/chi/CHI%20Interim%20Report%20FINAL%203–6–09.pdf

Linnan, L.A. (2010). The business case for employee health: What we know and what we need to do. *North Carolina Medical Journal 71* (1): 69–74.

Marx, E. and Wooley, S.F. (ed.) (1998). *Health is academic: A guide to coordinated school health programs.* New York: Teachers College Press.

Matthews, C.E., Chen, K.Y., Freedson, P.S. et al. (2008). Amount of time spent in sedentary behaviors in the United States, 2003–2004. *American Journal of Epidemiology 167* (7): 875–881.

National Association for Sport and Physical Education. (2009). *Reducing school physical education programs is counter-productive to student health and learning and to our nation's economic health.* Retrieved from www.blindbrook.org/cms/lib07/NY01913277/Centricity/Domain/61/REDUCING-SCHOOL-PHYSICAL-EDUCATION-PROGRAMS-IS-COUNTER-11-25–09-FINAL-2-3.pdf

National Association of Registered School Nurses. (n.d.). *School nurse certification.* Retrieved from www.nasn.org/RoleCareer/SchoolNurseCertification

Perkins, T. (2002). *Comprehensive community initiatives (CCI): A comparison of community implementation plans.* University of Nebraska Public Policy Center, Paper 71. Retrieved from http://digitalcommons.unl.edu/publicpolicypublica tions/71

Powell, L.H., Shahabi, L., and Thoreson, C.E. (2003). Religion and spirituality: Linkage to physical health. *American Psychologist 58* (1): 36–52.

Robert Wood Johnson Foundation (2013, February). *School district wellness policies: Evaluating progress and potential for improving children's health five years after the federal mandate.* Chicago: Bridging the Gap. Retrieved from www.bridgingthegapresearch.org/_asset/13s2jm.

van Sluijs, E.M.F., McMinn, A.M., and Griffin, S.J. (2007). Effectiveness of interventions to promote physical activity in children and adolescents: Systematic review of controlled trials. *BMJ 335*: 703.

Umberson, D. (1987). Family status and health behaviors: Social control as a dimension of social integration. *Journal of Health and Social Behavior 28*: 306–319.

US Department of Labor. (2011). *American time use survey.* Retrieved from www.bls.gov/tus/data files_2011.htm

Young Men's Christian Association. (2014). *About the Y.* Retrieved from www.ymca.net/about-us

CHAPTER 11

HEALTH PROMOTION-RELATED ORGANIZATIONS, ASSOCIATIONS, AND CERTIFICATIONS

Anastasia Snelling and Michelle Kalicki

This chapter introduces a number of different associations and organizations that broadly support health promotion. Most commonly, nonprofit health-related associations or organizations target the general public or a subset of the general public to advocate for a specific health condition or topic through fund-raising, sponsoring research, lobbying to advance legislation, and raising awareness about a health condition. Professional health associations specifically target professionals who work directly in the fields of health promotion, public health, and health education. Professionals in the field may become members of these associations, which offer continuing education through local, regional, and national conferences, newsletters, journals, and e-mail lists. Some associations or organizations focus exclusively on the publication of scholarly journals, providing critical information and research to health promotion practitioners and policymakers in the field. In addition, other organizations offer health-related certifications in the areas of exercise science, health coaching, nutrition education, or to become wellness specialists. These organizations may be national or international in scope. This chapter explores how these organizations and associations contribute to the field of health promotion.

One of the most frequently asked questions by any prospective health promotion student is, "Where do health promotion professionals work?" The truth is, health promotion is more visible than most people think. As described in chapter 10, health promotion activities are taking place in many different settings. Health promotion is an immensely prevalent field, focusing on many different behaviors and occurring in almost all communities across the country. Promoting healthy lifestyles is a field that has a long, interesting, and encouraging history. Many active organizations and associations have been contributing in different ways to the health of our nation for many decades.

LEARNING OBJECTIVES

After reading this chapter, the student will be able to:

- Describe how associations and organizations contribute to health promotion activities.

- Define the purpose of different associations and how they relate to health promotion.

- Identify the variety and role of certifications related to the field of health promotion.

- Discuss why and how an individual becomes a member of a certain organization or association.

- Summarize the benefits of joining a professional association.

Introduction to Health Promotion, Second Edition. Edited by Anastasia Snelling.
© 2024 John Wiley & Sons Inc. Published 2024 by John Wiley & Sons Inc.
Companion Website: www.wiley.com/go/snelling2e

These entities respond to our ever-changing health culture and play a critical role in moving our nation toward a healthier society.

Nonprofit Health Associations

nonprofit health organizations
associations that target the general public or a subset of the general public to advocate for a specific health condition or topic through fundraising, sponsoring research, lobbying to advance legislation, and raising awareness about a health condition

There are hundreds of **nonprofit health organizations** and associations aimed at promoting different aspects of health. Many are well known because of the popular events they regularly hold or the marketing they do to promote a specific health concern. Organizations such as the American Heart Association and the American Cancer Society are good examples of organizations that receive significant public attention because of their important role in raising money through various charitable events and funding critical medical research. As of this writing, heart disease and cancer are the top two leading causes of death in the United States, respectively. Fortunately, many, though not all, of the risk factors associated with the development of these diseases are preventable, or their prevalence can be reduced through living healthy lifestyles. The American Heart Association and American Cancer Society address these issues in terms that are more readily understood by the majority of Americans. These associations operate local chapters that serve communities around the nation. They are active, well-managed organizations that operate and support numerous programs and efforts to achieve their missions.

American Heart Association (AHA)

The mission of the American Heart Association (AHA) is to "build healthier lives, free of cardiovascular diseases and stroke." Recognizing the need for a national organization to share research findings and promote further study, six cardiologists representing several smaller groups founded the American Heart Association in 1924. To broaden its scope, the AHA reorganized in 1948 and brought in nonmedical volunteers with skills in business management, communication, public education, community organization, and fundraising.

The AHA focuses on addressing the many conditions that fall under the "heart disease" umbrella through numerous campaigns and continuous education. One AHA goal is to provide credible heart disease and stroke information for effective prevention and treatment. The National Wear Red Day initiative, started in 2002, is an official campaign to raise awareness and inform women about the risk factors of heart disease. The Start! campaign promotes walking and being active to support heart health. Life's Simple 7 Check—a program designed to help Americans get and stay healthy—promotes the use of a simple tool that quickly assesses a person's current health status and provides suggestions as to how to improve his or her score. The Simple 7 behaviors comprise getting active, controlling cholesterol, managing blood pressure, eating better, losing weight, reducing blood sugar, and quitting smoking. All of these behaviors are described in this textbook and are related not only to heart disease but also to other chronic diseases, including cancer and diabetes.

These are just a few examples of American Heart Association activities. Volunteers are paramount to the AHA's success, but there are also a variety of career positions available, from fund-raising to health services to marketing.

Other Nonprofit Health Organizations

There are many other nonprofit organizations that address a variety of chronic diseases at the national, state, and local levels. Organizations such as the AHA and the others listed in table 11.1 are valuable institutions in the realm of health promotion; they act as advocates for the public at large. These organizations strive to bridge that critical knowledge gap between the professional health community and the general public.

Professional Health Associations

Although the specific mission of each **professional health association** varies, they all share the common goal of advocating for and educating professionals by holding national conferences, regional and local meetings, and educational summits; publishing journals or periodicals; hosting webinars and facilitating discussions; and taking positions on public policy to promote health. For an extensive list of professional associations, see table 11.2.

This section identifies important professional health associations by aspects of health behaviors associated with chronic diseases, such as nutrition, physical activity, and health education. At this time, the field of health promotion does not have an association specific to the field; however, many organizations integrate the field of health promotion into their specific content area.

professional health association
an association that specifically targets and represents professionals who work directly in the fields of health promotion, public health, and health education

Nutrition

The overall imbalance of nutrition in the country correlates with our nation's rising chronic health problems. Food desert issues, the rise in type 2 diabetes, and the obesity epidemic are all aspects that can, at least in part, be attributed to nutrition. As discussed in chapter 5,

Table 11.1 Nonprofit Health Associations

Association	Website
American Heart Association	www.heart.org
American Diabetes Association	www.diabetes.org
American Lung Association	www.lung.org
National Osteoporosis Foundation	www.nof.org
Susan G. Komen Foundation	www.komen.org
American Cancer Society	www.cancer.org
Mental Health America	www.nmha.org
American Health Care Association	www.ahcancal.org
American Association of Retired Persons	www.aarp.org
Leukemia and Lymphoma Society	www.lls.org
The American Institute of Stress	www.stress.org
American Institute for Cancer Research	www.aicr.org
Stroke Foundation	www.stroke.org

Table 11.2   Select Health Professional Associations

Agency	Website
Nutrition	
Academy of Nutrition and Dietetics	www.eatright.org
American College of Nutrition	www.americancollegeofnutrition.org
Society for Nutrition Education and Behavior	www.sneb.org
Global Alliance for Improved Nutrition	www.gainhealth.org
National Association of Nutrition Professionals	www.nanp.org
School Nutrition Association	www.schoolnutrition.org
American Society for Nutrition	www.americannutritionassociation.org
Physical Activity	
SHAPE America	www.shapeamerica.org
American College of Sports Medicine	www.acsm.org
National Association for Health and Fitness	www.physicalfitness.org
National Coalition for Promoting Physical Activity	www.ncppa.orge-newsletters
National Health and Exercise Science Association	www.nhesa.org
Health, Education, and Wellness	
Wellness Council of America	www.welcoa.org
International Association for Worksite Health Promotion	www.iawhp.org
American Public Health Association	www.apha.org
Institute of Health and Productivity Management	www.ihpm.org
American College Health Association	www.acha.org
American School Health Association	www.ashaweb.org
National Wellness Institute	www.nationalwellness.org
Society for Public Health Education	www.sophe.org
International Union for Health Promotion and Education	www.iuhpe.org
Partnership for Prevention	www.prevent.org
American Health Care Association	www.ahcancal.org

trends in our nation's diet have changed dramatically since the 1950s. The role of nutrition-related associations is to organize and clearly disseminate timely information that is constantly being discovered and published regarding the role of nutrition in health.

Academy of Nutrition and Dietetics (AND)

The Academy of Nutrition and Dietetics, the world's largest organization of food and nutrition professionals (Academy of Nutrition and Dietetics, 2014), was founded in 1917 with a goal to improve the nation's health by empowering its members to become the leading figures in the field. The academy's primary activities in support of its mission are as follows:

- Providing reliable and evidence-based nutrition information for the public
- Accrediting undergraduate and graduate programs
- Credentialing dietetic professionals
- Advocating for public policy
- Publishing a peer-reviewed periodical

In order to become a member of the Academy of Nutrition and Dietetics, individuals must comply with very specific guidelines. This strict process ensures that only the most qualified individuals are awarded membership and become actively contributing members. The academy and its members work to provide the most accurate and up-to-date information about food and nutrition, disease management and prevention, food safety, and related topics to the general public.

American College of Nutrition (ACN)

Another prominent association in the world of nutrition education is the American College of Nutrition (ACN). The ACN works to "stimulate nutrition research and publication, elevate nutrition knowledge among researchers and clinicians, and provide practical guidance on clinical nutrition" (American College of Nutrition, 2014). The ACN provides a platform for professionals to come together and exchange knowledge, views, experiences in the field, and research findings to broaden their scope of understanding. A unique feature of the ACN is that they recognize the importance of nutrition education and research to the medical community. The ACN accepts no funding from for-profit corporations in an effort to provide the most accurate information without compromise.

Society for Nutrition Education and Behavior (SNEB)

The Society for Nutrition Education and Behavior (SNEB) is an international organization of nutrition professionals who work in a variety of different settings, including schools, government agencies, volunteer organizations, and the food industry. Founded in 1968, SNEB works toward bridging research findings and practitioner work in the field to promote nutrition behavior change. This is significant because changing behavior is also part of the underlying principle of health promotion. SNEB publishes the *Journal of Nutrition Education and Behavior* as a way to disseminate scientific research findings to interested parties worldwide.

Physical Activity

Nearly two-thirds of people in the United States are either overweight or obese due to poor nutrition and a lack of exercise. As technology and innovation have expanded, lives have become increasingly sedentary, as discussed in chapter 6. Organizations focused on promoting physical activity and encouraging active lifestyles among adults and children have become more prevalent. The role of these organizations is to educate people on the importance of regular physical activity and to encourage everyone to lead active lifestyles.

professional development
the combination of experiences, memberships, and connections one makes to advance his or her career

By offering continuing **professional development** and fostering the work of health promoters in the field, these associations are playing a huge role in the ongoing efforts to reverse the current health trends in the country.

SHAPE America

One of the most recognized and far-reaching associations in this area is the Society of Health and Physical Educators or SHAPE America, formerly known as the American Alliance for Health, Physical Education, Recreation, and Dance (AAHPERD). SHAPE America understands the importance of addressing health and physical activity from many different points, working "to advance professional practice and promote research related to health and physical education, physical activity, dance, and sport" (SHAPE America, 2014). The association hosts annual conventions, publishes a number of different journals, tenders accreditations, and offers a variety of educational opportunities.

SHAPE America was founded in 1885 as the Association for the Advancement of Physical Education (AAPE). At the time of its inception, AAPE consisted of forty-nine members, all physical educators. After going through multiple restructurings and name changes, SHAPE America is now twenty thousand members strong and consists of professionals involved in a multitude of areas related to achieving an active, healthy lifestyle, including physical education, physical activity, dance, sport, and more.

advocacy
a technique used by many health organizations to influence policy-making decisions

Historically, the organization's main roles have been to provide numerous professional development opportunities, maintain a strong **advocacy** presence, disseminate research in physical activity and health through its research council, and work to advance national standards and guidelines in the areas of health and physical education. However, as the landscape of health and physical activity continues to change, so does SHAPE America.

SHAPE AMERICA'S AREAS OF FOCUS

- Physical education
- Physical activity
- Health education
- Research
- Early childhood education
- Sport coaching
- Dance

On reorganizing in 2014, SHAPE America has added early childhood education to its repertoire. SHAPE America strives to maintain its leadership position in the area of physical activity and will continue to provide the latest tools for its members and their beneficiaries.

American College of Sports Medicine (ACSM)

Another prominent physical activity organization is the American College of Sports Medicine (ACSM). According to its mission, ACSM "advances and integrates scientific research to provide educational and practical applications of exercise science and sports medicine" (American College of Sports Medicine, 2014). ACSM members are professionals and students working and studying in scientific and clinical settings, academia, and the health and fitness industry. ACSM is considered the gold standard by many in the industry because their guidelines and positions on relevant policy issues are widely used and cited by professionals around the world, in addition to the quality of their certifications. ACSM initiatives focus on a range of issues, from antidoping in sports to childhood obesity. Although ACSM primarily focuses on sports medicine and exercise science, improving quality of life for all is a goal ACSM shares with all of the associations discussed in this chapter. ACSM holds conferences and summits, supports regional chapters, and has created interest groups to initiate discussion forums on topics such as aging, minority health research, and worksite health promotion, among many others. These interest groups are essentially subcommittees of ACSM that have a particular focus area and meet annually at the ACSM conference. ACSM is also widely recognized for its professional certifications, which are discussed later in this chapter.

Health, Wellness, and Education

The large number of professional health associations underscores the dynamic and all-encompassing field of health promotion. The organizations described in this section address broader health, wellness, and education efforts in a variety of settings.

American Public Health Association (APHA)

An emerging aspect of health promotion is its relationship with public health. Although the fields have distinct characteristics and goals, they do intersect, and it is important to recognize this fact. Historically, public health officials' emphasis was on the prevention of infectious disease and access to health care, as discussed in chapter 1. However, since the 1990s, this focus has expanded to include chronic conditions; currently, there is more overlap between health promotion and public health. With the growing obesity epidemic and its associated health complications, it is essential for all health professionals to collaborate to formulate solutions. The American Public Health Association (APHA) is the oldest public health association in the United States; APHA members have a rich history of striving to achieve the vision of "a healthy global society" (http://apha.org). Founded in 1872 with a goal to advance science to reveal the causes of communicable diseases, the APHA laid the foundation for the public health profession and for the infrastructure to support its work. From its inception, the APHA has been dedicated to improving the health of all US residents.

The APHA is composed of a diverse group of health professionals that includes educators, environmentalists, and policymakers whose aims are not only to prevent serious health threats but also to advocate for families and communities to receive proper health care, find adequate funding for health services, and eliminate health disparities. The association holds an annual meeting and exposition to provide its members the opportunity to connect face-to-face and enhance their knowledge of all aspects of public health. APHA achieves its goals with the help of state **affiliates**.

affiliates
state- or local-level subgroups of a national organization

As discussed in chapter 10 two major settings for health promotion are education settings and worksites. Programs in these settings focus on all aspects of health and wellness to encourage and facilitate lifestyle and behavior changes in students, staff, and worksite employees. Work in these settings is often associated with public health activities.

Society for Public Health Education (SOPHE)

For more than sixty years, the Society for Public Health Education (SOPHE) has served a diverse membership of health education professionals and students in the United States and other countries. The organization promotes healthy behaviors, healthy communities, and healthy environments through its membership, its network of local chapters, and its numerous partnerships with other organizations. Members work in a number of settings such as elementary and secondary schools, universities, voluntary organizations, health care settings, worksites, and local, state, and federal government agencies.

Wellness Councils of America (WELCOA)

The Wellness Councils of America (WELCOA) is a leading association for worksite health promotion in the United States. In the 1980s, WELCOA's founders were among the first to make the connection between health and well-being and its impact within the workplace. WELCOA bases its mission on the belief that a healthy workforce is essential to America's growth and that by investing in employee health and well-being, our nation will be more productive and health care costs will be better controlled. Healthy employees benefit a company or organization; WELCOA's members work to promote healthy worksites and worksite health promotion programs. WELCOA is a dominant source of information for worksite wellness programs in the United States.

American College Health Association (ACHA)

The American College Health Association (ACHA) may be of particular importance to health promotion students enrolled in this course. The mission of the ACHA is to provide advocacy, education, communications, products, and services, as well as promote research and culturally competent practices to enhance its members' ability to advance the health of all students and the campus community (American College Health Association, 2014). Members include two- and four-year institutions, individual health professionals and students, and corporations and nonprofits dedicated to college health.

American School Health Association (ASHA)

The American School Health Association (ASHA) and its members have never been more vital. ASHA's goals are to promote interdisciplinary collaboration between health and academic professionals, advocate for coordinated school health programs, offer professional development opportunities for its more than two thousand members around the world, support and disseminate research initiatives, and provide crucial resources to support its members and their mission. Members come from a wide range of backgrounds, including school administrators, counselors, health and physical educators, psychologists, nurses, and physicians, among others.

BENEFITS OF ASSOCIATION MEMBERSHIP

- Network with other professionals in similar positions or areas
- Stay current on research and best practices of the profession
- Network for job opportunities
- Attend local, regional, and national conferences for continuing education credits
- Learn more about the profession and the variety of jobs and opportunities
- Discounts on conference fees
- Opportunities to present information to colleagues in order to promote best practices

---

Most associations require an annual membership fee, so it is important to select the association most beneficial to you and your career.

Table 11.2 identifies health professional associations and lists their websites for additional information.

Scholarly and Professional Health Journals

In addition to nonprofit health organizations and health professional associations, there is a diverse array of **scholarly and professional health journals** to disseminate research and information on health promotion. These journals include publications covering a range of broad topics, such as the *American Journal of Health Promotion,* to more specific topics, such as the *American Journal of Clinical Nutrition.* Access to many of these journals is provided free of charge to students at academic institutions through university library databases. Peer-reviewed journals are considered the most accurate and desirable resources for papers, projects, and presentations because of the rigorous review process each article must undergo prior to publication. Upon submission, articles are critiqued for research content by multiple peer reviewers as well as editors for accuracy, clarity, and relevance. Thus, although many mainstream media outlets offer valid information, most have not been reviewed as thoroughly as articles published in peer-reviewed journals. Table 11.3 lists a selection of journals.

scholarly and professional health journals typically peer-reviewed publications that publish research articles and commentaries

Becoming familiar with these publications as a student, especially those of particular interest to you and your career, will assist you upon graduation; journals are a source of continuing education for professionals in the field.

Table 11.3   Select Scholarly Journals

Journal	Association	Website
Nutrition		
Journal of the Academy of Nutrition and	Academy of Nutrition and Dietetics	www.adajournal.org
Journal of the American College of Nutrition	American College of Nutrition	www.jacn.org
Journal of Nutrition Education and Behavior	Society of Nutrition Education and	www.jneb.org
Journal of Child Nutrition & Management (SNA)	School Nutrition Association	www.schoolnutrition.org
American Journal of Clinical Nutrition (ASN)	American Society for Nutrition	www.acjn.nutrition.org
Physical Activity		
American Journal of Health Education	SHAPE America	www.shapeamerica.org/publications/journals/
Journal of Physical Education, Recreation, and Dance		
Women in Sport and Physical Activity Journal		
Medicine & Science in Sport & Exercise	American College of Sports Medicine	www.acsm.org/access-public-information/acsm-journals
General Health Promotion and Education		
Health, Education, and Wellness		
American Journal of Public Health	American Public Health Association	http://ajph.aphapublications.org
Journal of Health and Productivity	Institute of Health and Productivity Management	www.ihpm.org/jhp/index.php
Journal of American College Health	American College Health Association	www.acha.org/Publications/JACH.cfm
Journal of School Health	American School Health Association	www.ashaweb.org/i4a/pages/index.cfm?pageid=3341
Health Education and Behavior	Independent	http://heb.sagepub.com
Health Promotion International and Global Health Promotion	International Union For Health Promotion and Education	http://heapro.oxfordjournals.org http://ped.sagepub.com
Childhood Obesity	Independent	https://home.liebertpub.com/publications/childhood-obesity/384/overview
Health Affairs	Project HOPE	www.healthaffairs.org
Health Communication	Independent	www.tandfonline.com/toc/hhth20/current
American Journal of Health Promotion	Independent	www.healthpromotionjournal.com
American Journal of Health Behavior	Independent	www.ajhb.org
International Journal of Occupational and Environmental Health	Center of Occupational and Environmental Health	www.ijoeh.com

Certifications

Obtaining a degree in health promotion is the first step to beginning a career in this exciting field. However, in a society that requires specific educational standards from its graduates, attaining a certification in the preferred field of interest may be a recommended next step. As the health industry expands, professional certifications are one of its fastest-growing aspects. **Certification** comes in all shapes and sizes for individuals, organizations, and institutions and is offered through many of the associations identified in this chapter. If an individual's career aspirations are to work in an academic setting or a public health department, becoming a certified health education specialist (CHES) may be a perfect fit. If an individual chooses to work in the field of personal training or fitness instruction, a fitness-based certification is usually a prerequisite for employment.

certification
an endorsement of qualifications obtained by an individual or organization showing a degree of expertise in a particular field

The following sections explore a few of the health promotion certifications available for various paths.

Health Promotion Certifications

The National Wellness Institute (NWI), founded in 1977, provides resources and services to support and foster health promotion and wellness professionals in their fields. The NWI offers a certified work-site wellness specialist (CWWS) certification to acquire the skills needed to run a successful worksite health promotion program and a certified worksite wellness program manager (CWWPM) certification for those pursuing a worksite wellness management role. Additionally, the NWI offers a general wellness practitioner certification for professionals dedicated to continuing their wellness education and leadership experience. For more information, check out the NWI website at www.nationalwellness.org.

Certified Worksite Wellness Specialist (CWWS)

The CWWS is the first step in NWI's worksite wellness certification programming and delivers the tools required to carry out a successful worksite wellness program. Program participants include worksite wellness coordinators and managers, human resource professionals, occupational health nurses, employee assistance professionals, insurance and benefit providers and brokers, and other individuals seeking training and certification in worksite wellness.

Certified Worksite Wellness Program Manager (CWWPM)

The CWWPM is geared toward professionals who are currently in a worksite wellness manager-supervisor role or who are working toward a manager-supervisor role. It is the next step in worksite wellness certification following completion of the CWWS program. The program covers critical competencies in managing the planning, design, implementation, and measurement of a comprehensive worksite wellness–health management program.

Certified Wellness Practitioner (CWP)

The certified wellness practitioner (CWP) is not specific to worksite wellness programs but is rather a designation for those who have strong academic and professional credentials and have shown a commitment to continuing their overall development. With the CWP designation, a professional in the field is certified to create and evaluate programs using sound health promotion models and theories and help to create "health-enhancing environments" (www.nationalwellness.org). To become a CWP, an individual has to either (1) apply and be selected by the review committee or (2) be a graduate of an NWI-accredited academic program.

Health Education Certifications

The objective of the National Commission for Health Education Credentialing (NCHEC) (2010) is to facilitate the enhancement of an upstanding health education system.

Certified Health Education Specialist (CHES)

The CHES designation is obtained by demonstrating competency with the standards issued by the NCHEC and passing the exam. To take the exam, an individual must have a bachelor's, master's, or doctorate's degree from an accredited institution and have an official transcript clearly showing a major in health education or an official transcript showing at least twenty-five semester hours of course work in the seven areas of responsibility for health education (see the sidebar). The certification is valid for five years, with the caveat that seventy-five hours of **continuing education** must be completed during that time. For more information, see the National Commission for Health Education Credentialing at www.nchec.org.

continuing education
a requirement for maintaining certifications; can be obtained through attending conferences, taking various classes, and so on

Health education specialists are professionals who design, conduct, and evaluate activities that help improve the health of all people. These activities can take place in a variety of settings that include schools, communities, health care facilities, businesses, universities, and government agencies. Health education specialists are employed under a range of job titles, such as patient educators, health education teachers, health coaches, community organizers, public health educators, and health program managers. (www.nchec.org)

SEVEN AREAS OF RESPONSIBILITY FOR HEALTH EDUCATION

Area 1: Assess needs, assets, and capacity for health education.

Area 2: Plan health education.

Area 3: Implement health education.

Area 4: Conduct evaluation and research related to health education.

Area 5: Administer and manage health education.

Area 6: Serve as a health education resource person.

Area 7: Communicate and advocate for health and health education.

Continuing education is required for certain certifications or degrees. Continuing education is usually completed through attending local or national conferences or reading articles published in journals.

Master CHES (MCHES)

Beyond the entry-level CHES certification is the Master CHES certification. Candidates for this exam are either current CHES recipients or non-CHES recipients. As a CHES recipient, candidates need to have five continuous years of health education employment. For a non-CHES recipient, candidates must have a master's degree or higher. Additionally, candidates must have five years of documented experience as a health education specialist. Similar to maintaining the CHES certification, continuing education credits are necessary for the MCHES.

Fitness-based Certifications

There are a number of fitness-based certifications available through a variety of associations. The focus, expertise, and prestige of each certifying organization are varied, so it is important to identify one's interests and specific professional requirements prior to committing to a certain certification. In general, a high level of comprehension of human anatomy and exercise physiology is necessary to pass the exam, as well as a strong knowledge of the specific guidelines for that organization's theory of best practice. For those individuals planning to work at a fitness facility or start an independent personal training company, the credibility provided through a formal certification process is essential. Additionally, many certifying organizations offer more than one certification option for personal training. Group fitness instructors, strength and conditioning specialists, and professionals focusing on certain age groups, such as seniors or youth, may also benefit from a certification or specific credential.

Some of the most recognizable and respected fitness-based certification organizations are listed in table 11.4.

Table 11.4   Fitness-Based Certification Organizations

Organization	Website
American College of Sports Medicine	www.acsm.org
National Strength and Conditioning Association	www.nsca.com
National Association of Sports Medicine	www.nasm.org
American Council on Exercise	www.acefitness.org
Aerobics and Fitness Association of America	www.afaa.com
American Fitness Professionals and Associates	www.afpafitness.com
National Exercise and Sports Trainers Association	www.nestacertified.com

Nutrition Certifications

Certified nutrition specialists (CNS) use medical nutrition therapy to combat obesity and the chronic diseases widely associated with poor nutrition habits. The Certification Board of Nutrition Specialists administers exams twice each year to interested and qualified candidates. A graduate degree in nutrition or a clinical health care–related field with specific course work in nutrition, biochemistry, physiology, and clinical, life, or physical sciences, and supervised nutrition experience are required to obtain the CNS credential.

As the health industry continues to grow, different organizations are offering nutrition specialist certifications as well. As a professional working more generally to help people improve eating habits or lose weight, certain certifications may be beneficial. As it becomes clearer that a combination of physical activity and better eating habits is the only proven formula for healthy living, many of the fitness-based organizations listed in table 11.4 have begun to offer nutrition or weight management certifications. A few of these certifications are described in the following:

- The American Fitness Professionals & Associates (AFPA) has multiple certifications that enhance one's knowledge and credibility in the field. AFPA offers a weight management consultant certification, a nutrition and wellness consultant certification, and a sports nutrition consultant certification.

- The National Association of Sports Medicine (NASM) offers a fitness nutrition specialist and weight loss specialist credential.

- The American Council on Exercise (ACE) offers a weight management specialist certification.

Again, as with any certification, these do not guarantee employment. Continuing education, broadening one's knowledge base, and professional experience will most benefit your career.

Health Coaching

Health coaching is another growing area in the field. Health coaching combines evidence-based practice interventions with the science of motivational interviewing in an effort to reduce costs, change behaviors, and improve health outcomes. The occupation initially appeared in the late 1990s and continues to evolve. Worksite health promotion programs are the primary employers of health coaches, along with health care organizations and human resources departments.

Table 11.5 shows some of the certifying agencies for health coaching and the specific requirements for each.

Academic Institute Certifications

academic institution
an educational body dedicated to teaching and research that also grants degrees

In addition to the aforementioned individual certifications, **academic institution** are also eligible to become accredited. The National Wellness Institute Council on Wellness Accreditation and Education (CWAE) provides recognition to health promotion programs

Table 11.5   Health Coaching Certification Organizations

Organization	Description	Website
International Coach Federation (ICF)	• Gold standard for coaching certifications • Evaluate other programs according to a specific criterion	www.coachfederation.org/ICF
Coach Training Alliance (CTA)	• Certified coach program • Teleconferencing, online media, and interactive software • Six months • ICF approved the course to be worth thirty-six hours	www.coachtrainingalliance .com
The Coaches Training Institute (CTI)	• ICF accredited • Two components: core curriculum and certification program • Telephonic, six months	www.thecoaches.com
Wellcoaches	• Telephonic course • Ten weeks • CHES accepts certification as continuing education hours	www.wellcoaches.com
National Society of Health Coaches (NSHC)	• Online program based on motivational interviewing • Created for health professionals who must have specific degrees to qualify	www.nshcoa.com

within a college or university. For schools, accreditation demonstrates that they have met or exceeded the standards issued by the CWAE, contributing to recognition in the academic community. For students, on graduation they are eligible to be an NWI-CWP as a result of the program's accreditation, and employers can hire these graduates with assurance that they are competent for entry-level positions in the field. More information on the National Wellness Institute's accreditations and certifications can be found at www.nationalwellness.org.

As mentioned previously, public health is increasingly involved in health promotion. The academic accreditation from the Council on Education for Public Health (CEPH) is recognized by the US Department of Education to accredit schools and programs of public health at the undergraduate and graduate levels. As with the CWAE accreditation, it is a great benefit for the school to attain a CEPH accreditation. Students graduating from CEPH-accredited universities or colleges can be expected to have a high level of public health knowledge based on the standards that must be met for accreditation, found at www.ceph.org.

Summary

This chapter identifies a variety of different associations that support the field of health promotion. Understanding that the field is diverse and overlaps with other fields, students might consider learning more about and joining a number of different associations. These associations provide many educational and networking opportunities that keep professionals current in their field. The chapter also introduced several different personal certifications that students might consider as they progress through their careers. The diverse certifications are for general worksite health promotion, health education, personal training, health coaching, and nutrition, among others. Each certification requires a different set of prerequisites, variable costs, and continuing education credits. The importance of associations, journals, conferences, and certifications will become more apparent as health promotion students and professionals develop their careers. Now is the time to explore these opportunities.

KEY TERMS

1. **Nonprofit health organizations:** associations that target the general public or a subset of the general public to advocate for a specific health condition or topic through fundraising, sponsoring research, lobbying to advance legislation, and raising awareness about a health condition

2. **Professional health association:** an association that specifically targets and represents professionals who work directly in the field of health promotion, public health, and health education

3. **Professional development:** the combination of experiences, memberships, and connections one makes to advance his or her career

4. **Advocacy:** a technique used by many health organizations to influence policy decision making

5. **Affiliates:** state- or local-level subgroups of a national organization

6. **Scholarly and professional health journals:** typically peer-reviewed publications that publish research articles and commentaries

7. **Certification:** an endorsement of qualifications obtained by an individual or organization showing a degree of expertise in a particular field

8. **Continuing education:** a requirement for maintaining certifications; can be obtained through attending conferences, taking various classes, and so on

9. **Academic institution:** an educational body dedicated to teaching and research that also grants degrees

REVIEW QUESTIONS

1. Why would someone join the Society of Nutrition Education and Behavior or the American Public Health Association?

2. If you wanted to attend a conference sponsored by the SOPHE, what would the registration cost be for members? Is there a special rate for students? Do they accept interns?

3. There are a number of personal training certifications available to consumers. What criteria would you use to select a personal training certification?

4. What is the role of nonprofit health associations in health promotion?

5. What is the overall importance of associations in the field of health promotion?

STUDENT ACTIVITIES

1. List the five leading causes of disease and identify two nonprofit organizations dedicated to reducing death and disability related to those condition.

2. Discuss the reasons why you might consider a certification in addition to receiving your bachelor's degree.

3. Find a job listing that includes the phrase "CHES preferred." Describe the position.

4. Select two personal certifications and compare and contrast the eligibility requirements for these two certifications.

5. Select two journals, find two articles of interest, and write an abstract for each journal article.

References

Academy of Nutrition and Dietetics (2014). *Who we are and what we do.*

American College Health Association (2014). *Who we are.*

American College of Nutrition (2014). *About the college.* Retrieved from http://americancollegeofnutrition.org/content/about-college

American College of Sports Medicine (2014). *Who we are.* Retrieved from www.acsm.org/about-acsm/who-we-are

National Commission for Health Education Credentialing (2010). *Health education profession.* Retrieved from http://nchec.org/credentialling/profession

SHAPE America (2014). *About us.* Retrieved from www.shapeamerica.org

CHAPTER 12

TRENDS IN HEALTH PROMOTION

David Hunnicutt

Although health promotion is still a relatively new concept and largely considered by many to be an emerging discipline, according to a variety of experts there's little question that this area will continue to grow in both need and popularity over the next several decades. In fact, several significant trends will drive the expansion of the field of health promotion. Specifically, there are ten trends, which have the potential to contribute to the growth of health promotion and prevention.

Trend #1: The Population Will Get Much Older in the Next Three Decades

Trend #2: As Americans Age, Our Collective Physical Health Status Will Steadily Decline If We Don't Do Things Differently

Trend #3: Physical Health Problems Won't Be Our Only Concern

Trend #4: Healthcare Costs Will Remain an Issue of Significant Concern Far into the Future

Trend #5: Because of Its Potential, Prevention Will Become a National Priority

Trend #6: Telehealth Will Gain Rapid Popularity

Trend #7: Physical Activity Will Become the Most Commonly Prescribed Medicine

Trend #8: Efforts to Curb Obesity Will Intensify Greatly

Trend #9: Wearables, Apps, Big Data, and AI Will Dominate the Wellness Arena

Trend #10: The Need for Talented Health Promotion Professionals Will Skyrocket

In the following paragraphs, it is the intention to provide documentation for each one of these emerging trends. In doing so, there will be numerous personal, professional, and societal implications that will emerge. In addition, a call to action will be issued at the conclusion of this chapter. As a result of reading this chapter, you should have a much better grasp as to what the future holds for health promotion, prevention, and wellness in the United States.

Trend #1: The Population Will Get Much Older in the Next Three Decades

Over the course of the next three decades, both the U.S. and the world's population will age rapidly. To provide the context for this phenomenon, it is important to understand the present makeup of the current U.S. population. At the time of this writing, there are presently some 333 million citizens in this country—and one the most significant segments of the population that will drive the country's aging phenomenon is that of the baby boomers (those born between 1946 and 1964) (U.S. Census Bureau, 2022).

Check this out.

According to the U.S. Census Bureau, there are roughly 56 million Americans who are presently sixty five years and older residing in the United States. By 2030, that number will grow to approximately 73 million; and by 2060, nearly one in four Americans will be sixty five years and older! What's more, the number of people aged eighty five will triple, and the country will add 500,000 centenarians! (U.S. Census Bureau, 2022).

Although it's hard to fathom, right now, one U.S. baby boomer is turning age sixty every eight seconds and that trend will continue for years into the future. Moreover, some 10,000 people are retiring *each day* in the US (Kessler, 2014).

But it's not just the Baby Boomers who are greying.

Believe it or not, in less than two decades, the profound aging of America across all groups will be inescapable. In fact, in 2034, older adults are projected to outnumber kids for the first time in U.S. history (U.S. Census Bureau, 2022).

Indisputably, this rapidly-aging wave of Americans will have a breathtaking transformational impact across many institutions and segments of society—not least of which will be the discipline of health promotion. Indeed, the unprecedented aging of the U.S. population will bring with it health and medical care issues that have never needed to be addressed in this country—until now.

In simpler terms, without good health, the aging of the American population could bring with it dire consequences for both individuals and our society at large. In fact, consider this quote from one of the nation's leading economists, Dr. Laurence Kotlikoff, in his book, "The Coming Generational Storm":

It's 2030 . . .you see a country where the collective population is older than that of Florida today. You see a country where people in wheelchairs will outnumber kids sitting in strollers. You see a country with twice as many retirees but only 18% more workers to support them. You see a country with large numbers of impoverished elderly citizens languishing in understaffed, overcrowded, substandard nursing homes. . ." (Kotlikoff & Burns, 2004)

So what does all this mean for aspiring health promotion professionals?

For starters, this country is going to need an army of health promotion and allied health professionals who are well-trained and motivated to keep an aging population healthy, happy, and productive. Moreover, we'll also need thousands upon thousands of personal health coaches who are willing to step up and embrace the responsibility for helping our country's citizens manage their own health and well-being.

The $64,000 question is whether or not we can start the engines fast enough to produce an adequate supply of talented and capable health promotion professionals who will, again, be required to adequately address what is sure to be an overwhelming need for better health practices in the United States.

Trend #2: As Americans Age, Our Collective Physical Health Status Will Steadily Decline If We Don't Do Things Differently

Now that we have a better understanding of how quickly our population is aging, it's time to start connecting the dots—and this brings us to Trend #2. As Americans age, our collective physical health status will steadily decline if we don't do things differently.

Although this an ominous forecast, this shouldn't come as a surprise to anyone who makes (or aspires to make) their living in this field.

In fact, for decades, some of the nation's preeminent health promotion researchers have been warning us of this stark reality: As people get older, they generally move from relatively good health to compromised health to poor health (Fries, 2005).

This bears repeating.

As people get older, they generally move from relatively good health to compromised health to poor health.

And, if you look closely at the epidemiological data supplied by the National Association of Chronic Disease Directors (Hoffman, 2022) that's exactly what's happening right now.

Consider the following:

- Nearly 60% of adult Americans have at least one chronic disease (and of those who have one, 40% have two or more).

- Chronic conditions are the leading cause of death in the United States. In fact, more than two-thirds of all deaths are caused by one or more of five chronic diseases: heart disease, cancer, stroke, chronic obstructive pulmonary disease, and diabetes.

- Evidence is mounting that one chronic illness has a negative impact on the risk of developing others—particularly as people age.

Almost implausibly, Kotlikoff's bold prediction (foreshadowed in the previous trend) of an elderly population languishing in understaffed, substandard nursing homes begins to make sense.

But could this really happen? Could an entire country—all of whom are getting old at the same time—potentially put such a strain on our society (and specifically our healthcare system) to bring us to our knees? Truth be told, it's already happening.

Consider for a moment just a few of the statistics related to type 2 diabetes alone that indicate our population is indeed migrating from low-risk to moderate-risk to high-risk health status.

At the time of this writing, 28.7 million people in the U.S. have type 2 diabetes. Add to that another 8.5 million of our citizens who are presently undiagnosed and that brings the total to 37.3 million people with type 2 diabetes in the U.S. But the real concern is the fact that some 96 million Americans (aged eighteen and older) are considered to be pre-diabetic and, if left unaddressed, these people will most assuredly progress to type 2 diabetes (Centers for Disease Control and Prevention, 2022).

Do the math. This means that, of our nation's approximately 333 million citizens, 130+ million are wrestling with type 2 diabetes alone. But there's more. If left unchecked, type 2 diabetes will most assuredly manifest itself in terms of heart disease, vascular problems, blindness, and amputations. Now consider this. There are approximately 208,000 primary care physicians in the US (Agency for Healthcare Research and Quality, 2022). Each physician already has somewhere in the ballpark of 3,000 patients (Michas, 2022). With potentially 100+ million Americans entering the healthcare system (because of their emerging chronic conditions), even experts agree that there is no way that the U.S. healthcare system can withstand the additional burdens caused by this tsunami of need.

As can be plainly seen, the potential catastrophic human, economic, and social consequences of an aging population (many of whom will be migrating from low-risk to high-risk status) only further solidifies the need for placing a greater emphasis on health promotion and better preventive practices for all.

And, make no mistake, with a greater emphasis being placed on developing and delivering new and exciting health-promoting protocols, there will also come a renewed interest in better understanding and mastering the various well-documented, theoretically-based, behavior change models such as Prochaska's Transtheoretical Model as well as Bandura's Social Cognitive Theory just to mention a few.

Trend #3: Physical Health Problems Won't Be Our Only Concern

Undoubtedly, recent events (e.g., the COVID-19 pandemic, political upheavals, the breakdown in race relations, financial crises, economic downturns, etc.) have all exacted a tremendous toll on our nation's citizens—especially in terms of mental health and emotional distress.

In fact, according to the CDC (National Center for Chronic Disease Prevention and Health Promotion, Division of Population Health, 2021), mental illnesses are now among the most common health conditions in the United States.

Although it's hard to fathom:

- More than 50% of Americans will be diagnosed with a mental illness or disorder at some point in their lifetime.

- one in five will experience a mental illness in any given year.

- one in five children, either currently or at some point during their life, will have a seriously debilitating mental illness.

- one in twenty five Americans is now living with a serious mental illness, such as schizophrenia, bipolar disorder, or major depression.

And this speaks nothing of mood disorders like transient depressive episodes (21 million adults had at least one depressive episode in 2020), anxiety (40 million adults have an anxiety issue of some kind in any given year), and stress (which we all experience from time to time). To be sure, all of these disorders profoundly affect how we feel, think, and behave (National Institutes of Mental Health, 2022).

To make matters worse, the U.S. is nowhere near having enough mental health professionals to treat everyone who is suffering. Already, roughly half of our population is living in federally designated mental health professional shortage areas. Astoundingly, more than half of U.S. counties don't have a single psychiatrist. And with mental health concerns on the rise, in just a few years, the country will be short tens of thousands of psychiatrists. In an attempt to pick up the slack, psychologists, social workers, and others will do their best to address these concerns, but without reinforcements, it's highly unlikely much progress will be made (Weiner, 2022).

So what does all this mean for aspiring health promotion professionals?

The need for motivated, talented, and well-educated allied health professionals—especially those who have expertise in advancing mental and spiritual well-being—will be greater than at any other time period in our nation's history.

Also, there will be certain U.S. populations that will be clamoring to secure the nation's best and brightest minds. These groups include those who serve children and adolescents, working Americans, incarcerated populations, couples and families, veterans, and those grappling with addiction.

What's more, healthcare, education, and workplaces will all be looking to hire qualified people who can help physicians, nurses, teachers, coaches, and corporate leaders avoid burnout and flourish in these extremely demanding times.

The urgency in this area cannot be understated.

In fact, if large segments of our population are unable to bring their "A" game, day-in and day-out, this country will struggle to compete in a global marketplace and the consequences could be felt for decades.

Trend #4: Healthcare Costs Will Remain an Issue of Significant Concern Far into the Future

When it comes to forecasting the societal implications of a rapidly aging population—of whom the vast majority are losing both their physical and mental health status all at the same time—it's impossible to have a well-rounded conversation without bringing up the issue of healthcare costs. And, as a result of the three previously aforementioned trends, a fourth significant trend will no doubt emerge—that being that healthcare costs will continue to remain an issue of significant concern far into the future.

Presently, the US spends $4.3 trillion annually on healthcare. This is six times the $714 billion spent in 1990 and over 16 times the $253 billion spent in 1980. To put this into perspective, the nearly $4.3 trillion healthcare expenditures in the United States represent about 18.3% of our economy's annual spending and is more than 5.5 times what we spend on national defense (Centers for Medicare & Medicaid Services, 2022).

Almost incomprehensibly, in 2021, healthcare spending was about $12,914 for every man, woman, and child in the U.S. (Centers for Medicare & Medicaid Services, 2022).

With respect to the future, experts predict that U.S. healthcare expenditures will increase to $6.2 trillion by 2028 (Centers for Medicare & Medicaid Services, 2022). Certainly these projected expenditures are not only mind-numbing but alarming as well as most Americans will be hard-pressed to afford access to quality healthcare if this trend remains unabated.

To address these expenditures, health promotion will become integral to how America conducts its daily affairs as chronic diseases—preventable things like heart disease, cancer, stroke, etc.—are now responsible for approximately 70+% of the 3.3 million annual deaths in America and consume perhaps as much of 90% of current healthcare spending (Buttorff, Ruder, & Bauman, 2017). To further build the case for better health-promoting practices, we know definitively that lifestyle-related chronic illnesses—heart disease, cancer, diabetes, and mental health concerns—are also the leading causes of disability in the U.S. Last but certainly not least, as far back as 2014, the CDC estimated that approximately 40% of all deaths in the United States are premature and, again, largely preventable with some 900,000+ deaths annually related to tobacco use, poor diet, sedentary lifestyle, misuse of alcohol/drugs, and accidents alone (National Center for Chronic Disease Prevention and Health Promotion, 2022).

Because a significant percentage of healthcare expenditures are estimated to be largely preventable, health promotion brings with it enormous opportunity to contain at least a portion of these escalating costs. Moreover, because lifestyle behaviors—things like smoking, exercise, and dietary choices—contribute to 50% of an individual's overall health status, it is reasonable to think that the rapid adoption of better health practices in the U.S. can bring with it numerous benefits—not least of which is the containment of healthcare costs. Indeed, by widely promoting better health practices, many believe it is possible to have a profound effect not only on two of the leading causes of death in the U.S.—heart disease and cancer—but on numerous other conditions as well.

Moreover, what is certain to emerge as a result of escalating healthcare costs is an increasing interest in approaches and methodologies that will demonstrate concrete return on investment for those who invest heavily in evidence-based health promotion interventions. This represents a significant opportunity for those who are preparing to enter the field of health and wellness as many employers, healthcare administrators, and public health leaders will be searching for talented individuals who are devoted to demonstrating such outcomes.

Trend #5: Because of Its Potential, Prevention Will Become a National Priority

There is little question that, when it comes to the health and well-being of our nation's citizens, we are standing at the crossroads. Without significant change and a much greater emphasis on health promotion and more intensive preventive practices, it is likely that many of our nation's citizens will suffer the devastating effects of ill health—much of which is, ironically, largely preventable. While individual consequences of poor health are tragic by themselves, it is far from the true impact that an aging population and increasing healthcare costs could have on this country's economic future.

Consider this.

The more than 140+ million Baby Boomers and Gen Xers who are now in their fifties and sixties are largely unprepared to meet the financial demands of retirement. In fact, at the time of this writing, the typical near-retiree has nowhere near enough saved for retirement (DeVon, 2022). To add fuel to the fire, healthcare costs in retirement are estimated to cost boomers more than $315,000 (Fidelity Viewpoints, 2022). These financial realities mean that a large percentage of the Boomer and Gen X populations will be required to work much longer than they had originally anticipated in order to make ends meet. In fact, because of poor planning, a global financial meltdown, a pandemic, and an impending recession, far too many people will have to work well into their seventies instead of retiring in their mid-sixties.

To meet the demands of having to work later into life, tens of millions of people will rely greatly upon their health status in order to keep working. To be sure, if one's health is failing, it is unlikely that they will be able to productively contribute at work—and even less likely that they will be able to hold down a job at all.

Not convinced?

In a landmark analysis of the Health and Retirement Study's (HRS) initial cohort conducted by Kathleen McGarry (McGarry, 2004), roughly 37% of those working at age fifty eight retired earlier than they were planning. Not surprisingly, health status was the single most important driver of early retirement (Munnell, Rutledge, & Sanzenbacher, 2019).

The ramifications of this scenario are profound and immediate. If an aging America is unable to work, who will provide for them? Will there be enough workers to keep our nation's economy moving forward? How will the already overburdened healthcare system absorb this additional demand?

With this in mind, unless we change how we address health and well-being in this country, the forecast is not a rosy one. However, to the contrary, if we as a nation are able to embrace the potential catastrophic realities of a people who loses its health status—and make sweeping changes in the very near term—there is a chance we can avert disaster.

In light of these realities, much of the population will immediately see the need for better health practices and embrace the value of good health. As a result, many employers, policymakers, and working Americans will begin to advocate for better health practices not just as a good idea but as a necessity to ensure that America will continue to be able to remain productive and a global economic superpower.

Trend #6: Telehealth Will Gain Rapid Popularity

To date, Americans have relied far too heavily on the U.S. healthcare system to address minor, self-treatable, health concerns—ailments like colds, upset stomachs, and minor aches and pains. In fact, recent research reveals that there were 143 million emergency room visits in 2019 (the most recent year for which data is available) (Barrett, Owens, & Roemer, 2022). These ER visits resulted in tens of millions of diagnostic tests—including millions of X-rays and CT scans. Astoundingly, the average cost of the typical ER visit was $1,389 (up 176% from previous decade) (Alltucker, 2019). But what's most interesting about these statistics is that out of the 140+ million ER visits, only 16.2 million resulted in hospital admission. Of those, only 2.3 million required admission to a critical care unit (National Center for Health Statistics, 2022a). This data suggests that an enormous percentage of ER visits are unnecessary. In fact, recent estimates confirm that more than 70% of emergency department visits from patients with employer-sponsored insurance coverage are for *nonemergency* conditions or conditions preventable through outpatient care (Gold, 2013).

Similarly, there were 860 million physician visits in 2018. The average median cost per visit was approximately $116 (National Center for Health Statistics, 2022b). Like ER visits, it's estimated by experts that approximately 30% of all physician visits were unnecessary (Moise, 2017). Moreover, seven in ten visits resulted in at least one prescription, or 2.7 billion prescriptions overall. As of 2010, it is estimated that approximately 130 million Americans take at least one prescription daily (Jacobson, 2022).

Because of Americans over self-reliance on the U.S. healthcare system, emergency rooms and hospitals are bursting at the seams. In fact, in 2020, 60+% hospitals reported overcrowding. What's more, at the time of this writing, depending on where you live in the U.S., it takes about sixty six days to schedule an appointment to see a primary care provider. Similarly, due to overcrowding, it can take hours to be seen in an emergency room (Bernstein, 2014).

Enter telehealth.

By definition, according to Gajarawala and Pelkowski, "Telehealth is a subset of e-health and is the use of telecommunications technology in healthcare delivery, information, and education. . .Telemedicine is considered to be under the umbrella of telehealth and refers specifically to clinical services. Telehealth and telemedicine cover similar services, including medical education, remote patient monitoring, patient consultation via videoconferencing, wireless health applications, and transmission of imaging and medical reports" (Gajarawala & Pelkowski, 2021).

And although not traditionally included in the vernacular of traditional health promotion programs and approaches, with the present state of overutilization of our healthcare system, telemedicine programs will gain in popularity.

This is so for two reasons.

First, Americans will have fewer disposable dollars available to offer up to unnecessary treatments—and insurance companies (and employers) will become increasingly stingy with reimbursing unnecessary treatments. Second, because of the enormous constraints on every healthcare practitioner's time, more providers will move to triage patients via the Internet.

And for the savvy health promotion practitioners who have strong tech skills and the ability to effectively communicate electronically, the career opportunities are virtually limitless.

Trend #7: Physical Activity Will Become the Most Commonly Prescribed Medicine

Let's cut to the chase.

According to the legendary Dr. Ken Cooper, "Physical activity is one of the greatest bargains the world has ever known. When people are fit and physically active the world is a different place—you can do the things you want and lead the kind of life that has purpose and meaning. There's no question that physical activity really is one of the central components necessary for living a productive life" (Cooper, 2010).

As to the power and efficacy of physical activity as a legitimate medical prescription, Dr. Steve Aldana states, "If you could take this component of exercise and sell it as a pill, it would be the single most effective medication ever devised in the history of mankind. Exercise affects so many conditions, and it impacts them so much that the dose would be considered the most powerful medication and the most beneficial medication ever devised. Is it a magic bullet? It's as close to a magic bullet as anything that we have" (Aldana, 2010).

Despite the overwhelming evidence as to the power of physical activity to improve human health and delay the onset of disease and disability, the message has been slow to catch on with the American populace. In fact, recent statistics from the CDC indicate that only a very small percentage of Americans get the recommended amount of physical activity during the course of any given day. To make matters worse, Dr. Wayne Wescott—a noted U.S. exercise scholar—revealed in a recent interview that our already dismal participation in physical activity might be significantly lower than current U.S. estimates indicate.

Alarmingly, Wescott and colleagues put accelerometers on two groups of 5,000 Americans of all ages and found that only 3.5% were getting thirty minutes of modest-level activity. States Westcott, "This is very disconcerting, as it's not a lot of activity. For those over sixty, it was less than 2.5%. . ." In an age of poor health and increasing costs, this is certainly discouraging—especially given the fact that walking thirty to forty five minutes on most, preferably all, days of the week will delay the onset of disability by ten to twelve years (Westcott, 2010).

In the years ahead, there's no question that physical activity will be the most commonly prescribed medicine that's available—and for good reason. In fact, according to Dr. Steven Blair, perhaps the most celebrated exercise physiologist in the world, "Physical activity and low fitness is perhaps the most important predictor of morbidity and mortality that we know of. Low fitness levels account for more sickness and death in the population than anything else that we've studied. . .The best insurance you can get to stay out of a nursing home where you become frail, feeble, and incontinent is to be physically active. Physical activity improves brain health, reduces the risk of senile dementia, and preserves your function so that you can continue on with life's activities" (Blair, 2010).

"If you look at it from a medical and a financial perspective," says Dr. Tyler Cooper, "The country simply cannot exist this way going forward. When we look at the issue of obesity and lack of physical activity, we will have a major fiscal and social problem in the country in the not-too-distant future" (Cooper, 2010).

As can be easily seen, given its benefits and high accessibility, physical activity will become the most commonly prescribed medicine in America.

Trend #8: Efforts to Curb Obesity Will Intensify Greatly

From 2000 to 2020, the prevalence of obesity in the U.S. increased from 30.5% to 41.9%. During the same time, the prevalence of severe obesity increased from 4.7% to 9.2% (Centers for Disease Control and Prevention, 2022). If that's not enough, nineteen states now have obesity rates over 35%, up from sixteen states in 2021 (Trust for America's Health, 2022).

Incomprehensibly, this translates into well over 100+ million U.S. adults and children who are struggling with carrying too much weight. Because obesity increases the risk of a myriad of health conditions including hypertension, adverse lipid concentrations, and type 2 diabetes, of most concern is the fact that the prevalence of obesity in the United States continues to escalate.

Hence, given the health risks of obesity and its high prevalence, it is imperative for health promotion professionals, policymakers, educators, physicians, food producers, scientists, drug-makers, venture capitalists, techies, and business leaders to continue to develop and implement aggressive strategies to combat this major public health concern.

To date, much of the effort to reduce the incidence and prevalence of obesity in the U.S. has centered on personal change efforts designed to modify individual behaviors. For example, diets based on interventions like Weight Watchers, Keto, Vegan, Mediterranean, and Paleo (not to mention scores of others) have attracted tens of millions of individuals seeking to shed pounds. Despite the popularity and appetite for these types of interventions, the outcomes have been disappointing at best.

So what's next?

Over the course of the next several decades strategies to reduce obesity among the U.S. population will evolve significantly. In fact, it is realistic to think that—given the potential seriousness of the problem—the obesity dialogue will begin to meaningfully engage the pharmaceutical industry, healthcare, restaurateurs, soda manufacturers, food producers, grocers, fast food, cities and municipalities, state and federal governments, and a whole host of others.

And while these partnerships are still too few and far between if you look hard you can begin to see signs that changes are coming.

For instance, at the time of this writing, The Nutrition Facts label (which appears on the majority of packaged foods and has been mandated by the FDA for over three decades) recently received an important update. Now included on all food labels is information about the link between diet and chronic diseases, such as obesity and heart disease. The updated label also makes it easier for consumers to make better-informed food choices (U.S. Food and Drug Administration, 2022).

While this may seem small by comparison to the size of the obesity problem, the majority of Americans use the Nutrition Facts label to guide their food choices. And with this new mandate, much of the mystery will now be eliminated from the decision-making process.

Certainly, this is but one example of a potential efficacious strategy that's being employed.

Optimistically, many others are also emerging.

For example, the FDA recently approved the medication Wegovy, a weight management drug that will be used in treating patients with obesity. According to leaders at Yale University, while "there is no magic pill that will cure obesity. . .there are new types of medicines that are potential game-changers" (Katella, 2022).

Hopefully, this will be one.

But, because the obesity issue remains such a serious one, there are some who are taking much more extreme measures.

Consider the approach implemented by leaders at the University of California at San Francisco.

In 2015, UCSF banned the sale of sugary beverages on its campus, and a group of researchers set out to measure the impact of the ban.

For the ban, UCSF removed sugar-sweetened beverages from cafeterias, food trucks, and vending machines across all campus sites and medical facilities. Fast food chains on campus also stopped selling the sugary drinks. The only exception to the ban was 100% fruit juices, which have no added sugar. In addition, UCSF installed more water stations to encourage more water consumption during the ban. (Advisory Board, 2019)

Ten months after the sales ban went into effect, across both groups, employees had cut their daily intake of sugar-sweetened beverages by almost in half, from 35 ounces per day to 18 ounces per day. The group that received the intervention reduced their daily sugary drink intake by an average of 25.4 ounces, while the control group reduced daily intake by 8.2 ounces. (Advisory Board, 2019)

At the conclusion of the study, the researchers found that about 70% of participants overall had a smaller waist size. (Advisory Board, 2019)

Moving forward, it's essential for the next generation of the nation's health promotion practitioners to continue to keep obesity on the radar screen. Judging by the pushback that this topic has generated over the last decade, it will not be easy. However, just because it's hard, doesn't mean it's not worthwhile. Moreover, because of the sheer magnitude of the problem, ample opportunities will be available—but those interested will need to have a very strong resolve.

Trend #9: Wearables, Apps, Big Data, and AI Will Dominate the Wellness Arena

Fitbit, the wirelessly-enabled wearable technology/activity tracker that records physical activity and monitors things like heart rate and overall quality of an individual's sleep, was introduced to the world in 2007 (Marshall, 2020). Since then, an avalanche of wearables and apps have followed suit and descended upon the wellness space.

Driven by the harnessing of big data (and the ability to synthesize that data), wearables and wellness apps have now become the rage. In fact, they've become so common that, at this point in history, it's highly likely that every American is using one in some form or another.

But this is just the beginning.

In fact, at the time of this writing, one of the largest companies in the history of the world suddenly changed its name from Facebook to Meta and, in 2022 alone, spent more than $10 billion dollars of its cash reserves with the hopes of creating a virtual reality headset that will allow users to enter the metaverse (Isaac, 2022).

By my many accounts, the metaverse is the future of the internet and, in essence, is a virtual reality (VR) platform that allows the user to immerse themselves in three-dimensional virtual worlds as well as augmented reality (AR) (Anderson & Rainie, 2022).

While still in its infancy, the metaverse wields enormous power for changing the world for the better. For instance, imagine if aspiring surgeons were able to virtually practice delicate operations thousands upon thousands of times before ever going live on a real patient. Now imagine if walkers could connect virtually with their social support group and walking clubs just by slipping on a headset before they dive into their workout (think Peleton on steroids!). What's more, consider how much more effective health coaches could be if they were able to practice important interactions with their "clients" before ever even having a real interaction with them.

Remarkably, in just the last few months alone, there are companies who have already launched VR/AR products and are now helping people successfully deal with anxiety disorders, ADHD, PTSD, pain management, and a whole host of other issues.

Again, if executed carefully and thoughtfully, the possibilities and potential for improving human health are endless.

But there's more.

AI or Artificial Intelligence is also taking hold. In a nutshell, AI is the simulation of human intelligence and is orchestrated by using computers and machines to expertly perform both routine and complex tasks. Perhaps the most powerful feature of AI is that it can iteratively improve itself by analyzing and synthesizing the information that is collected (Burns, 2022).

For example, interacting with a personal assistant like Apple's Siri or Amazon's Alexa is a simple example of how AI works. As you begin your initial interactions, both personal assistants begin to learn more about your favorite activities, preferences, and daily rhythms. The more you use them, the more refined they become. Over time, things begin to happen almost automatically (e.g., your alarm goes off at precisely the right time, your favorite playlist is magically activated, your coffee maker starts the brewing cycle, and your shower starts to stream at the ideal temperature).

Now let's take it a step further.

Imagine if there was a comfortable, temperature-efficient, wearable garment that you wore under your clothes that could measure your daily movements as well as your heart rate, your sleep patterns, the times you eat, and the amount of positive human interaction you get on a daily basis. Over time, this type of AI could make important health-promoting refinements to your daily pursuits and expertly guide you toward achieving optimal health.

Believe it or not, they're already in production (Brown, 2022).

The implications of AR, VR, and AI for a new generation of health promotion professionals are legion. In fact, it opens a number of brand new doors that have never existed including coding, programming, data management, algorithm development, manufacturing, venture capital, and entrepreneuring just to mention a few.

Trend #10: The Need for Talented Health Promotion Professionals Will Skyrocket

As we look to the future, one final thing becomes strikingly apparent—doing what we have done in the past will not get us to our desired destination. Treating disease after it has already taken hold has driven healthcare costs in the U.S. to unprecedented levels—not to mention the fact that the untold millions of individual health consequences have been heartbreaking.

In moving forward, health promotion and prevention will become a standard way of doing business in this country. In fact, the dominoes have already been kicked over and momentum is being gained on a variety of fronts. Hospitals and physicians are now making concerted efforts to address primary prevention in a system that has traditionally focused solely on treating disease. Health insurance companies are now beginning to reimburse for primary prevention practices. National legislation as witnessed by the passage of Barack Obama's Patient Protection and Affordable Care Act now incorporates significant incentives for prevention and healthier lifestyles. Millions of businesses in the U.S. are hard at work designing wellness initiatives in an attempt to contain costs, improve health, and create healthier cultures.

There's absolutely no question that a big part of the future of the U.S. centers on the notion of health promotion as it has become glaringly obvious to everyone that we need healthy citizens in order to compete on a global level. Indeed health promotion is no longer just an interesting idea—it has become a national imperative.

To sustain the momentum that has been achieved by the pioneers of this movement, it is essential that training programs be put into place to ensure that talented and effective professionals are available to step into the opportunities that are now emerging. To meet the demand, institutions of higher education, medical schools, community colleges, and a variety of other professional preparation programs will dedicate substantial resources toward developing capable men and women who will possess the knowledge, skills, acumen, and desire to step into these programs and lead the way to better health.

Summary

In this chapter, ten trends for the future of health promotion have been presented. When taken together, it is evident that there is still much work to be done if we are to keep our nation's citizens healthy and our country globally competitive. At the same time, it is also important to see that there are substantial opportunities for individuals to play meaningful and necessary roles that will not only help others remain healthy but provide long and satisfying careers for those who choose to accept the call.

References

Advisory Board (2019). *UCSF banned soda on campus 4 years ago. Did it work?* Retrieved from https://www.advisory.com/daily-briefing/2019/11/14/sugary-drinks on 10/07/2022.

Agency for Healthcare Research and Quality (2022). The distribution of the U.S. primary care workforce. Content last reviewed July 2018. Agency for Healthcare Research and Quality, Rockville, MD. https://www.ahrq.gov/research/findings/factsheets/primary/pcwork3/index.html on 06/24/2022.

Aldana, S. (2010). *Getting active: An expert interview with Dr. Steve Aldana.* Retrieved from https://www.welcoa.org/resources/getting-active/ on 11/14/2022.

Alltucker, K. 2019. *USA today: 'Really Astonishing': Average cost of hospital Er visit surges 176% in a decade, report says.* Retrieved from https://bettersolutionsforhealthcare.org/usa-today-really-astonishing-average-cost-of-hospital-er-visit-surges-176-in-a-decade-report-says/#:~:text=The%20average%20emergency%20room%20visit,IVs%2C%20drugs%20or%20other%20treatments on 08/16/2022.

Anderson, J. & Rainie, L. (2022). The metaverse will fully emerge as its advocates predict. *Pew Research Center.* Retrieved from https://www.pewresearch.org/internet/2022/06/30/the-metaverse-will-fully-emerge-as-its-advocates-predict/ on 06/15/2022.

Barrett, M.L., Owens, P.L., & Roemer, M. (2022). *Changes in emergency department visits in the initial period of the COVID-19 pandemic (April–December 2020), 29 states.* Retrieved from https://www.hcup-us.ahrq.gov/reports/statbriefs/sb298-COVID-19-ED-visits.jsp#:~:text=In%20the%20United%20States%20in,ED%20visits%20resulted%20in%20hospitalization on 11/02/2022.

Bernstein, L. (2014). Here's how long you'll wait for a doctor's appointment in 15 U.S. cities, by specialty. *The Washington Post.* Retrieved from https://www.washingtonpost.com/news/to-your-health/wp/2014/05/23/heres-how-long-youll-wait-for-a-doctors-appointment-in-15-u-s-cities-by-specialty/ on 12/01/2022.

Blair, S. (2010). *Taking a stand on sitting down: An expert interview with Dr. Steven Blair.* Retrieved from https://www.welcoa.org/resources/taking-stand-sitting-expert-interview-dr-steven-blair-dangers-sitting/ on 11/18/2022.

Brown, P. (2022). *The future of healthcare may reside in your smart clothes. Mouser electronics.* Retrieved from https://www.mouser.com/applications/healthcare-may-reside-in-smart-clothing/ on 12/02/2022.

Burns, E. (2022). *What is artificial intelligence (AI)? TechTarget.* Retrieved from https://www.techtarget.com/searchenterpriseai/definition/AI-Artificial-Intelligence on 05/05/2022.

Buttorff, C., Ruder, T., and Bauman, M. (2017). Multiple Chronic Conditions in the United States. Santa Monica, CA: Rand Corp.

Centers for Disease Control and Prevention (2022). *National Diabetes Statistics Report website.* Retrieved from https://www.cdc.gov/diabetes/data/statistics-report/index.html on 08/26/2022.

Centers for Disease Control and Prevention (2022). *Adult obesity facts.* Retrieved from https://www.cdc.gov/obesity/data/adult.html on 08/27/2022.

Centers for Medicare & Medicaid Services (2022). *National Health Expenditures Fact Sheet.* Retrieved from https://www.cms.gov/Research-Statistics-Data-and-Systems/Statistics-Trends-and-Reports/NationalHealthExpendData/NHE-Fact-Sheet#:~:text=Historical%20NHE%2C%202021%3A,17%20percent%20of%20total%20NHE on 12/17/2022.

Cooper, K. (2010). *Doctor's orders: An expert interview with Dr. Ken Cooper.* Retrieved from https://www.welcoa.org/resources/doctors-orders/ on 11/14/2022.

Cooper, T. (2010). *Making a big push for a little movement: An expert interview with Dr. Tyler Cooper.* Retrieved from http://2010.welcoatrainingsummit.com/resources/new-expert-interview-with-cooper-aerobics-now-available on 11/16/2012.

DeVon, C. (2022). *Here's how much Americans have saved for retirement at every age.* Retrieved from https://www.cnbc.com/2022/07/30/vanguard-how-much-americans-have-saved-for-retirement-by-age.html on 09/09/2022.

Fidelity Viewpoints (2022). *How to plan for rising health care costs.* Retrieved from https://www.fidelity.com/viewpoints/personal-finance/plan-for-rising-health-care-costs on 09/16/2022.

Fries, J.F. (2005). The compression of morbidity. *Milbank Q* 83 (4): 801–823.

Gajarawala, S. N. & Pelkowski, J. N. (2021). Telehealth benefits and barriers. *The Journal for Nurse Practitioners.* Retrieved from https://www.ncbi.nlm.nih.gov/pmc/articles/PMC7577680/ on 04/16/2022.

Gold, A. (2013). *70% of ER visits unnecessary for patients with employer-sponsored insurance.* Fierce Healthcare. Retrieved from https://www.fiercehealthcare.com/healthcare/70-er-visits-unnecessary-for-patients-employer-sponsored-insurance on 11/25/2022.

Hoffman, D. (2022). *Commentary on chronic disease prevention in 2022.* Retrieved from https://chronicdisease.org/wp-content/uploads/2022/04/FS_ChronicDiseaseCommentary2022FINAL.pdf

Isaac, M. (2022). Meta spent $10 billion on the metaverse in 2021, dragging down profit. *The New York Times.* Retrieved from https://www.nytimes.com/2022/02/02/technology/meta-facebook-earnings-metaverse.html on 06/06/2022.

Jacobson, A. (2022). *Prescription drug statistics 2022.* Retrieved from https://www.singlecare.com/blog/news/prescription-drug-statistics/#:~:text=More%20than%20131%20million%20Americans%20take%20at%20least%20one%20prescription%20medication on 11/07/2022.

Katella, K. (2022). Doctors say new treatments are effective in treating the disease. *Yale Medicine.* Retrieved from https://www.yalemedicine.org/news/new-medications-treat-obesity on 07/04/2022.

Kessler, G. (2014). Do 10,000 baby boomers retire every day? *The Washington Post.* https://www.washingtonpost.com/news/fact-checker/wp/2014/07/24/do-10000-baby-boomers-retire-every-day/

Kotlikoff, L.J. and Burns, S. (2004). The Coming Generational Storm: What You Need To Know About America's Economic Future. MIT Press. ISBN 0-262-11286.

Marshall, C. (2020). The story of Fitbit: How a wooden box was bought by Google for $2.1bn. *Wareable.* Retrieved from https://www.wareable.com/fitbit/story-of-fitbit-7936#:~:text=The%20beginning,board%20in%20a%20wooden%20box on 11/08/22.

McGarry, K. (2004). Do changes in health affect retirement expectations? *The Journal of Human Resources* 39 (3): 624–648.

Michas, F. (2022). *Number of patients U.S. physicians saw per day 2012–2018.* Statista. Retrieved from https://www.statista.com/statistics/613959/us-physicians-patients-seen-per-day/ on 08/07/2022.

Moise, I. K. (Ed.). (2017). *Overtreatment in the United States.* PLoS One. Retrieved from https://www.ncbi.nlm.nih.gov/pmc/articles/PMC5587107/ on 03/05/2021.

Munnell, A.H., Rutledge, M.S., & Sanzenbacher, G.T. (2019). *Retiring earlier than planned: What matters most? Issue in brief: Center for Retirement Research.* Retrieved from https://crr.bc.edu/wp-content/uploads/2019/01/IB_19-3.pdf on 05/01/2022.

National Center for Chronic Disease Prevention and Health Promotion (2022). *Health and economic costs of chronic diseases.* Retrieved from https://www.cdc.gov/chronicdisease/about/costs/index.htm on 11/2/2022.

National Center for Chronic Disease Prevention and Health Promotion, Division of Population Health (2021). *About mental health: Mental health basics.* Retrieved from https://www.cdc.gov/mentalhealth/learn/index.htm#:~:text=How%20common%20are%20mental%20illnesses,some%20point%20in%20their%20lifetime.&text=1%20in%205%20Americans%20will,illness%20in%20a%20given%20year on 07/15/2022.

National Center for Health Statistics (2022a). *Emergency department visits*. Retrieved from https://www.cdc.gov/nchs/fastats/emergency-department.htm on 10/31/2022.

National Center for Health Statistics (2022b). *Ambulatory Care Use and Physician office visits*. Retrieved from https://www.cdc.gov/nchs/fastats/physician-visits.htm on 11/02/2022

National Institutes of Mental Health (2022). *Major depression*. Retrieved from https://www.nimh.nih.gov/health/statistics/major-depression#:~:text=disorders%2C%20or%20medication.-,Prevalence%20of%20Major%20Depressive%20Episode%20Among%20Adults,8.4%25%20of%20all%20U.S.%20adults on 03/16/2022.

Trust for America's Health (2022). *State of obesity 2022: Better policies for a healthier America*. Retrieved from https://www.tfah.org/report-details/state-of-obesity-2022/#:~:text=Trust%20for%20America%27s%20Health%27s%20(TFAH,drivers%20of%20increasing%20obesity%20rates on 11/02/2022.

U.S. Census Bureau. (2022). U.S. World and Population Clock. Department of Commerce. Retrieved from https://www.census.gov/popclock/ on 12/12/2022; United States Census Bureau. (2023). Older Americans Month: May 2023. U.S. Department of Commerce. Retrieved from https://www.census.gov/newsroom/stories/older-americans-month.html on 05/09/2023.

U.S. Food and Drug Administration (2022). *Changes to the nutrition facts label*. Retrieved from https://www.fda.gov/food/food-labeling-nutrition/changes-nutrition-facts-label on 11/25/2022.

Weiner, S. (2022). *A growing psychiatrist shortage and an enormous demand for mental health services*. Association of American Medical Colleges. Retrieved from https://www.aamc.org/news-insights/growing-psychiatrist-shortage-enormous-demand-mental-health-services on 10/07/2022.

Westcott, W. (2010). *The good. The bad. And the just plain scary: An expert interview with Dr. Wayne Westcott*. Retrieved from https://www.welcoa.org/resources/wayne-westcott-good-bad-just-plain-scary/ on 11/18/2022.

Chapter 1: Health Promotion

American Public Health Association

www.apha.org/What-is-Public-Health

Centers for Disease Control and Prevention

www.cdc.gov/about/history/tengpha.htm

www.cdc.gov/nchs/fastats/lifexpec.htm

www.cdc.gov/chronicdisease

www.cdc.gov/socialdevterminants

Infectious Disease Society of America

www.idsociety.org/Index.aspx

National Association of Chronic Disease Directors

www.chronicdisease.org

Office of Disease Prevention and Health Promotion

http://odphp.osophs.dhhs.gov

Society of Public Health Education

www.sophe.org

US Department of Health and Human Services

www.hhs.gov/healthcare/rights

World Health Organization

www.who.org

www.who.int/westernpacific/about/how-we-work/programmes/health-promotion

Chapter 2: Health Behavior Change Theories and Models

Education

www.education.com/reference/article/social-cognitive-theory

Euromed Info

www.euromedinfo.eu/the-health-belief-model.html

Instructional Design

www.instructionaldesign.org/theories/social-learning.html

Pro-Change Behavior Systems

www.prochange.com/transtheoretical-model-of-behavior-change

Substance Abuse and Mental Health Services Administration

www.samhsa.gov/co-occurring/topics/training/change.aspx

Chapter 3: Program Planning Models

American College Health Association

www.acha.org/healthycampus/ecological_model.cfm

Centers for Disease Control and Prevention

www.cdc.gov/hrqol/featured-items/match.htm

www.cdc.gov/violenceprevention/overview/social-ecologicalmodel.html

www.cdc.gov/healthcommunication/healthbasics/whatishc.html

Making Health Communications Programs Work

www.cdc.gov/healthcommunication/

PRECEDE-PROCEED Model

www.lgreen.net/precede-proceed

Weinreich Communications

www.social-marketing.com/Whatis.html

Chapter 4: Tobacco Use

American Cancer Society

www.cancer.org

American Legacy Foundation

www.legacyforhealth.org

American Lung Association

www.lung.org

American Nonsmokers' Rights Foundation

www.anrf.org

Centers for Disease Control

www.cdc.gov/nchs/icd/icd10cm.htm

www.cdc.gov/tobacco/data_statistics/

www.cdc.gov/healthyyouth/stories/pdf/ss_booklet_1011.pdf

www.cdc.gov/tobacco/data_statistics/sgr/history/index.htm

www.cdc.gov/workplace healthpromotion/implementation/topics/tobacco-use.html

www.cdc.gov/tobacco/data_statistics/fact_sheets /smokeless/betel_quid/index.htm

Department of Health and Human Services

www.ncbi.nlm.nih.gov/

Food and Drug Administration

www.fda.gov/TobaccoProducts/GuidanceComplianceRegulatoryInformation/ucm297786.htm

www.fda.gov/tobacco-products/labeling-and-warning-statements-tobacco-products/cigarette-labeling-and-health-warning-requirements

www.fda.gov/tobacco-products/retail-sales-tobacco-products/tobacco-21

www.fda.gov/tobacco-products/products-ingredients-components/smokeless-tobacco-products-including-dip-snuff-snus-and-chewing-tobacco

www.fda.gov/tobacco-products/public-health-education-campaigns/every-try-counts-campaign

www.fda.gov/tobacco-products

National Cancer Institute

www.cancer.gov

www.cancer.gov/about-cancer

SmokeFree.gov

www.smokefree.gov

Smoking Cessation Leadership Center

http://smokingcessationleadership.ucsf.edu

Tobacco Free Kids

www.tobaccofreekids.org/what-we-do/us/statereport/

World Health Organization

www.who.int.org

Chapter 5: Eating Behaviors

America's Healthy Food Finance Initiative

www.investinginfood.com/about-hffi

Center for Science in the Public Interest

www.cspinet.org

Centers for Disease Control and Prevention

www.cdc.gov/nchs/data/hestat/obesity-adult-17-18/Estat-adults-fig.png

www.cdc.gov/workplacehealthpromotion/health-strategies/nutrition/index.html

www.cdc.gov/chronicdisease/resources/publications/factsheets/cancer.htm

www.cdc.gov/nutrition/data-statistics/sugar-sweetened-beverages-intake.html

www.cdc.gov/healthyweight/effects/index.html

Food and Drug Administration

www.fda.gov/food/new-nutrition-facts-label/added-sugars-new-nutrition-facts-label

www.fda.gov/food/food-labeling-nutrition/changes-nutrition-facts-label

Food Politics Blog by Marion Nestle of New York University

www.foodpolitics.com

International Food Information Council

foodinsight.org

National Heart, Lung, and Blood Institute (NHLBI) Portion Distortion

http://hp2010.nhlbihin.net/portion

Nutrition Source—Harvard School of Public Health

www.hsph.harvard.edu/nutritionsource

Dietary Guidelines for Americans

www.ncbi.nlm.nih.gov/books/NBK482514/S

www.ncbi.nlm.nih.gov/pmc/articles/PMC5902736/

The Food Trust

thefoodtrust.org/what-we-do/corner-stores/

thefoodtrust.org/what-we-do/corner-stores/

US Department of Agriculture

www.MyPlate.gov

www.myplate.gov/resources/graphics/myplate-graphics

www.dietaryguidelines.gov/sites/default/files/2021-03/Dietary_Guidelines_for_Americans-2020-2025.pdf

www.ers.usda.gov/topics/food-nutrition-assistance/wic-program/

www.fns.usda.gov/cnd/governance/legislation/nutritionstandards.htm

Yale Rudd Center for Food Policy and Obesity

www.yaleruddcenter.org/what_we_do.aspx?id=7

Chapter 6: Physical Activity Behaviors

Active Living Research

activelivingresearch.org/policies-and-standards-promoting-physical-activity-after-school-programs,

Alliance for a Healthier Generation

www.healthiergeneration.org

American Alliance for Health, Physical Education, Recreation, and Dance

www.aahperd.org

Centers for Disease Control and Prevention

https://www.cdc.gov/workplacehealthpromotion/index.html

www.cdc.gov/workplacehealthpromotion/data-surveillance/summary-report.html

www.cdc.gov/physicalactivity/activepeoplehealthynation/creating-an-active-america.html

www.cdc.gov/nccdphp/dnpao/state-local-programs/span-1807/span-1807-recipients.html

www.cdc.gov/nchs/fastats/exercise.htm

Community Preventive Services

www.thecommunityguide.org/pages/task-force-findings-physical-activity.html

Eat Smart, Move More North Carolina

www.eatsmartmovemorenc.com

Healthy Children

www.healthychildren.org/English/Pages/default.aspx

Let's Move!

www.letsmove.org

National Institute of Health

www.nhlbi.nih.gov/health/health-topics/topics/phys/types.html

President's Council on Fitness, Sport, & Nutrition

www.fitness.gov

Robert Wood Johnson Foundation

www.rwjf.org

Physical Activity Guidelines for Americans

health.gov/sites/default/files/2019-0

World Health Organization

www.who.int/news-room/fact-sheets/detail/physical-activity

www.who.int/news/item/04-04-2002-physical-inactivity-a-leading-cause-of-disease-and-disability-warns-who

Chapter 7: Stress, Emotional Well-Being, and Mental Health

American Institute of Stress

www.stress.org

www.stress.org/workplace-stress

American Psychiatric Association

www.psychiatry.org

American Psychological Association

www.apa.org

The Center for Mind-Body Medicine

www.cmbm.org

MentalHealth.gov

www.mentalhealth.gov

National Alliance on Mental Illness

www.nami.org

National Institute on Mental Health

www.nimh.nih.gov

www.nimh.nih.gov/health/statistics/mental-illness

The Substance Abuse and Mental Health Services Administration

www.samhsa.gov

Chapter 8: Clinical Preventive Services

American Health Insurance Plans

www.ahip.org

Centers for Disease Control and Prevention

www.cdc.gov

www.cdc.gov/coronavirus/2019-ncov/vaccines/safety/safety-of-vaccines.html

The Community Guide

www.thecommunityguide.org

National Institutes of Health—Office of Disease Prevention

http://prevention.nih.gov

National Prevention Strategy

www.surgeongeneral.gov/initiatives/prevention/strategy

Partnership for Prevention

www.prevent.org

US Preventive Services Task Force

www.uspreventiveservicestaskforce.org

www.uspreventiveservicestaskforce.org/uspstf/recommendation/brca-related-cancer-risk-assessment-genetic-counseling-and-genetic-testing

www.uspreventiveservicestaskforce.org/uspstf/recommendation/hypertension-in-adults-screening

Chapter 9: National and State Initiatives to Promote Health and Well-Being

Association of State and Territorial Health Officials

www.astho.org

Centers for Disease Control and Prevention

www.cdc.gov

Healthy People 2020

www.healthypeople.gov

National Association of City and County Health Officials

www.naccho.org

National Conference of State Legislatures

www.ncsl.org

National Institutes of Health

www.nih.gov

US Department of Agriculture

www.usda.gov

US Department of Health and Human Services

www.hhs.gov

Chapter 10: Settings for Health Promotion

American College Health Association

www.acha.org

American Community Garden Association

www.communitygarden.org

American School Health Association

www.ashaweb.org/

Centers for Disease Control and Prevention

www.cdc.gov/family

www.cdc.gov/nationalhealthyworksite/index.html

Coordinated School Health (CDC)

www.cdc.gov/HealthyYouth/cshp

Food and Nutrition Service, USDA

www.fns.usda.gov/cnd/governance/legislation/cnr_2010.htm

International Association for Worksite Health Promotion

www.acsm-iawhp.org

International Health, Racquet and Sport Association

www.ihrsa.org

National Association for Community Health

www.nachc.com

National Wellness Institute

www.nationalwellness.org

Wellness Councils of America

www.welcoa.org

YMCA

www.ymca.net

Chapter 11: Health Promotion–Related Organizations, Associations, and Certifications

The Academy of Nutrition and Dietetics

www.eatright.org

American Alliance for Health, Physical Education, Recreation, and Dance

www.aahperd.org

American Association of School Health

www.ashaweb.org

American College of Nutrition

www.americancollegeofnutrition.org

American College of Sports Medicine

www.acsm.org

American Heart Association

www.heart.org

American Public Health Association

www.apha.org

Institute of Health and Productivity Management

www.ihpm.org

Society for Public Health Education

www.sophe.org

Chapter 12: Trends in Health Promotion

Agency of Healthcare Research and Quality

www.ahrq.gov

American Health Insurance Plans

www.ahip.org

American Medical Association

www.ama-assn.org

Centers for Disease Control and Prevention

www.cdc.gov/diabetes/data/statistics-report/index.html.

Health Care Cost Institute

www.healthcostinstitute.org

Institute of Health and Productivity Management

www.ihpm.org

Kaiser Family Foundation

http://kff.org

National Business Group on Health

www.businessgrouphealth.org/

National Center for Health Statistics

www.cdc.gov/nchs

US Department of Labor

www.dol/gov

World Population on Aging

www.un.org

INDEX